# LONG-TERM
# PAEDIATRIC UROLOGY

*Dedicated to Anna*
*who has suffered more than any*
*in the writing of this book*

# *Long-term Paediatric Urology*

C.R.J. WOODHOUSE MB FRCS
Senior Lecturer in Urology, The Institute of Urology,
Honorary Consultant Urologist,
The Hospital for Sick Children, Great Ormond Street,
and St Peter's Hospitals;
Consultant Urologist,
St George's Hospital and
The Royal Marsden Hospital,
London

*With a chapter by*

C.J. MILLWATER
Senior Registrar in Nephrology,
St Peter's Hospitals

*and*

G.H. NIELD
Professor of Nephrology,
The Institute of Urology

OXFORD

BLACKWELL SCIENTIFIC PUBLICATIONS

LONDON EDINBURGH BOSTON

MELBOURNE PARIS BERLIN VIENNA

Editorial Offices:
Osney Mead, Oxford OX2 0EL
25 John Street, London WC1N 2BL
23 Ainslie Place, Edinburgh EH3 6AJ
3 Cambridge Center, Cambridge,
Massachusetts 02142, USA
54 University Street, Carlton
Victoria 3053, Australia

Other Editorial Offices:
Arnette SA
2, rue Casimir-Delavigne
75006 Paris
France

Blackwell Wissenschaft
Meinekestrasse 4
D-1000 Berlin 15
West Germany

Blackwell MZV
Feldgasse 13
A-1238 Wien
Austria



First published 1991

Set by Setrite Typesetters, Hong Kong
Printed and bound in Great Britain
by William Clowes Limited,
Beccles and London

DISTRIBUTORS

Marston Book Services Ltd
PO Box 87
Oxford OX2 0DT
(*Orders*: Tel: 0865 791155
Fax: 0865 791927
Telex: 837515)

USA
Mosby–Year Book, Inc.
11830 Westline Industrial Drive
St Louis, Missouri 63146
(*Orders*: Tel: (800) 633–6699)

Canada
Mosby–Year Book, Inc.
5240 Finch Avenue East
Scarborough, Ontario
(*Orders*: Tel: (416) 298–1588)

Australia
Blackwell Scientific Publications
(Australia) Pty Ltd
54 University Street
Carlton, Victoria 3053
(Orders: Tel: (03) 347–0300)

British Library
Cataloguing in Publication Data

Woodhouse C.R.J. (Christopher Richard James)
Long-term paediatric urology
1. Medicine. Urology
I. Title II. Millwater, C.J. III. Nield, G.H.
616.6

ISBN 0–632–02936–6

# Contents

# 1 *Introduction*

*There is nothing gives a greater check to the progress of an art, than to believe it is already perfected by those that have gone before us, and so to content ourselves with their determinations: for had our ancient artists been so supinely credulous, and thought it sufficient to have traced their predecessors, limiting their wits within other men's bounds, never had time brought to light such discoveries in our profession, nor had the mysteries of our art been so far communicated to posterity as they already are.*

Snape A. (1683) *The Anatomy of an Horse,* p. 3. M. Flesher, London.

When a baby is born with a gross congenital abnormality the parents are shattered. Their first thoughts after 'what did we do wrong?' and 'whose fault is it?' are usually concerned with the immediate prospects for life and for reconstruction. They are probably little concerned with thoughts of the baby's life as an adult. In 16 years time the baby will be grown up; will want a job, a sex-life, independence from home, a family, security in the remaining 60 or 70 years of life and all the other things that normal adults might expect.

The urogenital system is the seat of the largest number of congenital anomalies. The goals of the paediatric urologist are the saving of life, the saving of nephrons and functional reconstruction. Forty years ago the first two of these were of greatest importance and the third was a more remote consideration. The surgeons of that generation pioneered procedures that allowed the children to survive. Functional reconstruction is now an integral part of paediatric management, and is based on the lessons learned from the survivors of preceding generations.

This book is about the long-term consequences of urological diseases and their management in childhood. It might have been called 'Adolescent Urology' as a sequel to 'Paediatric Urology', but the consequences do not stop in adolescence. Long-term follow-up may mean 70 years.

It is not about urological diseases that begin in young adults except where a congenital anomaly presents late. Nor will much be found about conditions that are unequivocally cured in childhood except where that cure exposes the patient to a new and unsuspected problem.

By definition the patients were first diagnosed and treated many years ago. As paediatric urology is developing new treatments all the time and many are better treatments, some of the problems found here will soon disappear. However, some may be replaced by other, unanticipated problems.

Many of the patients described were originally treated by Sir David Innes Williams. It is to his great credit that the vast majority have grown through childhood so well. When his patients required long follow-up he saw them in his adult clinic. For 10 years, since his retirement, this clinic has been devoted exclusively to the care of 'grown-up children'. Children who outgrow the combined paediatric urology unit of The Hospital for Sick Children, Great Ormond Street, UK and The St Peter's Hospitals, UK are transferred to this clinic.

It is from these patients that I have learnt about adolescent urology. Much of this book is based on the experiences of this clinic and the work of people who have been associated with it. As such it is likely to contain some prejudices and some opinions that are not supported by independent sources. This is inevitable in a field that is relatively new and constantly changing.

I have tried to lay out the book in chapters and headings that would be familiar to readers of the paediatric urology literature. I have also assumed that the reader is familiar with the usual management of paediatric urology problems. Current management is only described if there have been radical changes which will alter or abolish the adolescent problems of the future.

I am most grateful to the many registrars, nurses and research fellows who have shared the care of the patients. All have contributed to our present knowledge and to this book. I am also happy to acknowledge the great help, over many years, of R.E. Bartholomew and The Department of Medical Illustration at The Institute of Urology.

C. R. J.W.

# 2 *Useful investigations in long-term follow-up*

## THE PAST

Most young adults who have had a lifetime's experience under paediatric urologists will have had repeated investigations that we would now consider unsophisticated. Most seem little the worse as a result. Urine was cultured and tested for protein. Full blood counts, electrolytes, urea and sometimes creatinine were measured. Intravenous urograms were done from which conclusions which we now know to be inappropriate were drawn: particularly that dilatation equalled obstruction and that poor concentration equalled poor function. When the significance of vesicoureteric reflux was realised, the micturating cystogram became standard.

These investigation protocols were the best available at the time and it is astonishing how much excellent surgery was based on their results.

However, there are some problems as a result. We are sometimes unsure of the original diagnosis. Was a urea within the normal range really an indication that the kidneys were normal at 3 years old? Was the dilated and non-refluxing ureter really obstructed? Does the persistent hydronephrosis mean that the pelvi-ureteric junction obstruction was incompletely repaired?

It may be that a patient arriving in the adult clinic for the first time has no sure diagnosis. Occasionally, though much less often in the adolescents of today, even the current urinary tract function may be uncertain.

## INVESTIGATIONS BEFORE TRANSFER TO THE ADULT CLINIC

It is certainly not the business of the adult urologist to tell the paediatric urologist how to investigate his patients. But, when the child grows up, the care of a complicated case will be passed to a doctor who has had no previous share of it. A doctor's summary, no matter how careful, can never convey the full amount of work that has been done. Even the full package of notes and X-rays may not be sufficient. It is helpful to have some firm baseline information.

**1** *Blood pressure.* Children with any significant abnormality of the urinary tract should have their blood pressure measured at every clinic visit.

**2** *Urine.* The stick-test of urine (e.g. N-Multistix, Ames ltd, UK) provides semi-quantitative information on seven parameters and qualitative information on another for negligible cost. It should be established whether patients habitually have blood or protein in their urine. If they have proteinuria, the 24-hour excretion should be measured.

In childhood doctors are usually pedantic about urine cultures. It is not always recorded by doctors or parents whether the presence of bacteriuria is actually associated with any symptoms. When an adult develops bacteriuria or cystitis having previously had sterile urine, it may indicate a change for the worse in the urinary tract. This is particularly true in systems which can produce few symptoms such as ileal conduits and the prune belly syndrome. It should be recorded when a culture was positive, whether there were symptoms and whether the result was considered significant.

**3** *Renal function*. Once the glomerular filtration rate (GFR) has dropped to around 40 ml/min the plasma creatinine is probably as good a monitor as any. However, there is a big gap between 40 and a normal of around 120 ml/min. If there has been any significant renal damage and particularly if there is chronic hydronephrosis, a formal measurement of the GFR is essential.

**4** *Imaging*. Urologists are fortunate in having so many modalities of imaging available to them. It is essential to choose the right one to answer the current question. However, there is still no substitute for the pictures of the intravenous urogram (IVU) that will tell more than a thousand words! Other modalities enable us to interpret the IVU pictures and may suffice for follow-up. So I find it most helpful to have an IVU that post-dates the most recent significant change in the patient's urinary tract.

## ADULT INVESTIGATIONS FOR ROUTINE FOLLOW-UP

The majority of patients attending for routine follow-up have no symptoms. The consultation should be thorough enough to detect silent progression of the basic disease and yet not unduly burdensome for the patient who may have more important things on his or her mind. The follow-up protocol will vary according to the disease but the essential ingredients of history, examination and investigation remain.

Ample time must be given to the interview. Even the symptomless patient will have questions. Arrival in the adult clinic marks the beginning of separation from the parents who previously have taken the responsibility for the illness. Although it is best to have a gradual handover of responsibility to the patient, the adult clinic must take a lead. This will probably be the first time that a doctor has explained the problem to the patient who is usually anxious to understand. It quickly becomes obvious that the newly grown-up child has different requirements and priorities to those assigned by the parents. Sexual function and fertility are amongst the first.

Unless there are specific problems, the examination is relatively uninformative. The most useful measurement is the blood pressure which must never be omitted in patients with any hint of renal disease. Family planning specialists must be reminded of this when they monitor girls starting to take the contraceptive pill.

### Urine investigations

The stick-test of urine gives so much useful information that it must remain the basis of routine follow-up. The most commonly detected abnormality is proteinuria which will trigger further investigations for renal deterioration.

Routine urine culture is only useful when the detection of asymptomatic bacteriuria would be a sign of impending trouble. The main groups include: the prune belly syndrome, patients with cutaneous diversions (see below), known stone-formers and pregnant women.

### Blood investigations

Patients with renal damage have an estimation of plasma electrolytes, urea and creatinine once a year. Patients who have urine in contact with bowel need special care because of the known metabolic problems and those that we have yet to dectect. It seems likely, for example, that metabolic acidosis is much more common a problem than had been thought (see Chapter 11). Annual plasma chloride estimation should be added as a minimum.

### Imaging

Routine imaging has been made much easier by

the advent of ultrasound. Urinary tract ultrasound is certainly the mainstay of routine imaging in my 'adolescent clinic' and it is greatly helped by having the same team all the time. The main exception is for stone-formers who are still followed by plain X-ray. Patients whose urinary systems are at risk of change are examined every 5 years and 3-yearly in puberty. Where the urinary tract is grossly abnormal, it is almost impossible to interpret the findings on ultrasound without some accurate foreknowledge; it is therefore inevitable that an IVU must be done from time to time and certainly when there has been a major reconstruction.

The ultrasound and radiographic appearances can only be compared with earlier studies if the examinations were done under exactly the same conditions. The degree of dilatation of the renal collecting system and ureters can vary with posture and with bladder filling. This point is illustrated by the series of films in Fig. 2.1. All are part of the same IVU. The early pictures are taken with the patient supine and the bladder full. The later pictures are taken when standing and then after micturition. The lessening of the dilatation of the pelvis and ureters is not due to miraculous relief of obstruction during the study.

It is more of a problem to know what to do when the ultrasound detects a change. The suspected diagnosis will give some indication of the next step. Most commonly the change is increased dilatation and the question of obstruction arises. Much has been written on the diagnosis of urinary tract obstruction and we are fortunate to have so many alternative investigations.

Patients whose upper urinary tracts have been dilated for many years have a special problem. In my experience it is unusual for a DTPA isotope renogram to be able to distinguish between sluggish emptying and frank obstruction even when frusemide is given. Obstruction is sometimes excluded by this test. If there has been a previous isotope scan and a definite change is found, especially in the differential function, the diagnosis may be made, though seldom with the confidence necessary to embark on yet another operation.

In these circumstances the antegrade pressure/flow test described by Whitaker is essential. Great care must be taken completely to fill the 'dead space' of the upper tract before starting the measurements.

For lower tract obstruction standard urodynamic tests, with or without video filming, are indicated. We have also found these tests useful for patients with continent urinary diversions both as a routine and when continence or renal function have deteriorated (see Chapter 11).

When the upper tracts are suffering and the cause is thought to lie in the lower tract it is essential to investigate both systems. We have found it helpful to look at them simultaneously. This is done by performing a DTPA isotope scan and standard cystometrogram together. Changes in the clearance of the isotope from the kidneys in response to changing bladder pressure can be seen on the gamma camera (P.J.R. Shaw, personal communication 1989).

## Renal function

As the years pass, the anatomy and physiology of the urinary tract may become very complicated. As the real object of care is to preserve renal function (rather than to correct dilatation or straighten out kinks), it is reasonable to measure that function directly. If the GFR remains steady it is unlikely that any serious harm is occurring. There are other important parameters of renal function which occasionally need to be measured, but the GFR remains the main guide.

The GFR should be measured in all patients with very complex anatomy, with long-standing bilateral ureteric dilatation or with uncertain prognosis. For most of these cases the measurement, by chromium EDTA clearance, is done annually for 2 years after an operation and then 5-yearly. Whenever a doubt arises, it is very comforting to repeat the measurement and to find it unchanged.

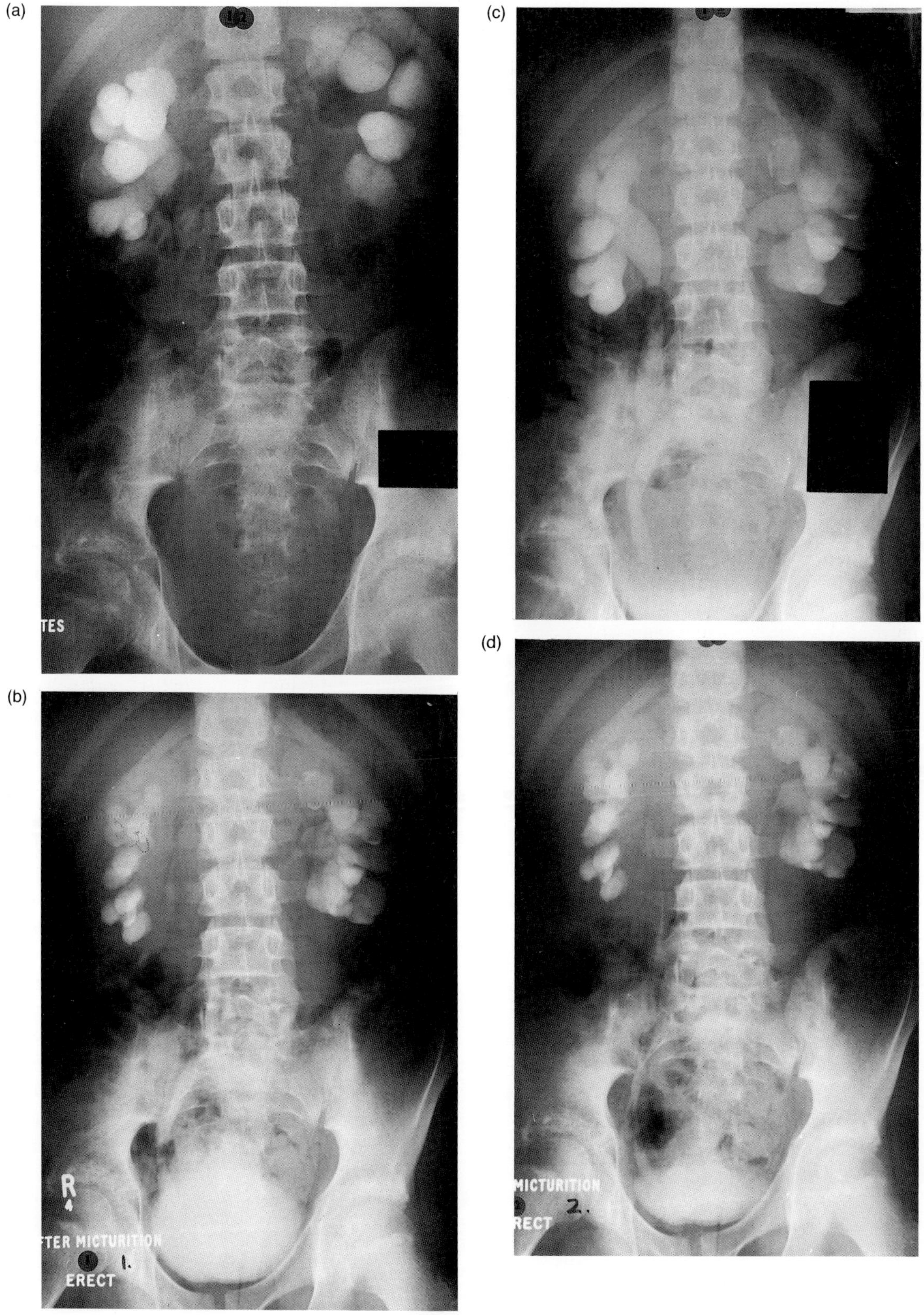
(a)
(b)
(c)
(d)
TES
R
4
FTER MICTURITION
ERECT
1.
MICTURITION
2.
RECT

## INVESTIGATIONS IN SPECIAL CIRCUMSTANCES

### Cutaneous diversions

In the days when ileal conduits were common in paediatric patients there was sometimes a tendency to think diversion cured all the patient's problems. Unfortunately it just exchanged one lot of problems for another. Many papers testify to the poor long-term results (see Chapter 10). Some poor results may be due to inadequate monitoring. The few remaining patients with cutaneous diversions are followed by a strict protocol (Table 2.1). Surprisingly, the main problem in this programme has been with the examination: patients are very resistant to allowing digital examination of the stoma. The clinic keeps a stock of all the commonly used bags so that 'I forgot to bring a spare' cannot be used as an excuse. The most common site of stomal stenosis is at abdominal wall level which will not be detected by looking at the outside of the stoma.

The significance of the catheter residual is uncertain. The ileum is supposed to be a 'conduit' and not a storage organ. Thus, although the residue may vary in different circumstances, one that is consistently above 15 ml does imply some measure of poor drainage. When combined with infection it is particularly worrying as renal deterioration has been associated with high antibody titres to *Escherichia coli* (see Chapter 10).

This regime (Table 2.1) has detected many complications at an early stage. In the last 10 years only one case of progressive renal damage has been seen in a man who developed end-stage renal failure from a GFR of 45 ml/min from one annual visit to the next.

**Table 2.1** Routine follow-up protocol for patients with ileal or colonic conduits.

| |
|---|
| *Every year*: |
| Blood pressure |
| Inspection and digital examination of stoma |
| Catheterisation of stoma to measure residual urine |
| Culture of catheter urine |
| *Every 5th year* (or with abnormalities of the above): |
| Urinary tract imaging |

The same problems with the choice of imaging modality apply in these as in other patients. In diagnosing obstruction the ascending loopogram is helpful: if there is free reflux to the kidney I assume that there is no obstruction. Although obstruction and reflux can co-exist in the same ureter, in practice it does not seem to happen.

### Ureterosigmoidostomy

The long-term dangers of this diversion are well known (see Chapter 10). However, it remains an attractive form of diversion in some circumstances. A few exstrophy patients still fail to achieve a working bladder; many patients in developing countries have little access to stoma services; these and a few other groups may be grateful for it. Furthermore, even with the availability of continent diversions I have yet to find a patient with a ureterosigmoidostomy who will volunteer for change, even knowing the cancer risks.

All patients who have ever had their urinary and faecal streams mixed and who retain the anastomosis must have an annual colonoscopy from the 8th year onwards. The cancer risk is not removed by a change of diversion unless the anastomotic site is completely removed.

**Fig. 2.1.** An IVU of a patient whose kidneys drain largely by gravity. (a) Supine film taken 30 min after contrast injection. (b) Film taken after standing for 15 min (i.e. 45 min after contrast injection) showing pooling of the contrast in the calyces but some filling of the ureters and bladder. (c) Film taken after the first attempt at micturition showing less calyceal dilatation and partial bladder emptying. (d) Film taken after second micturition showing further emptying of the upper tracts and a smaller bladder residue.

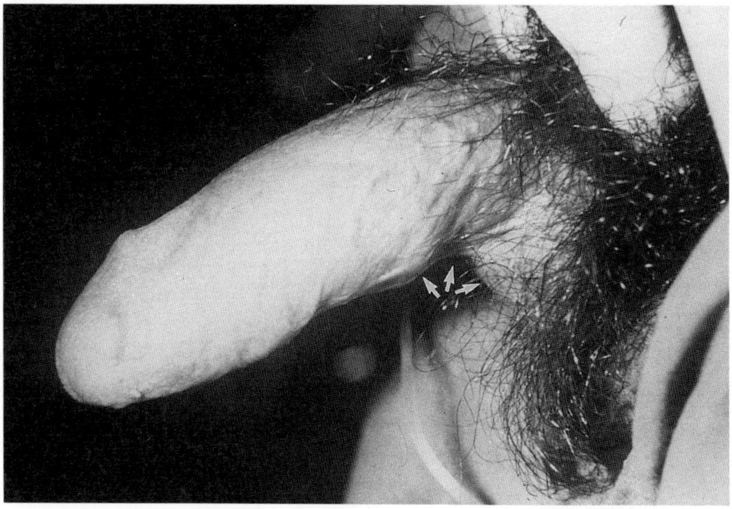

**Fig. 2.2** Clinical photograph taken during an infusion cavernosogram showing a ventral chordee of nearly 90° close to the base of the penis. This deformity would have been missed had the erection been obtained with a tourniquet around the base of the penis.

The other follow-up is the same as for cutaneous diversions. The plasma chloride should be measured annually. Even with this simple screen we have found a 50% incidence of hyperchloraemic acidosis with new cases turning up even after many years of apparent normality.

## Investigations of sexual function

Impotence is very rare in these patients. Even with gross genital anomalies it is striking how normal are the libido and sexual achievement. In many instances there is erectile deformity, especially in exstrophy and hypospadias (see Chapters 13 and 15). Some young males lack the confidence or knowledge to describe the abnormality. For them, some form of artificial erection is required, and as the defect often involves the buried portion of the corpora it is helpful to do a cavernosogram. The infusion method first described by Herzberg (see Chapter 13) gives the most useful information; putting a tourniquet around the base of the penis and injecting contrast into the distal corpora may miss a chordee arising in the perineum (Fig. 2.2).

Fertility in either sex does not feature prominently in the thoughts of the adolescent but requests for 'fertility tests' and genetic counselling are still common. It is surprising what strange ideas patients will have picked up during their passage through childhood. I am sure that mature patients should be told the truth (so far as it is known) about their potential fertility. Certainly men who are azoospermic and women who have absent uterus or ovaries should not be told that natural fertility is possible. There are no tests in either sex that will prove fertility. In females the monthly temperature chart should show whether ovulation is occurring. In males semen analysis will at least show whether or not sperm are made. Serum luteinising hormone (LH), follicle-stimulating hormone (FSH) and testosterone levels give further information on the pituitary–testicular axis. The results of these tests should be given to the patients with appropriate guidance on their interpretation.

Some help may be available from a knowledge of earlier cohorts of patients with the same diagnosis. As one patient with prune belly syndrome put it: 'you mean no prune has ever fathered a child!' However, even this information must be interpreted with caution: techniques of treatment in early life change and may improve the prognosis and, of course, the diagnosis may be wrong. I have recently encountered a male with micropenis apparently due to male pseudohermaphroditism who had been considered infertile. It came as a surprise to discover, on testicular biopsy, that he had Johnson counts of 9 and 8 on the two sides.

# 3 *Renal function in patients with congenital urological abnormalities*

## INTRODUCTION

Congenital urological abnormalities often lead to renal damage and sometimes to progressive impairment of renal function culminating in end-stage renal failure. A consideration of the possible mechanisms of renal damage is important in order that effective strategies can be planned, ideally to prevent such damage occurring in early childhood (or even *in utero*) but at least to minimise any further damage once it has begun.

Obviously there is a wide spectrum of congenital urological abnormalities, but only a small percentage of these consistently lead to impaired renal function. The more common causes, taken from a series of 54 patients referred for treatment of end-stage renal disease, are listed in Table 3.1 (Warshaw *et al.* 1982). Other rare causes seen at St Peter's UK include bladder exstrophy and prune belly syndrome, but any congenital abnormality should be considered as a potential cause of renal damage. It is therefore very important to monitor renal function closely and accurately in all such patients.

## PATHOPHYSIOLOGY OF RENAL DAMAGE

Apart from primary vesico-ureteral reflux (VUR) very little research has been done into the mechanisms of renal damage in this group of patients. Intuitively one imagines that most of the initial damage is secondary to either obstruction or reflux, with or without infection. This in fact may well be the case, but does little to explain the continuing deterioration in renal function which occurs in those patients in whom these problems have been to a large extent treated or excluded. Recent experimental research into the mechanisms of the progression of chronic renal failure has produced a theory that 'hyperfiltration' in remaining nephrons may be responsible for the continuing damage (Brenner *et al.* 1982, Fine 1988, Klahr *et al.* 1988), and this may well play a part in this group of patients.

It is important to remember that this is a heterogeneous group of patients and different factors may have more or less importance in particular individuals. Some of the factors which may contribute to the pathophysiology are listed in Table 3.2, and more details of their possible individual roles will now be discussed.

### Primary VUR

The past 20 years have seen intensive investigation in both animals and humans of the pathophysiology of reflux nephropathy. Fig. 3.1 shows a summary of the current concept of the natural history of primary reflux. The primary anatomical defect appears to be at the vesico-ureteral

**Table 3.1** Common abnormalities leading to end-stage renal failure (from Warshaw *et al.* 1982).

| Abnormality | Numbers |
|---|---|
| Bladder neck obstruction | 3 |
| Posterior urethral valves | 20 |
| Vesico-ureteral reflux or obstruction | 23 |
| Pelvi-ureteric junction obstruction | 4 |
| Neurogenic bladder | 3 |
| Undefined | 1 |
| Total | 54 |

**Table 3.2** Possible causes of renal damage.

| |
|---|
| Vesico-ureteral reflux and intrarenal reflux |
| Urinary tract obstruction |
| Renal dysplasia |
| Glomerular hyperfiltration |
| Infection |
| Hypertension |
| Acute tubular necrosis |
| Drugs |

junction. The lateral position of the ureter within the bladder leads to a short sub-mucosal section of ureter, and this allows urine to reflux freely from the bladder into the ureter. Damage to the kidney results initially from formation of discrete renal scars. At a later stage, usually when both kidneys are moderately or severely scarred, significant and sometimes nephrotic range proteinuria develops associated with progressive renal failure and progressive focal and segmental sclerosis in the remaining glomeruli, unrelated to further scar formation.

*Renal scar formation*

The scars occur in a radial pattern and consist of an area of cortical atrophy associated with a dilated calyx. The scar contains atrophic tubules with fibrotic interstitium and a few focal mononuclear cell infiltrates. There are often areas of cystic dilatation and colloid casts (Bailey 1988). The renal tissue between scars is normal in the early stages of the natural history. Work in both the human and the pig model of reflux nephropathy has shown these scars to be concentrated at the poles of the kidney, and to occur only in areas where urine is able to reflux freely into the ducts of the collecting system and so into the tubules of the individual nephrons (intrarenal reflux) (Rolleston *et al.* 1974, Hodson *et al.* 1975). Both the human and pig kidneys contain two types of papillae: simple and compound. Only the latter type will allow intrarenal reflux to occur, and the concentration of

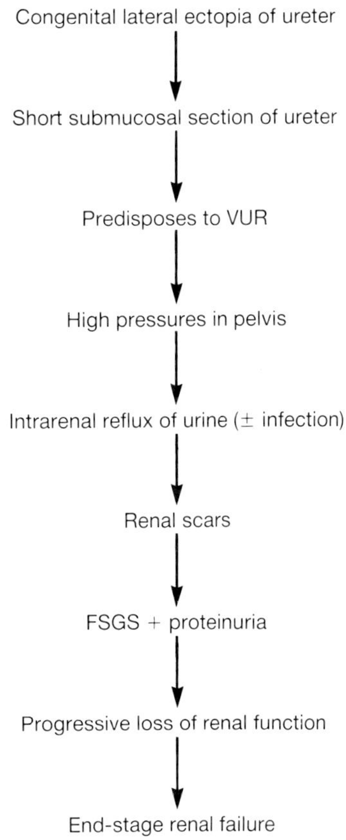


**Fig. 3.1** Natural history of reflux nephropathy.

compound papillae at the poles of the kidney correlates with the observed tendency for scars to form in this area (Ransley & Risdon 1974, Ransley & Risdon 1975a, b, Bourne *et al.* 1976, Funston & Gremin 1978).

A large number of studies have now examined the natural history of scar formation in VUR (Rolleston *et al.* 1970, Rolleston *et al.* 1975, Smellie *et al.* 1975, Shimada *et al.* 1988). Three general observations can be made.

**1** The majority of scar formation in primary VUR seems to occur at a very young age, usually in the first year of life. A minority of new scars may still occur up to the age of 5, and there have been rare reports of new scar formation up to the age of 10 (Smellie 1986). The reasons for this are still uncertain. Certainly part of the reason may be that reflux often ceases in early infancy, but a significant number of people continue to reflux into adult life with no apparent new scar formation. However scar formation may occur in adolescence or adult life in those such as paraplegics for instance, who have abnormal bladders and secondary VUR (Arnold *et al.* 1984).

**2** The amount and severity of the scarring correlates to some extent with the severity of the reflux (Rolleston *et al.* 1975, Smellie *et al.* 1975, Shimada *et al.* 1988). Those with grade 3 and 4 reflux seem most likely to develop scarring. Those with grade 1 and 2 reflux are much less at risk. Even so, scar formation has been recorded in significant numbers in infants with grade 1 and 2 reflux, and therefore all children with any degree of VUR remain at risk.

**3** Recurrent urinary tract infections (UTI) are a common problem in children and adults with VUR and are often the first presentation of children with this problem. Conversely, many adults who first present with end-stage renal failure secondary to reflux nephropathy have no history of symptomatic UTIs. A considerable controversy still remains over whether concurrent infection is necessary for scar formation. Recent studies have suggested that new scar formation in children with primary VUR is almost always associated with a preceding UTI (Smellie & Normand 1985, Smellie 1986). However this does not necessarily prove that scar formation cannot occur in the absence of infection. Certainly one can envisage that high pressure intrarenal reflux of urine may be enough of an insult alone to lead to damage and scar formation. Indeed it has been demonstrated in the pig model that high pressure sterile reflux does lead to scar formation and reflux nephropathy (Heptinstall & Hodson 1984, Hodson & Twohill 1984, Ransley *et al.* 1984). The problem remains unresolved, but it would seem that in primary VUR infection is usually (but perhaps not always) necessary for scar formation to occur. The situation may be different in those with high pressure bladders and VUR, in which high pressure sterile reflux may cause scarring even in the absence of infection.

Increasing interest is now being shown in the investigation of bladder function in patients with primary VUR. Hitherto it has been assumed that these individuals have normal bladders and that their propensity to renal damage is only related to the abnormality at the vesico-ureteral junction. Recent studies have suggested that there may be a sub-group of these patients with detrusor instability, and resolution of reflux may be helped by treatment with anticholinergic agents (Taylor *et al.* 1982, Koff & Murtagh 1983). It is interesting to speculate that bladder dysfunction may be more important than has previously been realised in all patients with primary VUR.

### *Proteinuria, hyperfiltration and glomerulosclerosis*

Some patients develop renal scarring secondary to primary VUR during infancy, but then continue normally into and throughout adult life with no new scar formation and with stable renal function. However, another group of patients go on to develop significant proteinuria associated with a progressive decline in renal function, often culminating in end-stage renal failure. Renal biopsy in these patients demonstrates a glomerular lesion identical to that seen in patients with primary or secondary focal and segmental glomerulosclerosis (FSGS) (Bhathena *et al.* 1980, Torres *et al.* 1980, Cotran 1982). This occurs in areas of the cortex otherwise unaffected by renal scarring, and indeed can occur in the contralateral otherwise completely normal kidney in patients with unilateral VUR and reflux nephropathy (Bailey *et al.* 1984b).

The pathogenesis of the glomerular lesions remains unknown. The two main possibilities are:

*Immunological injury to bacterial antigens or autologous antigens.* The presence of IgM and C3 in the sclerotic areas and mesangium of more than 50% of the patients with FSGS raises the possibility of an immune reaction (Zimmerman *et al.* 1973). The lesions could be caused by the deposition of circulating immune complexes or by *in situ* formation of immune complexes. With the exception of the demonstration of a coiled structure and spherical particles thought to represent altered bacterial forms in the glomerulus by one investigator (Kincaid-Smith 1979), other studies have failed to identify bacterial antigens in the glomeruli of patients with reflux nephropathy. Tamm–Horsfall protein is a possible endogenous antigen and is found in the renal interstitium in both experimental and human reflux nephropathy (Zager *et al.* 1978, Cotran & Hodson 1979). However, so far experiments have failed to localise Tamm–Horsfall protein in the mesangium of these patients.

*The hyperfiltration theory.* The second possibility is that the glomerular changes are similar to those found in many other renal diseases where loss of renal function from whatever cause leads to proteinuria, FSGS changes on renal biopsy and progressive loss of renal function. Experimental work mainly in the rat has led to the hypothesis that the glomerular changes are secondary to altered glomerular haemodynamics leading to increased glomerular capillary pressure or 'glomerular hypertension' and to an increased single nephron glomerular filtration rate. The concept of a glomerulus with a higher filtration rate than normal leading to subsequent structural damage has led to the label 'hyperfiltration' to describe the phenomenon (Brenner *et al.* 1982).

The simplest model of hyperfiltration in the rat is that of the sub-total nephrectomy where up to seven-eighths of total functioning renal tissue is removed surgically. The remaining renal tissue hypertrophies and the single nephron GFR in remaining nephrons is increased. This can be seen as an initially advantageous response to allow the remaining renal tissue to replace as far as possible the function of the lost nephrons. However, in the long-term it seems that the high glomerular capillary pressure necessary to increase single nephron GFR leads to structural damage to the glomerulus and to the changes of focal and segmental glomerulosclerosis. The details of how and why the haemodynamic changes lead to the pathological changes seen in the glomerulus remain uncertain and it may be that other mechanisms such as platelet aggregation and intraglomerular coagulation contribute to the damage (Diamond & Karnovsky 1988, Klahr *et al.* 1988). The idea that proteinuria itself may be responsible for the progressive damage has been raised, but it is also possible that this is the result of the structural change rather than the main cause.

A similar mechanism can be imagined in reflux nephropathy in which loss of functioning renal tissue through renal scarring leads to hyperfiltration in the remaining nephrons and subsequent glomerular damage.

## Secondary VUR

Apart from primary VUR, where the only abnormality is the failure of the vesico-ureteric junction to prevent reflux of urine from the bladder into the ureter, reflux may also occur as part of a spectrum of other congenital abnormalities. In particular it often occurs in the presence of a high pressure bladder from whatever cause. Two examples which commonly lead to secondary VUR are posterior urethral valves, or other causes of bladder outflow obstruction, and neuropathic bladder. Obviously the same mechanisms of renal damage may apply in secondary VUR as they do in primary VUR. However, as discussed above, it may be that in this particular group sterile reflux could play a more important role in renal scar formation. It is also important to note that in patients with spinal injuries, radiological studies show that renal scarring may occur *de novo* in adolescent and adult life (Arnold *et al.* 1984). It may be that the higher intravesical pressures in patients with secondary as opposed to primary reflux lead to transmission of higher pressure to the renal pelvis and therefore a higher propensity to cause renal damage with or without the presence of infection.

## Obstruction

It is well-recognised that urinary tract obstruction at all ages and from whatever cause may lead to renal damage and impaired renal function. The severity, time course and reversibility of the effects on the kidney depend on a number of factors includng whether it is:

**1** Acute or chronic.
**2** Partial or complete.
**3** Unilateral or bilateral.
**4** High or low obstruction.
**5** With or without infection.
**6** With or without other complicating factors.

Obstruction may certainly play a part in the pathophysiology of renal damage in a large number of congenital urinary tract abnormalities. Macroscopic examination of kidneys damaged by exposure to chronic urinary tract obstruction reveals widely dilated pelvis and calyces, complete destruction of the medulla and only a thin rim of cortex. Microscopically there is tubular dilatation and atrophy, interstitial fibrosis and inflammation, with hyalinisation of the glomeruli (Wilson 1988). Similarities may be recognised with the pathology of the renal scars of reflux nephropathy, except that the damage is widespread rather than localised. Interestingly, the pathology of some kidneys exposed to gross VUR is indistinguishable from that of kidneys exposed to long-term chronic obstruction (Bailey 1988).

The pathophysiology of the renal damage in urinary tract obstruction has not been completely unravelled (Wilson 1980, Klahr 1983), but important factors are:

**1** Transmission of high pressures to the renal tubules leading to pressure atrophy of tubular cells.
**2** Intrarenal reflux of urine as in reflux nephropathy with similar mechanisms of damage. It is possible that urine may leak into the interstitium which leads to inflammation and fibrosis.
**3** Urinary stasis predisposes to infection which may potentiate the damage to the kidney as in reflux nephropathy.
**4** There has been very little experimental work on the effects of long-term partial obstruction on the kidney, but a large body of work on the effects of acute complete ureteral obstruction in experimental animals suggests that ischaemia secondary to decreased renal blood flow may be important in the ensuing renal damage.

Much of that which we know about the effects of urinary tract obstruction comes from work in adults or experimental animals, but in the absence of much work on the effects on the kidney in children with obstruction we can only assume at present that similar principles may apply.

## Renal dysplasia

Some children as well as having congenital abnormalities of their urinary tract are also born with dysplastic kidneys. Debate has centred on whether dysplasia is part of the general spectrum of congenital abnormality, or whether it is due to damage from obstruction or reflux *in utero* as occurs in the adult. Experiments in sheep where the ureter was tied off *in utero* have suggested that the latter possibility is more likely (Beck 1971). Either way, the child born with one or two dysplastic kidneys will already have some impairment of renal function and if the hyperfiltration hypothesis is correct, may suffer continuing damage in the remaining functioning renal tissue.

## Infection

Patients with congenital urological abnormalities are prone to recurrent UTI for various reasons, the most important being the predilection to urinary stasis. Not only may they contribute to renal damage as mentioned in the preceding discussion, but they may lead to a temporary decrease in renal function in patients with non-obstructed and non-refluxing systems. Whether infections in this setting can lead to permanent renal damage is still the subject of debate, but it seems unlikely.

### Hyperfiltration

In the above discussion on the pathogenesis of reflux nephropathy the development of proteinuria and FSGS in these patients was shown often to presage the development of chronic progressive renal failure, and the possible importance of hyperfiltering glomeruli as the causative factor was discussed. No one has looked at whether a similar pathological lesion occurs in patients with other forms of congenital anatomical abnormalities. However our experience suggests that the majority of these patients who develop progressive chronic renal failure do develop significant proteinuria. Logically therefore it would seem attractive to postulate that the same mechanism operates in such patients.

### Hypertension

As with many causes of renal disease, patients with renal damage secondary to congenital anatomical abnormalities often develop hypertension. Two important factors are thought to be excess salt and water retention and increased renin secretion (de Wardener & MacGregor 1988). As in other renal diseases, this may contribute to further renal damage if it is not controlled.

A special case which warrants further discussion is that of patients with unilateral renal disease who have a small scarred kidney (Bailey *et al.* 1984a). The question arises of whether the hypertension in these patients is due to excess renin secretion by the damaged kidney and whether the hypertension can be cured by surgical removal of the kidney. The past 50 years has provided a wealth of literature on the subject although the number of good prospective controlled trials is small. The conclusion remains that surgical removal is undoubtedly successful in some of these patients but not in others. Therefore attention has centred on ways of predicting those who would benefit from the procedure. One obvious way of doing this would be to find those people in whom excess renin production by the damaged kidney was responsible for their hypertension. Unfortunately neither peripheral plasma renin measurement nor the more invasive differential renal vein renin measurement has proved useful in most studies. The procedure should therefore be kept as a last resort for patients whose hypertension is uncontrollable medically, particularly as angiotensin-converting enzyme inhibitors should produce a similar effect without surgery.

### Conclusion

Some of the possible factors which may contribute to renal damage in those patients with congenital urological abnormalities have been discussed above. One of the points that comes out of the discussion is that the microscopic pathology of the damaged kidney is similar in cases of damage from either reflux or obstruction, though it is more localised to the renal scars in pure reflux nephropathy. We would therefore postulate that the initial damage can be viewed as due to a spectrum ranging from primary reflux through high pressure secondary reflux to pure obstruction, depending on the specific urological abnormality. This may be modified according to the presence of other factors such as infection, hypertension or renal dysplasia. Whatever the initial injury, the loss of functioning renal tissue eventually leads to hyperfiltration in the remaining nephrons and the development of FSGS, proteinuria and progressive renal failure. Obviously if it is possible to interrupt this process early enough this final end-point may not be reached, and renal function may remain stable though impaired. This process is represented diagrammatically in Fig. 3.2. We would however stress that this hypothesis remains unproven and indeed it may not be possible to explain such a wide variety of abnormalities using one such theory. Even so it remains useful as a focal point for looking at ways of protecting renal function in these patients.

## PRACTICAL MANAGEMENT

### Assessment of renal function

The four commonly used measures of renal function are: plasma urea, plasma creatinine, creatinine clearance and glomerular filtration rate (GFR) measured by isotopic $^{51}$Cr-EDTA clearance. The plasma urea varies according to diet and is therefore an unreliable indicator of renal function. The creatinine is a fairly sensitive indicator of change in function once over 200 μmol/l, but may remain within the laboratory 'normal' range despite marked deterioration in renal function. The plasma creatinine is also affected by the muscle mass and thus a given level may have a very different significance in a small frail man compared to a muscular young man (as a rough guide, a figure of 45–75 in the former and 80–110 in the latter could be considered as indicating similar levels of renal function). It is vital to understand that by the time both the urea and creatinine are above 'normal', renal function is reduced by at least 50%, i.e. the GFR is 40–60 ml/min.

A creatinine clearance gives a reasonable idea of renal function when it is measured accurately. The period of the completed collection must be accurately noted. Creatinine clearance has a coefficient of variation of 30%. It becomes inaccurate when function is poor and tends to overestimate glomerular filtration rate. This is because, as renal function deteriorates, creatinine is increasingly excreted by tubular secretion. The most accurate measure of function is given by an isotopic $^{51}$Cr-EDTA clearance — this is an accu-

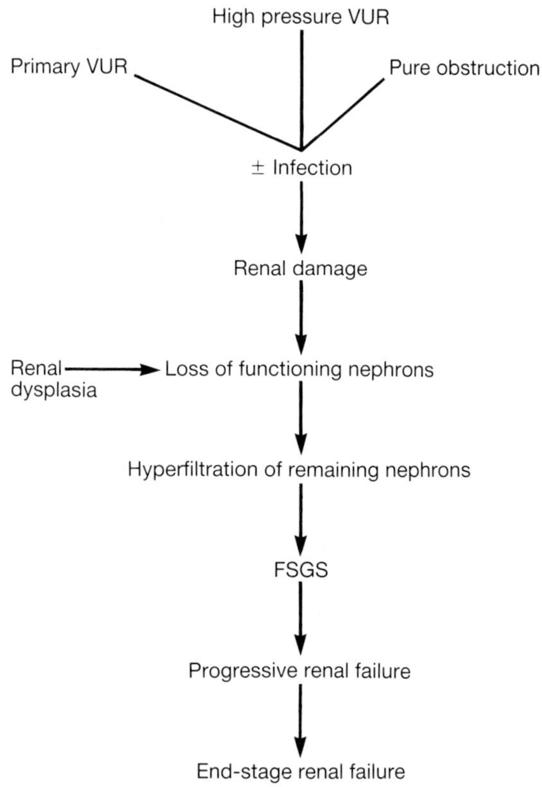


**Fig. 3.2** Natural history of urological renal failure.

rate reflection of GFR until function becomes very poor. The most important point to stress is that a 'normal' creatinine does not imply normal renal function, and a large fall in GFR occurs before the plasma creatinine falls outside the normal range.

The question has been raised (McCance 1959) as to whether the high growth rate during childhood may relieve the excretory burden on the kidney because of the requirement of dividing and growing cells for amino acids and electrolytes. If this is so, it is interesting to speculate that passing through puberty and going from a period of high growth to a period of little or no growth may reveal more severe renal impairment than was previously apparent if plasma urea and electrolytes are relied on as a measure of renal function — however this would not affect the creatinine clearance or isotopic GFR as a more accurate index of renal function.

Another important marker of renal pathology is proteinuria. This can be measured qualitatively by dipstick testing of the urine which should be a regular part of the assessment at every out-patient attendance. A 24-hour urine collection for protein excretion provides a quantitative measure of protein excretion and should be arranged at regular intervals on all these patients. Significant proteinuria may be the first indication that FSGS changes and progressive deterioration in renal function have developed.

## Assessment of the urinary tract

### *Renal parenchyma*

Assessment of the remaining renal parenchyma gives an idea of how much renal function may be salvageable after an insult to the kidney such as chronic obstruction. This is most easily measured by ultrasound examination. A more accurate assessment of the extent of renal scarring in primary or secondary reflux nephropathy may be given by an IVU or by isotopic DMSA scans, but anatomical detail becomes increasingly poor when the creatinine is above 200 μmol/l.

### *Urinary tract anatomy and assessment of obstruction*

The anatomy of the renal tract is still best assessed by an IVU, although renal ultrasound, plain abdominal X-ray and isotopic DTPA renogram can provide useful information. The assessment of obstruction within the urinary tract remains a difficult problem. The initial investigations in any patient in whom obstruction is suspected should be an ultrasound and DTPA renogram. The former will show dilatation of the pelvicalyceal system in gross obstruction. Unfortunately a grossly dilated pelvicalyceal system may occur in the absence of obstruction, particularly in patients who have been obstructed for long periods in the past. Comparison with previous ultrasound scans can be useful in this situation. Conversely a non-dilated pelvicalyceal system can be compatible with significant obstruction. A DTPA renogram can give useful information in cases of suspected obstruction. Unfortunately the sensitivity of the investigation relies strongly on the presence of a high urinary flow rate and poor drainage may be due either to obstruction or to a poor urinary flow. The sensitivity can be improved by the use of a diuretic (such as frusemide) to ensure a good urinary flow rate. Similarly a normal scan cannot absolutely exclude a degree of obstruction and the investigation becomes unreliable when renal function is poor (creatinine >200 μmol/l). When these two investigations are inconclusive an antegrade nephrostogram with pressure studies (Whitaker test) may become necessary. The demonstration of free flow of contrast and normal pressures makes significant obstruction very unlikely.

Even if all these investigations are completely normal we believe it is possible that some degree of functional obstruction not detectable by current criteria may contribute to the renal dysfunction in this group of patients. It is interesting to speculate that abnormalities in ureteric peristalsis may contribute to functional obstruction. Certainly the ureter is not just a passive structure linking the collecting system of the kidney to the bladder. Isotopic studies of ureteric peristalsis are now becoming available and may contribute useful information to this problem.

### *Urodynamics*

A formal discussion of urodynamics is outside the scope of this chapter, but it is becoming increasingly evident that good bladder function is very important in the preservation of normal renal function. It is well recognised for instance that high pressure bladders can play an important part in producing functional obstruction and VUR in patients with posterior urethral valves. It is also becoming evident that patients with primary VUR may have abnormal bladder function and this may contribute to renal dysfunction and damage.

## Basic investigations

A list of the minimal baseline investigations is summarised in Table 3.3. How often these individuals should attend for follow-up from the renal point of view will obviously depend on the urological abnormality, the degree of renal damage at presentation, and the potential for new or continuing renal damage in the future. They should certainly all have creatinine, urea and electrolytes, lying and standing blood pressures and urine dipstick testing at all out-patient visits. We would also recommend yearly GFR and 24-hour urine collections for protein in anyone with declining function. Yearly ultrasounds and DTPA renograms may also be useful depending on the underlying problem.

If a deterioration in renal function occurs then the first step is to exclude an obvious reversible cause such as obstruction, infection or desalination. Consideration should also be given to nephrotoxic drugs such as aminoglycoside antibiotics, tetracyclines, non-steroidal anti-inflammatory agents and radiocontrast media.

Desalination is a very important cause of an acute deterioration in renal function and these patients are particularly prone to this pre-, peri-, and postoperatively. Unless they are obviously fluid overloaded they should all receive intravenous fluids preoperatively. Postoperatively they should all be kept well-hydrated. Clinical assessment remains the best measure of hydration, and all doctors should become practised at assessing the fluid status of the patient. Daily weights where possible are also very useful at demonstrating changes in fluid balance. Desalination should also not be forgotten as a cause of an acute deterioration in renal function in the out-patient department.

A consideration of the relative merits of medical and surgical treatments of VUR in preventing reflux nephropathy in infants is outside the scope of this chapter, however the authors do not believe that continuing reflux in the adolescent or adult contributes to declining renal function and therefore antireflux operations are not indicated specifically to prevent this decline (see Chapter 8). If no reversible factors are found we must look at how remaining renal function may best be preserved in these patients.

**Table 3.3** Minimal baseline investigations for patients with impaired renal function and urological abnormalities.

| |
|---|
| Blood pressure |
| Urine dipstick testing |
| Creatinine, urea and electrolytes |
| Full blood count |
| Albumin |
| Calcium, phosphate and alkaline phosphatase |
| Plain abdominal X-ray |
| Isotopic GFR ($^{51}$Cr-EDTA) |
| Ultrasound kidneys, ureters, bladder, before and after micturition |
| Isotopic renogram ($^{99}$Tc-DTPA) |
| 24-hour urine for protein and creatinine clearance (×2) |

## Preservation of renal function

Patients with impaired renal function can conveniently be divided into two groups. The first group consists of those with impaired but stable renal function. This group has suffered renal damage in the past and has been left with a reduction in functioning renal tissue, but the damaging factor has now been removed. They usually have <1 G proteinuria/24 hours and a creatinine of <200. In this group the most important thing is to prevent further insults to the kidney. The blood pressure should be aggressively monitored and controlled with standard antihypertensive medication, and the diastolic blood pressure should be kept below 80 mmHg if possible in most patients.

The second group consists of those with progressively declining renal function with usually >1 G proteinuria/24 hours. The creatinine may be only minimally elevated initially, but continues to rise despite the absence of any obviously reversible factors. It is this group that we believe have developed FSGS secondary to hyperfiltration. What this fails to explain is why some patients with creatinines of 100–200 develop hyperfiltration, while others with creatinines of 200–300 retain stable renal function. This group provides the possibility of more specific therapy to try to arrest or slow down the progressive decline in renal function.

### *Blood pressure control*

As in patients with stable renal dysfunction, control of systemic hypertension has been shown to be critically important in slowing down the progression of renal dysfunction. This can be done with standard antihypertensive therapy, but as explained below there may be advantages in the use of angiotensin-converting enzyme (ACE) inhibitors as first-line therapy.

### *Prevention of hyperfiltration and glomerular injury*

As discussed in the section on hyperfiltration there are at least theoretical reasons why reduction of intraglomerular hypertension may slow down or arrest glomerular damage and progressive decline in renal function. Reduction of systemic hypertension by conventional therapy may in fact be effective in protecting renal function by reducing intraglomerular hypertension. However there are several ways in which we can specifically try to limit further glomerular damage.

*ACE inhibitors.* Angiotensin II constricts both the afferent and efferent arteriole of the glomerulus. However its effect is relatively greater on the efferent arteriole compared with the afferent side, and it therefore causes a rise in the intraglomerular pressure. ACE inhibitors prevent the conversion of angiotensin I to angiotensin II and therefore cause a decrease in intraglomerular pressure by relaxing the efferent arteriole. According to the hyperfiltration theory this should protect the glomerulus from further damage. There is no question that ACE inhibitors can reduce the amount of proteinuria in certain types of renal disease. Whether this reduces the progression of renal failure remains uncertain. Our experience suggests it does so in diabetic patients. The effect in patients with urological renal failure is not proven, but at present it is our policy to use them in all these patients with hypertension and/or significant proteinuria.

*Restriction of dietary protein.* Studies have shown that low protein diets are effective in reducing glomerular damage in hyperfiltering rats. Several studies in humans have suggested that low protein diets are effective in slowing progression of renal failure (Brenner *et al.* 1982, Fine 1988). Dietary protein restriction also has the effect of lowering intraglomerular pressures, but the mechanism is unknown. Conversely high protein diets increase GFR and cause hyperfiltration. We advise patients not to take too much protein and recommend 1 G protein/kg body weight/day. Low protein diets mean a restriction to 0.6 G protein/kg and may result in a significant and unwelcome fall in body weight.

*Anticoagulants and platelet inhibitors.* Intraglomerular coagulation may contribute to the progression of glomerular sclerosis according to animal experiments (Diamond & Karnovsky 1988, Klahr *et al.* 1988). The effect of anticoagulants and platelet inhibitors in the progression of renal disease in humans is at present uncertain.

*Restriction of dietary lipids.* Similarly there are theoretical reasons why the reduction of serum lipid levels may help protect against glomerular damage (Moorhead *et al.* 1982, Diamond &

Karnovsky 1988, Klahr *et al.* 1988). Lipid-lowering drugs are being evaluated, but the effect in humans remains unknown at present.

*Tubular and interstitial function*

The knowledge that calcium deposits commonly occur in the interstitium of chronically diseased kidneys led to the proposal that lowering of the calcium–phosphate product may be important in preventing the progression of chronic renal disease. Low phosphate diet and phosphate binders in rats have been shown to reduce the rate of progression of renal disease (Lumertgul *et al.* 1986, Fine 1988). Whether this is also true in humans is uncertain, but lowering serum phosphate protects against metabolic bone disease and is therefore a worthwhile objective. Reduction of protein intake will reduce plasma phosphate. Once plasma phosphate is at the upper limit of normal we control it with phosphate binders — currently either aluminium hydroxide or calcium carbonate (1–2 tablets or capsules taken with each meal). The alkaline phosphatase is raised in adolescents and this is not the usual assistance in assessing bone disease, nevertheless alphacalcidol should be prescribed to keep plasma calcium in the normal range. Acidosis may also contribute to progressive renal failure and metabolic bone disease and should therefore be controlled by administration of sodium bicarbonate.

## End-stage renal failure, dialysis and transplantation

However carefully these patients are managed, a number of them will eventually develop end-stage renal failure and require renal replacement therapy. Either haemodialysis or chronic ambulatory peritoneal dialysis (CAPD) may be suitable for these patients, and the reader should refer to standard nephrology texts or recent reviews for consideration of the relative merits of the two modalities (Gokal 1987, Maher 1989, Maiorca *et al.* 1989). We tend to prefer CAPD in most patients although this may often not be possible if they have had multiple abdominal operations or have an ileal conduit. Renal transplantation is the ultimate aim in all these patients whether it is a live-related transplant or a cadaver transplant. One of the most important considerations is whether the bladder function is suitable for maintaining long-term transplant function and this is considered in detail in Chapter 5.

## REFERENCES

Arnold E.P., Fukui J., Anthony A. *et al.* (1984) Bladder function following spinal cord injury: a urodynamic analysis of the outcome. *Br. J. Urol.* **56**, 172–9.

Bailey R.R. (1988) Vesicoureteric reflux and reflux nephropathy. In: Schrier G.W. & Gottschalk C.W. (eds) *Diseases of the Kidney*. Little, Brown & Co., Boston, pp. 747–83.

Bailey R.R., Lynn K.L. & McRae C.U. (1984a) Unilateral reflux nephropathy and hypertension. *Contr. Nephrol.* **39**, 116–25.

Bailey R.R., Swainson C.P., Lynn K.L. & Burry A.F. (1984b) Glomerular lesions in the 'normal' kidney in patients with unilateral reflux nephropathy. *Contr. Nephrol.* **39**, 126–31.

Beck A.D. (1971) The effect of intra-uterine urinary obstruction upon the development of the fetal kidney. *J. Urol.* **105**, 784–8.

Bhathena D.B., Weiss J.H., Holland N.H. *et al.* (1980) Focal and segmental glomerular sclerosis in reflux nephropathy. *Am. J. Med.* **68**, 886–92.

Bourne H.H., Condon V.R., Hoyt T.S. & Nixon G.W. (1976) Intrarenal reflux and renal damage. *J. Urol.* **115**, 304–6.

Brenner B.M., Meyer T.W. & Hostetter T.H. (1982) Dietary protein intake and the progressive nature of kidney disease: the role of hemodynamically mediated glomerular injury in the pathogenesis of progressive glomerular sclerosis in aging, renal ablation, and intrinsic renal disease. *N. Engl. J. Med.* **307**, 652–9.

Cotran R.S. (1982) Glomerulosclerosis in reflux nephropathy. *Kidney Int.* **21**, 528–34.

Cotran R.S. & Hodson C.J. (1979) Extratubular localisation of Tamm–Horsfall protein in experimental reflux nephropathy in the pig. In: Hodson C.J. & Kincaid-Smith P. (eds) *Reflux Nephropathy*. Masson Publishing USA Inc., New York, pp. 213–19.

de Wardener H.E. & MacGregor G.A. (1988) Blood pressure and the kidney. In: Schrier G.W. & Gottschalk C.W. (eds.) *Diseases of the Kidney*. Little, Brown & Co., Boston, pp. 1543–72.

Diamond J.R. & Karnovsky M.J. (1988) Focal and segmental glomerulosclerosis: Analogies to atherosclerosis. *Kidney Int.* **33**, 917–24.

Fine L.G. (1988) Preventing the progression of human renal disease: have rational therapeutic principles emerged? *Kidney Int.*, **33**, 116–28.

Funston M.R. & Cremin B.J. (1978) Intrarenal reflux — papillary morphology and pressure relationships in children's necropsy kidneys. *Br. J. Radiol.* **51**, 665–70.

Gokal R. (1987) Continuous ambulatory peritoneal dialysis — ten years on. *Quart. J. Med.* **63**, 465–72.

Heptinstall R.H. & Hodson C.J. (1984) Pathology of sterile reflux in the pig. *Contr. Nephrol.* **39**, 344–57.

Hodson C.J., Maling T.M.J., McManamon P.J. & Lewis M.G. (1975) Reflux nephropathy. *Kidney Int.* **8**, S50–S58.

Hodson C.J. & Twohill S.A. (1984) The time factor in the development of sterile renal scarring following high-pressure vesicoureteral reflux. *Contr. Nephrol.* **39**, 358–69.

Kincaid-Smith P. (1979) Glomerular lesions in atrophic pyelonephritis. In: Hodson C.J. & Kincaid-Smith P. (eds) *Reflux Nephropathy*. Masson Publishing USA Inc., New York, pp. 197–212.

Klahr S. (1983) Pathophysiology of obstructive nephropathy. *Kidney Int.* **23**, 414–26.

Klahr S., Schreiner G. & Ichikawa I. (1988) The progression of renal disease. *N. Engl. J. Med.* **318**, 1657–66.

Koff A.S. & Murtagh D.S. (1983) The uninhibited bladder in children: effect of treatment on recurrence of urinary infection and on vesicoureteral reflux resolution. *J. Urol.* **130**, 1138–41.

Lumertgul D., Burke T.J., Gillum D.M. *et al.* (1986) Phosphate depletion arrests progression of chronic renal failure independent of protein intake. *Kidney Int.* **29**, 658–66.

Maher J.F. (1989) *Replacement of renal function by dialysis*. Kluwer Academic Publishers, Boston.

Maiorca R., Cancarini G.C., Camerini C. *et al.* (1989) Is CAPD competitive with haemodialysis for long-term treatment of uraemic patients? *Nephrol. Dial. Transplant* **4**, 244–53.

McCance R.A. (1959) The maintenance of chemical stability in the newly born: Chemical exchange. *Arch. Dis. Child.* **34**: 361–65.

Moorhead J.F., El-Nahas M., Chan M.K. & Varghese Z. (1982) Lipid nephrotoxicity in chronic progressive glomerular and tubulo-interstitial disease. *Lancet* **ii**, 1309–11.

Ransley P.G. & Risdon R.A. (1974) Renal papillae and intrarenal reflux in the pig. *Lancet* **ii**, 1114.

Ransley P.G. & Risdon R.A. (1975a) Renal papillary morphology in infants and young children. *Urol. Res.* **3**, 111–13.

Ransley P.G. & Risdon R.A. (1975b) Renal papillary morphology and intrarenal reflux in the young pig. *Urol. Res.* **3**, 105–9.

Ransley P.G., Risdon R.A. & Godley M.L. (1984) High pressure sterile vesicoureteral reflux and renal scarring: An experimental study in the pig and minipig. *Contr. Nephrol.* **39**, 320–43.

Rolleston G.L., Maling T.M.J. & Hodson C.J. (1974) Intrarenal reflux and the scarred kidney. *Arch. Dis. Child.* **49**, 531–9.

Rolleston G.L., Shannon F.T. & Uttley W.L.F. (1970) Relationship of infantile vesicoureteric reflux to renal damage. *Br. Med. J.* **1**, 460–3.

Rolleston G.L., Shannon F.T. & Utley W.L.F. (1975) Follow-up of vesico-ureteric reflux in the newborn. *Kidney Int.* **8**, S59–S64.

Shimada K., Matsui T., Ogino T. *et al.* (1988) Renal growth and progression of reflux nephropathy in children with vesicoureteral reflux. *J. Urol.* **140**, 1097–100.

Smellie J.M. (1986) Urinary tract infection, vesicoureteral reflux, and renal scarring. *Sem. Urol.* **4**, 82–5.

Smellie J.M., Edwards D., Hunter N. *et al.* (1975) Vesico-ureteric reflux and renal scarring. *Kidney Int.* **8**, S65–S72.

Smellie J.M. & Normand I.C.S. (1985) Urinary infections in children. *Postgrad. Med. J.* **61**, 895–905.

Taylor C.M., Corkery J.J. & White R.H.R. (1982) Micturition symptoms and unstable bladder activity in girls with primary vesicoureteral reflux. *Br. J. Urol.* **54**, 494–8.

Torres V.E., Velosa J.A., Holley K.E. *et al.* (1980) The progression of vesicoureteral reflux nephropathy. *Ann. Intern. Med.* **92**, 776–84.

Warshaw B.L., Edelbrock H.H., Ettenger R.B. *et al.* (1982) Progression to end-stage renal disease in children with obstructive uropathy. *J. Pediatr.* **100**, 183–7.

Wilson D.R. (1980) Pathophysiology of obstructive uropathy. *Kidney Int.* **18**, 281–92.

Wilson D.R. (1988) Urinary tract obstruction. In: Schrier R.W. & Gottschalk C.W. (eds) *Diseases of the Kidney*. Little, Brown & Co., Boston, pp. 715–46.

Zager R.A., Cotran R.S. & Hoyer J.R. (1978) Pathologic localisation of Tamm–Horsfall protein in interstitial deposits in renal disease. *Lab. Inv.* **38**, 52–7.

Zimmerman S.W., Uehling D.T. & Burkholder P.M. (1973) Vesicoureteral reflux nephropathy: evidence for immunologically mediated glomerular injury. *Urology* **2**, 588–9.

# 4 Consequences of chronic renal failure in childhood

## INTRODUCTION

Throughout the chapters in this book, there are records of patients dying in childhood from renal failure. Some were born with insufficient renal parenchyma to support life, for example the severely affected prune belly patient. It seems unlikely, even with our present knowledge, that many such infants can be saved by neonatal dialysis and transplantation. Older children would not have died had they been born 10 or 15 years later because they would have been dialysed.

For babies born in the late 1960s and 70s, treatment for end-stage renal failure was available. The first survivors who were dialysed and transplanted are now arriving in adulthood and the long-term effects can be judged. On balance the results are very good, in some ways better than could have been hoped. However, there have been many problems.

## SURVIVAL

Until the 1960s, children with end-stage renal failure died. Although transplantation was widely practised in adults, it was generally held to be unsuitable for children. Aside from the poor survival, the burden on the child and its family was thought to be unsupportable. Surprisingly, transplantation for children began before dialysis.

Definitive treatment for children began in 1963. The survival results for the first 10 years at Guy's Hospital, UK gave an actuarial 5-year survival of 76% later rising to 90%. Survival was best on hospital dialysis programmes with a 5-year survival of around 95% (Chantler *et al.* 1980, Henning *et al.* 1988). However, it will be seen later that the price of survival was high.

The 5-year survival after transplantation was around 70% to 86%. However, in some cases there was a deliberate decision not to put a child back on dialysis when a transplanted kidney was rejected so that death was from a theoretically preventable cause. It is noticeable that results improved during those early years, but so far only about half of all children with end-stage renal failure have survived into adult life (67% in the series at Guy's) though death is sometimes from unrelated causes such as traffic accidents (Chantler *et al.* 1980, Najarian *et al.* 1986, Henning *et al.* 1988). In the small number of patients who were transplanted 15 or more years ago the patient and graft survival are 74 and 43% respectively (Najarian *et al.* 1986).

The majority of children have a live related donor who is likely to be young. The fate of the donor's remaining kidney over, say, 40 to 50 years is a cause of concern. Hyperperfusion of surviving nephrons (discussed in Chapter 3) might lead to progressive renal failure. No donors have run so long a course yet, but present information is that the donors do not suffer renal deterioration. A review of 27 patients who had a unilateral nephrectomy in childhood at a mean follow-up of 23 years showed that the average creatinine clearance was 84 ml/min. This figure was the equivalent of 74% of the clearance in healthy controls with two kidneys. More importantly it was the same clearance as donors have 3–6 months after their nephrectomy (Robitaille *et al.* 1985). In reviewing the literature, Spital concluded that the remaining kidney deteriorated at the rate expected for normal ageing (Spital *et al.* 1986). Perhaps the longest donor follow-up has been achieved by Bohannon who records a transplant between identical twins aged 12 in 1959: at 27-year follow-up the recipient had a GFR of 116 and the donor of 88 ml/min with normal renal biopsies (Bohannon *et al.* 1988).

Although there have been occasional reports of postoperative deaths, there seems every reason to encourage the practice of live related donation.

The age at which treatment for renal failure is considered worthwhile is getting younger. If a baby's other systems are normal, dialysis and transplantation are indicated in carefully selected cases. In the University of Minnesota 13 infants from 6 to 11 months old have been treated since 1978, all receiving an adult kidney. There were eight survivors at the latest follow-up (So *et al.* 1987).

## FACTORS AFFECTING SURVIVAL

The primary cause of renal failure, the relationship of the donor to the recipient and the ages of patient and donor affect the outcome of transplantation. All of these factors and the survival of the transplant also affect the survival of the patient.

### Cause of renal failure

In cadaveric transplants graft survival is closely related to the primary cause of renal failure. The most favourable group have renal disease or a surgical cause of renal failure that is unlikely to recur in the graft. This group includes reflux nephropathy, Alport's syndrome and medullary cystic disease. The 5-year graft survival is around 70%.

An intermediate group for survival includes glomerulonephritis, renal dysplasia and hypoplasia and cystinosis. The 5-year graft survival is 40–50%.

The worst group have a 'surgical' cause of renal failure which may well affect the transplanted kidney. This includes obstructive uropathies especially posterior urethral valves. The 5-year graft survival is a dismal 30–40%. It is in this group that there is the greatest prospect for improvement. The mechanisms of renal destruction are now better understood. Fewer such patients should develop renal failure in future and better management of their lower urinary tracts should protect the grafts (Churchill *et al.* 1988).

### Relationship of donor and recipient

As in every group of renal failure patients, the more closely related are the donor and recipient, the better is the long-term survival. The 10-year graft survival is about 70% with a live related donor. However, when this figure is broken down it is found that for human leukocyte antigen (HLA) identical donors and recipients, 10-year graft survival is 90% while for mismatched but related donors it is 52%.

In all cadaveric transplants the 10-year graft survival is between 40 and 50%. The number of matches on the HLA A and B loci does not appear to make a significant difference (Najarian *et al.* 1986).

There is general agreement that live related donation is best for children (Spital *et al.* 1986). The survival advantage of live related but mismatched donations over cadaveric ones is not great though it is said to be statistically significant. The risk to donors is small but ever present and it is therefore essential that selection meets the most stringent criteria: although 94% of transplant centres have not had a donor death, the obvious corollary is that 6% of centres have had one or more deaths (Spital *et al.* 1986).

### Effects of age

The original view was that the very young child should not be treated for renal failure, should not be transplanted and should not be a donor.

There is conflict even now about the first two of these views. In children under 5 years old several authors have reported unacceptably poor results (Rizzoni *et al.* 1980, Moel & Butt 1981, Churchill *et al.* 1988). In the most recent publication, for example, the cadaveric graft survival at 4 years of age was 70% for 2 to 5 year olds and only 50% for the under 2s; graft loss usually led to death of the child.

If it is true that younger patients have a higher mortality, it would at least seem that the death rate flattens out with time: Sheldon's group report few deaths beyond the age of 2 and none beyond 3 from transplantation. Conversely, there is a steady loss of grafts all the time with children returning for second and third grafts having had good growth and development while the first was working (Sheldon *et al.* 1987).

On the other hand Najarian has reported little difference in graft or patient survival with age even in patients under a year old. The only relatively poor result was in under 1 year olds receiving a cadaveric graft where 5-year graft survival was 50% against 60% for patients over 2 years old. More importantly loss of the graft did not usually lead to the patient's death (Najarian *et al.* 1986).

In view of this conflict and lack of knowledge about the outcome in adult life, of such early treatment, it seems sensible for the work to be done in a few specialist centres.

The age of the donor is also important in graft survival. Aside from the ethical question of live donation by minors, young kidneys have a high rate of early loss, mainly due to thrombosis. Kidneys under 2 years old have a 30% vascular failure rate against 5% for kidneys over 15 years old (Churchill *et al.* 1988).

## EFFECTS OF DIALYSIS

The general and short-term effects of dialysis are well known. The long-term outcome is little reported: it can be difficult to separate the effects of dialysis from those of the renal failure. The number of children remaining on dialysis over many years is small as the aim is usually to transplant a kidney.

### Growth

Children with end-stage renal failure are small at the time of entry to a dialysis programme, up to 40% being below the third percentile for height. At best, dialysis allows patients to maintain their positions on the percentile graph but many fall further behind and a few have virtual growth arrest. Only one-third of patients are likely to achieve normal growth on dialysis. The younger the onset of renal failure, the worse are the prospects for growth (Chantler *et al.* 1980, Fine 1985). In Chantler's series 11 of 12 children presenting at less than 12 years old fell further behind their expected growth on the percentile chart; 11 of 14 presenting at 12 years or later fell further behind but the fall was less marked. Only one child moved up the percentile chart on haemodialysis (1980).

A consistent feature of children in chronic renal failure is retarded bone age. Percentile charts for weight and height are drawn up according to chronological age of normal children. When the growth of renal failure patients is assessed by bone age, the picture is not quite so gloomy. Ultimate growth is better than expected from the position on the percentile chart in childhood though achievement of the final height is delayed.

### Sexual development and fertility

The onset of puberty is delayed by dialysis, especially in boys. It has been suggested that there is testicular insensitivity to luteinising hormone. On dialysis, libido is low though better than in untreated renal failure. Males have infrequent erections and females infrequent menstruation. In a few males complete impotence has required the insertion of penile prostheses. Four children in Chantler's series had priapism on dialysis and two became impotent as a result (1980).

These problems, common to all renal failure patients, are compounded in adolesence. The adolescent is very 'image conscious' and, obviously, is developing sexuality. Frustration in relationships with peers and in sexual inadequacy may show itself as unwillingness to be bound by the constraints of the illness. Such behaviour produces a high incidence of hyperkalaemia, hypertension and congestive cardiac failure all of which make the frustration worse (Fine 1985).

Pregnancy in severe renal failure, even on dialysis, is rare with about 15 cases reported in the literature. In those not on dialysis at the time, renal failure is accelerated. The pregnancies are complicated by hypertension, electrolyte disturbances, urinary infection and premature labour. However, the babies are normal and behave as other premature babies (Brem *et al.* 1988).

### Psychosocial problems

Adolescence is a difficult time to have any illness. Renal failure, especially when treated by dialysis puts a heavy burden on the whole family. The burden may be destructive or cohesive.

A year on haemodialysis may be acceptable to 80% of children but to only 50% of families. The burden is worse on home dialysis although compared to other measures it is the better system. In spite of the anxieties of surgery and graft rejection, transplantation is generally regarded as the ultimate goal by most patients.

Specific problems usually centre around denial of the illness and refusal to be constrained by it. Such behaviour worsens both the known complications of dialysis and the family problems. Peritoneal dialysis is better tolerated by the adolescent because of the greater freedom that is possible (Fine 1985).

### Education

Chronic renal failure impairs cognitive function in children and keeps them away from school. Patients have a lower IQ and achieve less than their peers. In Chantler's series no child on hospital dialysis was able to attend school full time; on home dialysis 80% were attending full time which compares well with other reported figures of 50–80% (1980). In many centres hospital dialysis is only used for patients with special medical or social problems or for a short period before transplantation, factors which also contribute to the lack of school attendance.

When IQ is measured formally, patients with renal failure fare badly in all parameters both compared to matched controls and to an identical twin with normal renal function. The worse the renal function and the earlier the onset of renal failure, the worse is the loss of IQ. Dialysis allows some improvement (Fennell 1984).

### Surgical complications

Even with an apparent 'medical treatment' patients are not free of surgical problems. When the native kidneys are of no use for urine production they may be a source of infection or hypertension. Our own experience has been that about one-third of adolescents with a 'urological' cause of renal failure (reflux, posterior valves, etc.) require upper tract clearance. Chantler records that 15 children in his series had native nephrectomies for hypertension. Upper tract clearance alone may lead to improved growth, appetite and general health (Chantler *et al.* 1980). Now that erythropoietin is becoming available for therapeutic use the problem of anaemia may be more easily managed.

The most common difficulty for dialysis patients is loss of access. In the long-term children require an average of one operation per year for such complications.

## EFFECTS OF TRANSPLANTATION

In spite of the risks of surgery and immunosuppression, transplantation remains the objective of most children and adolescents with renal failure. Their willingness to undergo second and third transplants after rejection of the first testifies to its value in the management. The ideal is transplantation before dialysis is needed, with a kidney from a well matched relative. Virtually all of the effects of chronic renal failure are corrected best by transplantation. In patients who have had both dialysis and transplantation it may be difficult to determine the effects of each individually.

## Growth

Transplantation allows much catching up in growth especially in prepubertal boys. The difficulties in the use of percentile charts mentioned above may make the picture seem worse than it should be. In Chantler's series seven of 10 children presenting before 12 years old maintained or improved their percentile position after transplantation; in those presenting after 12 only three of 10 did so. It is very interesting to note, however, that in a small sub-group of three patients who were dialysed for at least a year before transplantation growth velocity was not improved by the transplantation, in fact in two it was worsened (Chantler *et al.* 1980).

Although transplantation does allow some catching up, it is not complete. Only about one-third to a half of children receiving transplants will ultimately achieve normal adult height (Fine 1985). Transplantation during puberty is particularly damaging to growth. However, because bone maturation is delayed, growth may go on for longer than normal. Final adult height has been achieved at a mean of 20.3 years in boys and 18.7 years in girls transplanted in childhood or adolescence (van Diemen-Steenvoorde *et al.* 1986). By a mean age of 22, after dialysis and transplantation, 14 of 26 patients from Guy's Hospital, UK had a final height more than 2 SD below the mean (Henning *et al.* 1988).

In the very short follow-up that is available for treated infants, the growth is better than might have been expected. Six boys increased their lengths from a mean of 2.7 SD below normal by a mean of 1.4 SDs with one achieving normal length; three girls (all with oxalosis) hardly improved their growth at all. The infants all had microcephaly at presentation and successful treatment led to normal skull development, disappearance of fits and normal motor development (So *et al.* 1987).

## Sexual development and fertility

It is generally recognised that puberty is delayed in renal failure. However, the start of sexual development is related to bone age and not chronological age. Thus in 14 transplanted girls the menarche was between 13.4 and 17.7 years of chronological age, with a mean of 15.3 (peer normal: 11.7–15.0, mean: 13.4). However, in years of bone age, the menarche was between 10.5 and 14.0 years (mean: 12.9) which is the same as for the peer group. Once started, regular periods were established within a year (van Diemen-Steenvoorde *et al.* 1987).

In boys it is more difficult to judge the time of onset of puberty. Chronologically it is delayed to the same extent as in girls. When related to bone age, there seems to be a normal pattern with all of 29 boys being at Tanner stage 2 by bone age 11 (van Diemen-Steenvoorde *et al.* 1987).

The incidence of infertility in women on dialysis is unknown. Those with a normally functioning graft and regular periods do not seem to have any special difficulty. In practical terms it should certainly be assumed that all are fertile until proved otherwise.

In a relatively early survey of pregnancy after transplantation 244 pregnancies were reported with a stillbirth and neonatal death rate of 6.1%. Several survivors had a rather stormy time in the first few weeks of life (Rudolf *et al.* 1979).

Prospects have improved considerably. In 24 pregnancies in 20 women, all babies were born alive with no malformations at a mean of 37.8 weeks (Marushak *et al.* 1986). Davidson and

Lindheimer (1982) have listed criteria for low and high risk post-transplant pregnancies (Table 4.1). Applying these prospectively, Marushek found excellent correlation, especially in intrauterine growth retardation which was 25% in the high risk group but only 9% in the low risk. The rate of caesarean section is usually high, though perhaps only because obstetricians sometimes feel that previous transplantation is an indication in its own right! Even in the high risk group there does not appear to be an adverse effect on rejection episodes or renal function.

**Table 4.1** Criteria for low risk in pregnancy after renal transplantation (Davidson & Lindheimer 1982).

| Low risk patients |
|---|
| Transplantation to pregnancy interval >2 years |
| No proteinuria |
| Normotensive |
| No rejection episodes |
| Normal IVU |
| Normal renal function (creatinine >180 mmol/l) |
| Current prednisolone dose >15 mg/day |
| Current azothioprine dose >3 mg/kg |

*Note*: High risk patients have an abnormality of one or more of the above.

## Psychosocial development

The greater freedom that comes with transplantation allows near normal development. However, the problem of 'image' is still present. Steroids for immunosuppression alter the facial appearance and at least one teenager has given up the drugs allowing rejection to occur rather than accept her changed appearance. Cyclosporin should make this less of a problem in future.

Delayed growth and puberty put a great burden on the teenager. The news that both are more related to bone than chronological age is little consolation. Furthermore, bone disease may have its own complications; for example Henning found that four of 31 transplanted children could not run when reviewed at mean age of 22 years.

When assessed by questionnaire, Henning's patients listed driving restrictions, limitation on sporting activity, restricted foreign travel and inability to attend organised social events as their main complaints. Patients tended to live with their parents for longer than usual and to have difficulty establishing sexual relationships. When the renal failure patients were compared to a group of age-matched diabetics (without renal failure), the differences were striking: the diabetics were more independent, more likely to be married and did not have anxiety about body image. The diabetics did have similar restrictions on their social lives (Henning *et al.* 1988).

## Education

After transplantation children attend school more regularly: in Chantler's series 64% of transplanted children were attending full time and a further 8% were attending full time but with some limitation on their activities (1980).

With such a severe and demanding illness, limited education is inevitable. About 10% complete secondary education to a high standard ('A' level in the UK) and 33% to a medium level (GCSE level). However, 38% leave school with no formal qualifications

In a prospective study renal failure patients have been compared to matched controls with the same intelligence. When assessed 1 month after transplantation it was found that renal failure patients had improved all aspects of their IQ to a greater extent than the controls had done over the same period of time. The improvement was most marked in mathematics and non-verbal problem solving. In other words, transplantation had allowed the renal failure patients to do some catching up. One year after transplantation the controls and patients had improved their scores by similar amounts reflecting maturation and experience.

The same results were found in identical twins, only one of whom had renal failure. After transplantation the affected twin caught up with its sibling to some extent. At 1 and 3 years after transplantation the differences remained.

In children the damage most affects the acquisition of new information and problem solving capability. Recall of previously learned material and verbal skills are least affected. In children attention and vigilance are not much affected though they are in adults (Fennell *et al.* 1984).

It seems that chronic renal failure produces impairment of cognitive function in children at two levels. In one, the illness prevents adequate schooling and learning by normal experience and may cause some reversible brain damage. This is reversed fairly quickly by transplantation. In the other there is brain damage which is not reversible and which is more severe with early onset of renal failure.

## Recurrence of original disease

The risk of recurrence depends on the nature of the disease and the length of survival. When the cause of renal failure is 'urological' the risk is considerable unless the problem has been corrected. Reflux nephropathy does not reccur in transplanted kidneys. However, when a bladder has been responsible for the destruction of the native kidneys (as for example in posterior urethral valves) there is a good chance that it will destroy the transplant unless its abnormality has been corrected (see Chapter 5).

Some metabolic diseases, both congenital and acquired, also affect transplanted kidneys. In some cases the risk is so high that transplantation may be contraindicated. There have been several

| Disease | Effect on transplant |
|---|---|
| *Very high risk*: | |
| Dense deposit disease | Often severe |
| Primary hyperoxaluria | Usually severe |
| *High risk*: | |
| IgA nephropathy | Minor |
| Henoch–Shoenlein purpura | Often minor |
| *Moderate risk*: | |
| Focal segmental glomerulonephritis | Often severe |
| Membranoproliferative glomerulonephritis | Often severe |
| Membranous nephropathy | Minor |
| Crescentic glomerulonephritis | Minor |
| Progressive systemic sclerosis | Minor |
| *Low risk or rare*: | |
| Anti-GBM nephritis | Minor |
| Wegener's granulomatosis | Minor |
| Polyarteritis nodosa | Minor |
| Amyloidosis | Minor |
| Haemolytic uraemic syndrome | Minor |
| Hereditary nephritis | Insufficient data |
| Systemic lupus erythematosuis | Minor |
| Diabetes | Usually minor |
| Cystinosis | Usually minor |

**Table 4.2** The risks of recurrence of the original cause of renal failure in a transplanted kidney (from Sheldon *et al.* 1987).

reports of recurrence of glomerulonephritis in grafted kidneys. The risks of recurrence of the original disease in the transplant are shown in Table 4.2.

Sometimes the cause of graft loss cannot be determined. It is, therefore, useful to identify groups which have a poor record for graft survival (see above).

### Infective complications

It is well known that transplant recipients are prone to conventional and opportunistic infections. *Escherichia coli, Pseudomonas* and *Klebsiella* cause infection in the urinary tracts of at least half the patients. Measles, *Staphylococcus aureus, S. tuberculosis* and *S. varicella* cause generalised infection. Several viruses including cytomegalovirus and herpes cause opportunistic infections though normally only in the immediate post-transplant period or during rejection.

It should not be forgotten that some patients come from, or will travel to, tropical areas and may become infected with common but unfamiliar illnesses. Cases of bilharzia have been reported in transplant patients and in live or cadaveric donors. In one case the infestation appeared to have been unwittingly transplanted with the kidney (Weeden *et al.* 1982, Hefty & McCorkell 1986). In transplant patients the inflammatory reaction to the ova may be minimal and microscopy of urine may be negative so that only a bladder biopsy will make the diagnosis (Hefty & McCorkell 1986).

### Surgical complications

In a most comprehensive review of 1000 transplants in adults and children a surgical complication rate of 12.5% was reported: 95% of the complications were obstructions or fistulae. Virtually all occurred in the early months after transplantation. The long-term complications could arise from non-urological sources and included tuberculosis (one case) and malignancy (two cases). The late renal complications included stone formation and bladder outflow obstruction from benign prostatic hypertrophy (Mundy *et al.* 1981).

In a review of the literature it has been shown that 'urological' complications occurred in only 0.013% of 3084 transplants after 3 months. The worrying feature was the insidious onset and the delay in diagnosis (Thomalla *et al.* 1985).

## REFERENCES


Bohannon L.L., Barry J.M., Newman D.J. & Bennett W.M. (1988) Renal function 27 years after unilateral nephrectomy for related donor transplant. *J. Urol.* **140**, 810–11.

Brem A.S., Singer D., Anderson L., Lester B. & Abuelo J.G. (1988) Infants of azotaemic mothers: a report of 3 live births. *Am. J. Kid. Dis.* **12**, 299–303.

Chantler C., Carter J.E., Bewick M. *et al.* (1980) 10 years experience with regular haemodialysis and renal transplantation. *Arch. Dis. Child.* **55**, 435–45.

Churchill B.M., Sheldon C.A., McLorie G.A. & Arbus G.S. (1988) Factors influencing patient and graft survival in 300 cadaveric pediatric renal transplants. *J. Urol.* **140**, 1129–33.

Davidson J.M. & Lindheimer M.D. (1982) Pregnancy in renal transplant recipients. *J. Reprod. Med.* **27**, 613–21.

Fennell R.S., Rasbury W.C., Fennell E.B. & Morris M.K. (1984) Effects of kidney transplantation on cognitive performance in a pediatric population. *Pediatrics* **74**, 273–8.

Fine R.N. (1985) The adolescent and end stage renal disease. *Am. J. Kid. Dis.* **6**, 81–5.

Hefty T.R. & McCorkell S.J. (1986) Schistosomiasis and renal transplantation. *J. Urol.* **135**, 1163–6.

Henning P., Tomlinson L., Rigden S.P.A., Haycock G.B. & Chantler C. (1988) Long term outcome of treatment of end stage renal failure. *Arch. Dis. Child.* **63**, 35–40.

Marushak A., Weber T., Bock J. *et al.* (1986) Pregnancy following kidney transplantation. *Acta Obstet. Gynecol. Scand.* **65**, 557–9.

Moel D.I. & Butt K.M.H. (1981) Renal transplantation in children less than 2 years of age. *J. Pediatr.* **99**, 535–9.

Mundy A.R., Podesta M.L., Bewick M., Rudge C.J. & Ellis F.G. (1981) The urological complications of 1000 renal transplants. *Br. J. Urol.* **53**, 397–402.

Najarian J.S., So S.K.S., Simmons R.L. *et al.* (1986) The outcome of 304 renal transplants in children. *Ann. Surg.* **204**, 246–58.

Rizzoni G., Malekzadeh M.H., Pennisi A.F. *et al.* (1980) Renal transplantation in children less than 5 years of age. *Arch. Dis. Child.* **55**, 532–6.

Robitaille P., Mongeau J.G., Lortie L. & Sinnassamy P. (1985) Long term follow-up of patients who underwent unilateral nephrectomy in childhood. *Lancet* **i**, 1297–9.

Rudolf J.E., Schweizer R. & Bartus S.R. (1979) Pregnancy in renal transplant patients. *Transplantation* **27**, 26–9.

Sheldon C.A., McClorie G.A. & Churchill B.M. (1987) Renal transplantation in children. *Paediatr. Clin. N. Am.* **34**, 1209–32.

So S.K.S., Chang P-N., Najarian J.S. *et al.* (1987) Growth and development in infants after renal transplantation. *J. Pediatr.* **110**, 343–50.

Spital A., Spital M. & Spital R. (1986) The living kidney donor — alive and well. *Arch. Int. Med.* **146**, 1993–6.

Thomalla J.V., Lingeman J.E., Leapman S.B. & Filo R.S. (1985) The manifestation and management of late urological complications in renal transplant recipients. *J. Urol.* **134**, 944–8.

van Diemen-Steenvoorde R., Donckerwolcke R.A., Brackel H., Wolff E.D. & de Jong M.C.J.W. (1987) Growth and sexual maturation in children after kidney transplantation. *J. Pediatr.* **110**, 351–6.

Weeden D., Hopewell J.P., Moorhead J.F., Sweny P. & Fernando O.N. (1982) Schistosomiasis in renal transplantation. *Br. J. Urol.* **54**, 478–9.

# 5 Transplantation with abnormal lower urinary tracts

## INTRODUCTION

The proportion of patients in end-stage renal failure from a 'urological' cause varies according to the centre and the number of children on the programme. In the dialysis population as a whole the patients with primary renal disease predominate. In the paediatric group, 'urological' causes of renal failure are common. In major centres of paediatric dialysis various forms of primary renal disease account for 30 to 40% of patients; those whose renal failure could, theoretically, have been prevented by early detection and surgery are 40 to 60% (Chantler *et al.* 1980, Najarian *et al.* 1986, Churchill *et al.* 1988).

Aside from provoking regret that these children were not saved from dialysis, the figures have important implications for long-term management. Three main questions arise:

**1** Should the native upper tracts be removed to prevent further trouble?

**2** Will a lower urinary tract, particularly a bladder, that has destroyed two native kidneys do the same to a transplanted kidney?

**3** If the bladder is not usable for drainage of a renal transplant, what is the best alternative?

## FATE OF THE NATIVE UPPER TRACTS

Even in advanced uraemia the kidneys may have valuable residual function. Many continue to produce useful amounts of erythropoietin to keep a reasonable haemoglobin. This role may be of lesser importance when commercially produced erythropoietin is generally available. Many, also, produce good volumes of urine even though the quality is poor: the young adult appreciates the greater freedom of fluid intake that this allows.

Thus, unless there is some special problem, the native kidneys should be retained. If they must go, their removal should be delayed to a time as close to the transplant as possible.

Our own indications for native nephrectomy are uncontrolled infection or hypertension. In 40 patients with abnormal lower urinary tracts recently reviewed only two had nephroureterectomies, both with reflux.

Fairly similar figures are given for a group with all diagnoses in whom 14 of 198 patients required native nephrectomy. In eight of nine patients with abnormal lower urinary tracts the indication was infection. In five with normal lower urinary tracts, three had persistent pyelonephritis. Three patients had major complications and three had minor complications (including the clotting of two fistulae), experience that discourages such surgery if possible (Sheinfeld *et al.* 1985).

The Cleveland Clinic group advise native nephrectomy when a transplant is to be drained into a cutaneous diversion (MacGregor *et al.* 1986).

A particularly difficult group are those with polycystic kidneys. They may have pain, persistent haematuria or have uncomfortably large masses both for the patient and the transplant surgeon. One or both kidneys have often been removed in the past though in 1990 the indications are fewer and the operation is seldom done (Chapter 6).

The timing of native nephrectomy is controversial. The worst time is in the immediate transplant period. If a live donor is to be used the native nephrectomy may be done shortly before the planned transplant. For cadaveric donation only a guess can be made at the right time.

In two recent patients awaiting transplantation we have had difficulty in treating recurrent pyocystis in dry bladders. In both we eventually used repeated cycling with saline through a suprapubic catheter with good result. The patients managed the treatment at home without difficulty.

## VESICO-URETERIC REFLUX (VUR)

When reflux nephropathy has caused renal failure there are no special problems with transplantation except the possibility that the upper tracts may have to be removed. Assuming that the reflux is primary and not secondary to bladder dysfunction, the transplanted ureter is anastomosed to the bladder in the normal way.

Nineteen adult patients in our group fall into this category and have received 22 transplants. The 2-year graft survival was 70% ($n$=20) and 5-year was 60% ($n$=12). These figures are not significantly different from the graft survival in our total group of 160 transplants. Five patients had recurrent urinary infections and had a higher plasma creatinine at 1 year than the non-infected patients (134 μmol/l ± 36 *v.* 108 ± 24). Two patients with persistently infected urine had post-transplant upper tract clearance. No grafts were lost through bladder dysfunction.

Similar results have been reported in children. Reinberg had a 5-year graft survival of 73% in refluxers compared to 75% in age-matched controls with renal failure due to primary renal disease (Reinberg *et al.* 1988). Churchill found that refluxers fell into the best of his three diagnostic categories for graft survival with 65% at 5 years compared to 35% for his worst groups (Churchill *et al.* 1988, see Chapter 4).

## TRANSPLANTATION INTO CUTANEOUS DIVERSIONS

From the earliest days of transplantation some centres were adventurous enough to include on their programmes patients with cutaneous diversions even though most would have rejected them. The results of transplantation into an ileal conduit were not promising: three of seven patients in one report died and follow-up of the survivors was 2 to 40 weeks (Kelly *et al.* 1966).

Results have improved considerably and in 1990 there is general agreement that, although less satisfactory than even a reconstructed bladder, cutaneous diversion can be used for transplantation. Indeed in our recent review of 40 patients with abnormal lower urinary tracts, the eight patients with diversions did best: the 2-year graft survival was 84% and 5-year ($n$=4) was 75%.

Ileal and colonic conduits and cutaneous ureterostomies can all be used. MacGregor emphasises the need to ensure that the diversion is satisfactory and, if not, to revise it before transplantation (MacGregor *et al.* 1986). Although most surgeons would only use an existing conduit or form one in anticipation of transplantation, some surgeons are prepared to make a conduit at the time of transplantation. At least one patient has a graft draining into a ureterosigmoidostomy with good result at 5 years (Institute of Urology Consensus Conference 1988).

In a review of the literature from 1971–1985, 36 of 68 patients had functioning grafts with a cutaneous diversion. The most common complication was infection, known to have occurred in 18 and proving fatal in nine (Glass *et al.* 1985). However, most patients had persistent bacteriuria and that has been our experience in seven of eight patients.

Stones are a recognised complication of conduits and the risk seems to be increased after transplantation: four patients are quoted in the literature review. Our solitary, but rather dramatic, example is shown in Fig. 5.1.

Three pregnancies have been reported after transplantation into an ileal conduit. All were complicated by ureteric obstruction and deterioration of graft function. Two were electively terminated at 10 and 22 weeks. The third ran to 35 weeks and a normal infant was delivered by caesarean section (Hein *et al.* 1978).

## ASSESSMENT OF THE BLADDER FOR TRANSPLANTATION

Experience with urinary undiversion has taught a good deal about bladder assessment and established the concept of a 'safe bladder'. At an Institute of Urology Consensus Conference on transplantation with an abnormal lower urinary tract, indications for investigation and criteria for 'safety' were discussed (1988). It is clearly impractical to investigate all patients, though all males could do a urinary flow rate with little inconvenience and occasional benefit. Children and adults should have bladder evaluation if:

**1** Renal failure is known to be due to lower tract obstruction.

**2** There is any history of voiding dysfunction, especially in association with reflux.

**3** There is doubt about the aetiology of renal failure.

**4** There have been urological complications during the management of renal failure, especially repeated urinary infections or urethral stricture.

The programme of investigation is largely unchanged from that suggested by Marshall (1982). Under anaesthetic the patient has a cysto-urethroscopy. Minor strictures are incised and suspicious bladder lesions biopsied. A 5 fG suprapubic catheter and an epidural catheter are

(a) (b)

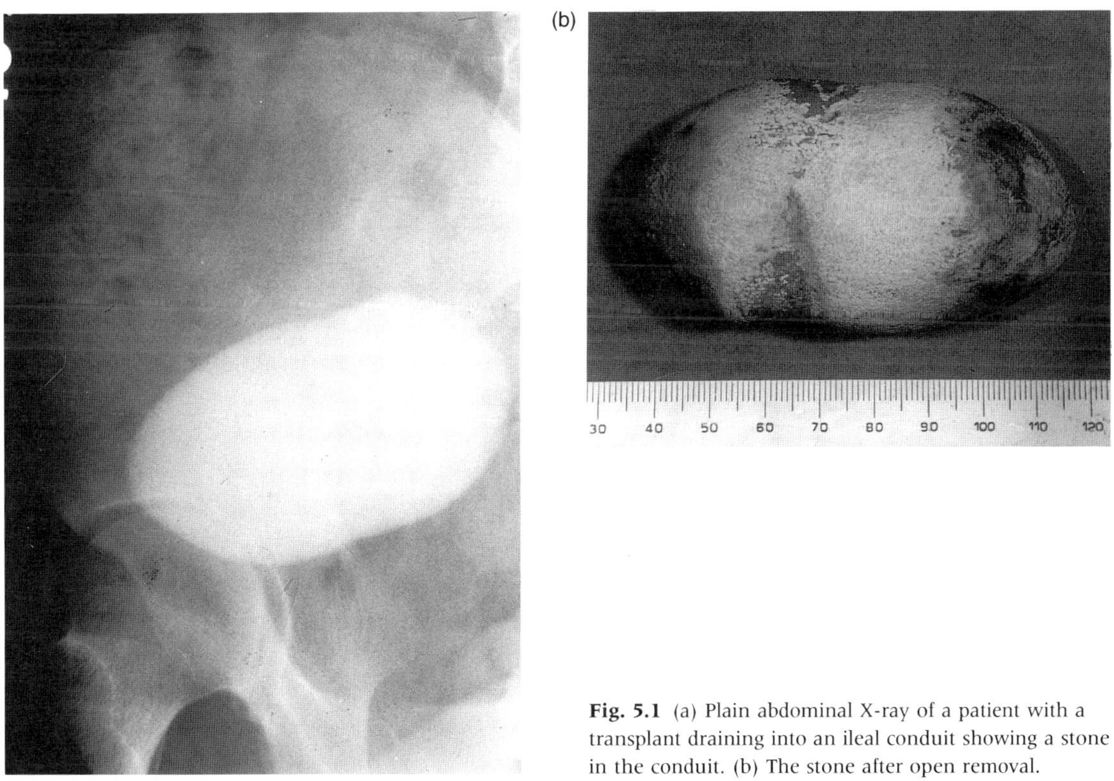


**Fig. 5.1** (a) Plain abdominal X-ray of a patient with a transplant draining into an ileal conduit showing a stone in the conduit. (b) The stone after open removal.

put into the bladder percutaneously and the position checked with the cystoscope: if the catheters are too low they may come down the urethra. When the patient has recovered a synchronous video cystometrogram is done (after bladder cycling if the bladder is dry).

The criteria for a 'safe' bladder are:

**1** A volume of at least 300 ml.

**2** An end-filling pressure of less than 30 cm $H_2O$.

**3** Absence of systolic detrusor contractions and normal compliance.

**4** A flow rate of at least 18 ml/second.

Neither continence nor complete bladder emptying is essential. Continence may be achieved by reconstruction of the bladder outlet or by insertion of an artificial sphincter. Bladder emptying may be achieved with intermittent clean self-catheterisation (ICSC).

Patients with paraplegia from spina bifida have been considered unsuitable for dialysis and transplantation. However, it would be reasonable to consider them, taking into account all of their handicaps including the bladder dysfunction. A series from Scotland included 12 spina bifida patients treated by dialysis and transplantation. Many had been referred late resulting in worse renal function which might have been prevented by more timely reconstruction. The criteria for acceptance onto the programme were not given. Home and hospital dialysis, peritoneal dialysis and cadaveric transplant were used with good results. A rather poor 3-year patient survival reflects the many problems faced by such patients (Muralikrishna *et al.* 1989).

## Timing of reconstruction

If these criteria are not met, a choice must be made between cutaneous diversion and reconstruction. The same considerations apply as in patients for undiversion or in whom diversion may be considered with normal renal function (Chapter 11). In general, any closed system is better than any cutaneous diversion and it will be seen later that almost every type of reconstructed lower urinary tract has been used for transplantation.

Patients presenting for transplantation with an unsuitable bladder in use must be reconstructed before transplantation. Those with a cutaneous diversion should, if they wish, be undiverted before transplantation. Such surgery does not worsen renal function and may, occasionally, improve it to delay transplantation (Cumming *et al.* 1988). Patients with suitable but dry bladders and a diversion may have the transplant ureter put into the bladder; the kidneys and conduit can then be removed when the transplant has proved successful.

## Use of the reconstructed bladder

The various techniques of reconstruction are discussed in Chapter 11. None seem to be contra-indicated for transplantation, although the numbers are small and the follow-up short. Mitchell particularly recommends the sigmoid colon for its simplicity and because of the little retroperitoneal dissection that is needed (Thomalla *et al.* 1989).

In two series 12 patients aged 11 to 40 years were reported with transplants draining into reconstructed bladders. Eight were functioning well at 6 months to 10 years of follow-up. Four were lost by rejection but three were poorly matched cadaveric grafts. At least one patient voided spontaneously but most were on self-catheterisation (Barnett *et al.* 1987, Thomalla *et al.* 1989).

There has been a case report of transplantation into a Kock pouch. The pouch was constructed 'dry' as the patient was anuric. It was tested and maintained expanded by 'cycling' with saline until a cadaveric transplant was performed. The patient and graft were well, without complications, at 6 months (Hertier *et al.* 1989).

## ICSC

Barnett reported eight patients who required temporary or permanent self-catheterisation after transplantation and also reviewed 13 patients from the literature. In total only 15 patients have been followed on self-catheterisation for more than 6 weeks. The longest reported is 4 years (Kogan *et al.* 1986) though one of our patients has been followed for 5 years. In these patients there is no evidence of any harm coming to the graft. Graft loss has always been from rejection rather than infection. However, infective complications are common: in Barnett's series covering only 85 months of patient follow-up, five patients had six infections, three of which required hospitalisation (Barnett *et al.* 1985).

It therefore seems a little early to conclude that ICSC is a satisfactory way of draining the bladder or that it is safer than ileal conduit diversion. Emotionally, all urologists will feel that anything is better than a bag, but we must accept that proof is lacking in this context.

### Artificial urinary sphincters

One case of transplantation has been reported where the graft ureter was anastomosed to a bowel augmented bladder controlled by a Brantley–Scott sphincter. The reconstruction had been done 42 months earlier. The sphincter was activated but the patient could not empty his bladder and used intermittent catheterisation. The transplant operating field was kept clear of the sphincter and its apparatus. The system worked well until the graft was lost at 6 months from renal artery stenosis. The patient took prophylactic antibiotics throughout.

It is interesting to note that the same group had transplanted a patient with an inflatable penile prosthesis. Its track was violated at the operation and the ensuing infection of the prosthesis contributed to the death of the patient (Thomalla *et al.* 1988).

## POSTERIOR URETHRAL VALVES

Our own studies on patients with posterior urethral valves have shown that late renal failure is common and the bladder function is particularly poor (Chapter 14). Correction of the bladder outflow obstruction is not always enough to render the bladder 'safe' either for the native kidneys or for a transplant.

The difficulties of evaluating the valve bladder for transplantation were first pointed out by Marshall and it is noteworthy that two of his four patients did not have transplants (Marshall *et al.* 1982). Our experience in six patients has been similar.

There seem to be no special problems with the operative technique or the early results. The long-term results are poor. It can be difficult precisely to attribute the cause of graft loss. Whatever the cause, valve patients have been shown to have a 5-year graft survival of only 35% after cadaveric transplant and 50% after transplantation from all sources (Churchill *et al.* 1988, Reinberg *et al.* 1988).

In Churchill's system, three cadaveric graft survival groups are described. The best group includes patients with normal bladders and non-recurring renal disease who have a 70% 5-year graft survival. The worst group includes patients with valves and other forms of obstructive uropathy who have a 30–35% 5-year graft survival (Churchill *et al.* 1988).

Reinberg compared the results of all grafts in valve patients with matched patients in other diagnostic groups. The 5-year graft survival was 50% for valve patients and 75% for others (Reinberg *et al.* 1988).

## COMPLEX URINARY TRACT PROBLEMS

In some patients especially with congenital abnormalities, the original diagnosis is lost in the mists of time (if it was ever known), or there may be multiple urinary tract problems. We have 10 such patients in the transplant programme with more than 2 years of follow-up. Diagnoses include prune belly syndrome, tuberculosis, imperforate anus and an isolated rectal bladder after cystectomy, among others.

It is difficult to draw conclusions from such different patients but we have learnt some lessons. Two grafts were lost from early rejection. Thereafter there were no problems for 2 years. I believe that bladder dysfunction destroyed two grafts and another was lost through a cerebrovascular accident during pregnancy.

Five grafts survive 2 to 5 years. Four are draining into a low pressure and compliant bladder or rectum. One drains into a dangerous high pressure bladder but the patient has refused reconstruction.

The clearest message is that however abnormal the urinary tract, transplantation can still be done if the bladder pressure is low and the wall compliant.

## REFERENCES

Barnett M., Bruskewitz R., Glass N., Sollinger H., Uehling D. & Belzer F.O. (1985) Long-term clean intermittent self-catheterisation in renal transplant recipients. J. Urol. **134**, 654–7.

Barnett M., Bruskewitz R., Sollinger H., Uehling D. & Belzer F.O. (1987) Ileocecocystoplasty bladder augmentation and renal transplantation. J. Urol. **138**, 855–8.

Chantler C., Carter J.E., Bewick M. *et al.* (1980) 10 years experience with regular haemodialysis and renal transplantation. *Arch. Dis. Child.* **55**, 435–45.

Churchill B.M., Sheldon C.A., McLorie G.A. & Arbus G.S. (1988) Factors influencing patient and graft survival in 300 cadaveric renal transplants. *J. Urol.* **140**, 1129–33.

Cumming J., Cox R. & Woodhouse C.R.J. (1988) Urinary undiversion in young adults. *Br. J. Urol.* **61**, 40–4.

Glass R., Uehling D., Sollinger H. & Belzer F. (1985) Renal transplantation using ileal conduits in 5 cases. *J. Urol.* **133**, 666–8.

Hein P.R., Jansen J.L.J. & Debruyne F.M.J. (1978) Successful pregnancy after renal transplantation in a patient with a urinary diversion. *Eur. J. Obstet. Gynec. Reprod. Biol.* **8**, 129–32.

Hertier Ph., Perraud Y., Relave M.H. *et al.* (1989) Renal transplant and the Kock pouch. *J. Urol.* **141**, 595–6.

Kelly W.D., Merkel F.K. & Markland C. (1966) Ileal urinary diversion in conjunction with renal homotransplantation. *Lancet* **i**, 222–7.

Kogan S.J., Weiss R., Hanna M. & Levitt S.B. (1986) Successful renal transplantation in a patient with a neurogenic bladder managed by clean intermittent catheterisation. *J. Urol.* **135**, 563–5.

MacGregor P., Novick A.C., Cunningham R. *et al.* (1986) Renal transplantation in end stage renal disease in patients with existing urinary diversion. *J. Urol.* **135**, 686–8.

Marshall F.F., Smolev J.K., Spees E.K., Jeffs R.D. & Burdick J.F. (1982) The urological evaluation and management of patients with congenital lower urinary tract anomalies prior to renal transplantation. *J. Urol.* **127**, 1078–81.

Muralikrishna G.S., Rodger R.S.C., MacDougall A.I. *et al.* (1989) Renal replacement treatment in patients with spina bifida or spinal cord injury. *Br. J. Med.* **299**, 1506.

Najarian J.S., So S.K., Simmons R.L. *et al.* (1986) The outcome of 304 primary renal transplants in children *Ann. Surg.* **204**, 246–58.

Reinberg R., Gonzalez R., Fryd D., Mauer S.M. & Najarian J.S. (1988) The outcome of renal transplantation in children with posterior urethral valves. *J. Urol.* **140**, 1491–3.

Sheinfeld J., Linke C.L., Talley T.E. & Linke C.A. (1985) Selective pre-transplant nephrectomy: indications and perioperative management. *J. Urol.* **133**, 379–82.

Thomalla J.V., Mitchell M.E., Leapman S.B. & Filo R.S. (1988) Renal transplantation in a patient with an artificial urinary sphincter device. *J. Urol.* **139**, 573–4.

Thomalla J.V., Mitchell M.E., Leapman S.B. & Filo R.S. (1989) Renal transplantation into the reconstructed bladder. *J. Urol.* **141**, 265–8.

# 6 *Renal anomalies and diseases*

## ANOMALIES OF DEVELOPMENT

### Solitary kidney

A solitary but normal kidney is of no clinical importance on its own unless it should be injured. Some solitary kidneys are complicated by abnormal drainage. It has been suggested that there is a high risk of complications. Emanuel, for example, found that only 33 of 74 patients escaped a major long-term complication (Emanuel *et al.* 1974). However, these patients were already selected as they had been admitted to hospital with 'solitary kidney' as their diagnosis; in other words, some complication had already occurred. In the community at large the risk is much lower.

Absence of a kidney may, however, be associated with other mesodermal abnormalities on that side. In males there may be absence of testicular development. More importantly, in females, there may be uterine or vaginal abnormalities: bicornuate uterus, vaginal septum or vaginal agenesis.

A solitary kidney is most often found in infancy through investigation of other congenital anomalies. When the diagnosis is suspected in later life it is important to confirm that a kidney that is non-functioning on IVU is truly absent. In most circumstances absence may be confirmed by ultrasound examination. Further confirmation may be necessary, and most surgeons would accept absence of the hemitrigone, as seen on cystoscopy, as proof, as this would only exclude cases of single ectopic ureter.

### Horseshoe kidney

Horseshoe kidney is the most common developmental abnormality of the kidney. It is of no clinical importance unless some other complication is present.

The horseshoe kidney may develop any of the conditions that normal kidneys have. There is almost certainly an increased incidence of pelviureteric junction (PUJ) obstruction. Whether there is an increased incidence of other conditions can be disputed. When a problem arises in a patient with horseshoe kidney it is memorable and may even be recorded in the literature while the same condition in a normal kidney is forgotten. Thus a review of the literature gives an entirely false impression of the relative incidence. Horseshoe kidney may occur in one in 400 people and most are symptomless.

In patients who present themselves for treatment at major urological institutions, 80% have been shown to have vesico-ureteric reflux, 33% infection, 21% stones and 16% PUJ obstruction (Segura *et al.* 1972, Pitts & Muecke 1975). This is not evidence that any of these conditions are more common than in the rest of the population.

In the longer term there may be concern about an increased risk of cancer. Again, the evidence is insubstantial, relying on reviews of the world literature. On such evidence it has been claimed that there is an increased risk of adenocarcinoma (Patoir 1959, Blackard & Mellinger 1968). As the literature review only found 52 cases the increased risk must be minimal or non-existent. In the Institute of Urology series of 147 patients with renal adenocarcinoma, none had a horseshoe kidney (Woodhouse *et al.* 1985).

In the case of transitional cell carcinoma, three cases were found in horseshoe kidneys in a series of 224 from the Mayo Clinic, USA (Murphy & Zincke 1982). This is hardly a greater number than would be expected in a secondary referral institute.

The increased risk, if any, of these conditions is certainly not great enough to require special surveillance of known cases. When a horseshoe kidney requires an operation, the surgeon should be aware of the peculiarities of the anatomy which are well known.

## CYSTIC DISEASE

A classification of cystic disease is shown in Table 6.1. Most of the conditions are rare and only those that are likely to be seen by a urologist will be considered.

**Table 6.1** Classification of cystic disease of the kidneys (from Glassberg *et al.* 1987).

| |
|---|
| *Genetic* |
| Autosomal dominant (adult) polycystic kidneys |
| Autosomal recessive (infantile) polycystic kidneys |
| Juvenile nephronophthisis/medullary cystic disease |
| Juvenile nephronophthisis (autosomal recessive) |
| Medullary cystic disease (autosomal dominant) |
| Congenital nephrosis (autosomal recessive) |
| Cysts plus multiple anomalies (e.g. tuberose sclerosis) |
| *Non-genetic* |
| Multicystic kidney (multicystic dysplasia) |
| Multilocular cyst (multilocular cystic dysplasia) |
| Simple cysts |
| Medullary sponge kidney |
| Acquired cystic disease on dialysis |
| Caliceal diverticulum (pyelogenic cyst) |

### Adult dominant polycystic kidney disease (ADPKD)

The term polycystic disease should be reserved for the two genetic diseases of the kidneys. The more common form is inherited as an autosomal dominant trait and was formerly called adult polycystic kidney. As it can be manifest in childhood (and the recessive disease can be manifest in adults) it is recommended that the 'adult' be dropped (Glassberg *et al.* 1987).

The condition was first described by Bartholomaeus Eustachius (1513–1574). The pattern of inheritance has been known at least since 1957 (Daalgard 1957). Nearly 10% of patients on dialysis suffer from it. It is, therefore, very disappointing to find that so few patients are aware of its hereditary nature. As a result, in one survey, only 18% of patients had had appropriate genetic counselling and only 9% of their offspring had had renal ultrasounds performed (Sahney *et al.* 1981). Identification of affected individuals would not, of course, alter the progressive development of cysts. But it would allow proper control of blood pressure which precedes renal deterioration in 92% of patients. The renal deterioration would be slowed and complications from the many extrarenal manifestations (especially berry aneurysms) might be avoided (Zeier *et al.* 1988). It has been suggested that derooting or aspirating cysts, especially around the hilum, improves symptoms and reduces blood pressure, though there is no evidence that it alters the course of the disease (Frang *et al.* 1988).

Affected individuals can be identified by ultrasound. Sensitivity of detection is about 22% under 10 years old, 68% under 20 and 86% under 30 years old (Watson *et al.* 1990). Identification of genetic markers makes it possible to identify an affected fetus *in utero* or a child before cysts have developed. In the case diagnosed *in utero* by Reeders an abortion was performed. The fetal kidneys appeared to be grossly normal but multiple cysts were seen on microscopy (Reeders *et al.* 1986a, b).

The progress of the disease is very variable. Not all patients develop renal failure, a few patients do so in childhood. Overall, about 25%

of patients will have developed end-stage renal failure by the age of 50 (Churchill *et al.* 1984). In those that do develop renal failure, the mean age at first elevation of creatinine is 38 years in females and 39.2 in males (Zeier *et al.* 1988). Thereafter, end-stage renal failure develops in about 4 years.

Polycystic kidneys may be painful, either spontaneously or through complications. In uncomplicated cases, pain is generally associated with cysts over 3 cm in diameter. Open decompression of the large cysts may damage renal function but percutaneous aspiration may be helpful. Surgical intervention should be reserved for patients in whom other therapy has failed (Editorial 1987).

The urologist will first encounter the patient with ADPKD when renal failure requires dialysis and transplantation. It has been common practice in the past to remove polycystic kidneys. This practice now seems to be unnecessary and possibly dangerous. A kidney should only be removed for a specific indication and preparation for transplantation is not one of them. It has been shown that nephrectomy does not affect the outcome of transplantation. In a series of 26 patients 5-year graft survival was 64% with previous bilateral nephrectomy and 56% without, but 5-year patient survivals were 77% and 83% (Mendelssohn *et al.* 1988). It must also be noted that in this series four of the 21 patients who had a nephrectomy had serious complications and two of them died. It is unusual for a polycystic kidney to produce uncontrollable symptoms and the evidence for a predisposition to adenocarcinoma is poor (Zeier *et al.* 1988).

ADPKD patients do well on dialysis with a 5-year survival rate of 77%. The majority of deaths are due to the cerebrovascular and coronary artery complications (Mendelssohn *et al.* 1988). Transplantation has equally good results with a graft survival of 73% to 88% at 1 year and 49% at 5 years. Overall graft and patient survival are similar to those in all other patients allowing for the vascular deaths. ADPKD has not occurred in the graft at up to 9 years' follow-up (Cook & Takiff 1986, Ho-Hseieh *et al.* 1987).

### Recessive polycystic kidney disease

This much rarer condition is only manifest in homozygotes. The most severe cases present early, with renal failure in the immediate post-natal period. In less affected cases renal failure develops in childhood or sometimes as late as 20 years old. They do not have the extrarenal manifestations of ADPKD such as berry aneurysms; however they do have hepatic fibrosis which is more severe in those with the better kidneys (Glassberg *et al.* 1987).

### Medullary cystic disease/familial juvenile nephronophthisis complex

Medullary cystic disease (MCD) and familial juvenile nephronophthisis (FJN) are diseases which share clinical and pathological features but differ in their heredity. In addition, FJN is associated with retinal abnormalities. In both conditions, in spite of the name, cysts are not an essential feature and may be absent in up to 25% of cases. The primary abnormality is probably metabolic and the cysts, when present, are secondary. MCD is an autosomal dominant condition and FJN is an autosomal recessive. Sporadic examples of both are seen. FJN is a common cause of renal failure in adolescents. Patients present with slowly progressive renal failure, commonly with salt loss. The kidneys are small, granular and usually contain medullary cysts on ultrasound examination.

### Multicystic kidneys

This condition normally affects only one kidney (bilateral disease is not compatible with life). It is now diagnosed on prenatal ultrasound. It appears to be more common than was thought when presentation was with an abdominal mass in the neonatal period. The current estimate is one in

4300 live births (Gordon *et al.* 1988). The kidney is cystic and functionless, the ureter is absent or atretic. When the ureter is absent the ureteric orifice is also absent or only a dimple, otherwise the ureteric orifice is normal. In cases that present with symptoms the contralateral kidney is abnormal in 75% of cases though usually has adequate function (Pathak & Williams 1964). In series diagnosed largely by prenatal ultrasound about 75% of contralateral kidneys are normal.

The early diagnosis of multicystic kidney has shed new light on the natural history of the condition. Not only is it more common than was once thought, but in many cases the kidney involutes and may disappear altogether (Avni *et al.* 1986, Gordon *et al.* 1988). The long-term outcome depends on the contralateral kidney. In early series the prognosis was poor, only 58% surviving early childhood in Pathak's series for example. However, this must reflect the type of case that came to the attention of specialist units at that time. Now that the real incidence is known it is likely that the prognosis of all cases will turn out to be good.

Views are also changing on the management of the multicystic kidney itself. In the past the kidneys were usually removed either for symptoms or 'prophylactically'. In considering whether this is necessary it must be remembered that the kidney contains no functioning tissue, is not connected to the rest of the urinary tract and probably has a natural tendency to shrink.

Symptoms that have been attributed to multicystic kidneys include pain, haematuria, infection and generalised symptoms such as failure to thrive. Many patients, even with large masses, may have no symptoms. If the mass is painful and tender, it is probably best removed. Other symptoms should be carefully evaluated as many will turn out to be from other causes. This was so in all of 14 cases in Gordon's series (Gordon *et al.* 1988).

In the longer term, it has been thought that malignancy and hypertension were potential complications. In reviewing the literature, Gordon was able to find only six cases of malignancy associated with multicystic kidney (two nephroblastomas, three adenocarcinomas and one adult embryonal tumour). This association seems hardly more than coincidence. Similarly, he found only nine cases of hypertension in the literature. Large series of patients with multicystic kidneys had only occasional cases of hypertension. Conversely, series of hypertensives seldom contained patients with definite multicystic kidneys. When the association was found, the hypertension seldom improved after nephrectomy (Gordon *et al.* 1988).

Multicystic kidneys should not be removed unless they are the cause of definite symptoms. The case for 'prophylactic' removal is weak.

## Medullary sponge kidney (MSK)

Medullary sponge kidney is a rare condition in which the collecting tubules show diffuse cystic dilatation. The cysts fill with contrast early during an IVU and are also filled by retrograde and antegrade pyelography. The condition is segmental so that large areas may not be affected at all. It is, by definition, confined to the medulla and pyramids. The appearances on IVU and ultrasound are characteristic. The original description only dates to 1939 though many cases (both before and after) were mistaken for renal tuberculosis.

There is a well known association with congenital hemihypertrophy of the body. When the renal lesion is confined to one side, the hemihypertrophy may affect either side of the body; similarly hemihypertrophy can occur even when both kidneys are affected (Harrison & Williams 1971).

The presence of MSK by itself is of no importance. Presumably more symptomless cases will be identified with wider use of ultrasound, though this problem has yet to be reported. Most cases come to light because of recurrent urinary infection or renal stones in young adults. The cysts have a high incidence of calcium deposition from which small stones are subsequently formed and released into the renal pelvis. MSK was the third most common diagnosis (13.4%) in 708 patients in the metabolic stone clinic at St Peter's Hospitals, UK on whom it was possible to make a definitive diagnosis (G.A. Rose, personal communication 1990).

Although local stasis of urine in the cysts might be an explanation for the calcification, there has always been the suspicion that renal function was abnormal in MSK. Most authors have undertaken extensive tests on the patients in their care. As many patients have only relatively small areas of the kidney involved, tests of overall function are likely to be near normal even if the urine passing through the affected tubules is grossly abnormal.

Steyn investigated three patients with moderately extensive MSK. He found normal glomerular filtration rates and blood calcium. One had consistently raised urine calcium, in one it was raised on one occasion and in the third it was normal. Tests of tubular function gave variable results (Steyn & Logie 1964). Other investigators, usually investigating only one aspect of function, have concluded that glomerular filtration rate remains normal until there is extensive destruction of the medulla by calcification and infection. In cases that have only small areas affected by MSK, the renal damage will never be extensive enough to produce measurable deterioration in function as the cyst formation is not progressive.

Investigations of tubular function have produced inconsistent results. Harrison found no cases of acidification defects though four of nine patients had hypercalciuria (Harrison & Williams 1971). Others have found impaired acidification (Granberg *et al.* 1971).

Good evidence that some patients have renal tubular acidosis (RTA) has now been put forward. In a series of 13 patients eight were found to have distal RTA (two complete and six partial) and one had proximal RTA. All the patients had a long history of stone formation and 12 had bilateral and, apparently, extensive MSK changes (Osther *et al.* 1988). RTA can be corrected by giving oral sodium bicarbonate.

On this evidence it seems reasonable to conclude that tubular function can be impaired in MSK. RTA may play a part in recurrent stone formation. Even so, there does not seem to be enough evidence to investigate or treat all patients found to have MSK, especially if it involves only small areas of kidney. Tubular function should be investigated in those with extensive involvement or who have formed stones.

## PELVI-URETERIC JUNCTION OBSTRUCTION

Pelvi-ureteric junction (PUJ) obstruction is a fine subject for urological debate. The hydronephrosis that is not accompanied by hydroureter is another example of the observation that dilatation does not necessarily equate with obstruction or functional deterioration. These arguments will not be repeated here. The concerns in long-term follow-up are twofold: firstly, if a kidney is hydronephrotic but not obstructed, is there any harm in leaving it alone? Secondly, if the PUJ is obstructed, what are the results of surgical correction?

The extensive literature attests to the difficulties in deciding whether or not obstruction is present. In some cases even the most intensive investigations may give the wrong answer. In other cases obstruction may be present at some times and in some circumstances but not at others (Fig. 6.1). If a dilated kidney that was not obstructed was, nonetheless, at risk of losing function, surgical correction might save it. There would then be no point in doing elaborate investigations to establish the presence of obstruction. If, however, dilatation alone is harmless, there is every reason to make the correct diagnosis as surgery can be avoided.

There is little evidence in the literature to help in answering the first question. Clinical experience shows that some patients, particularly

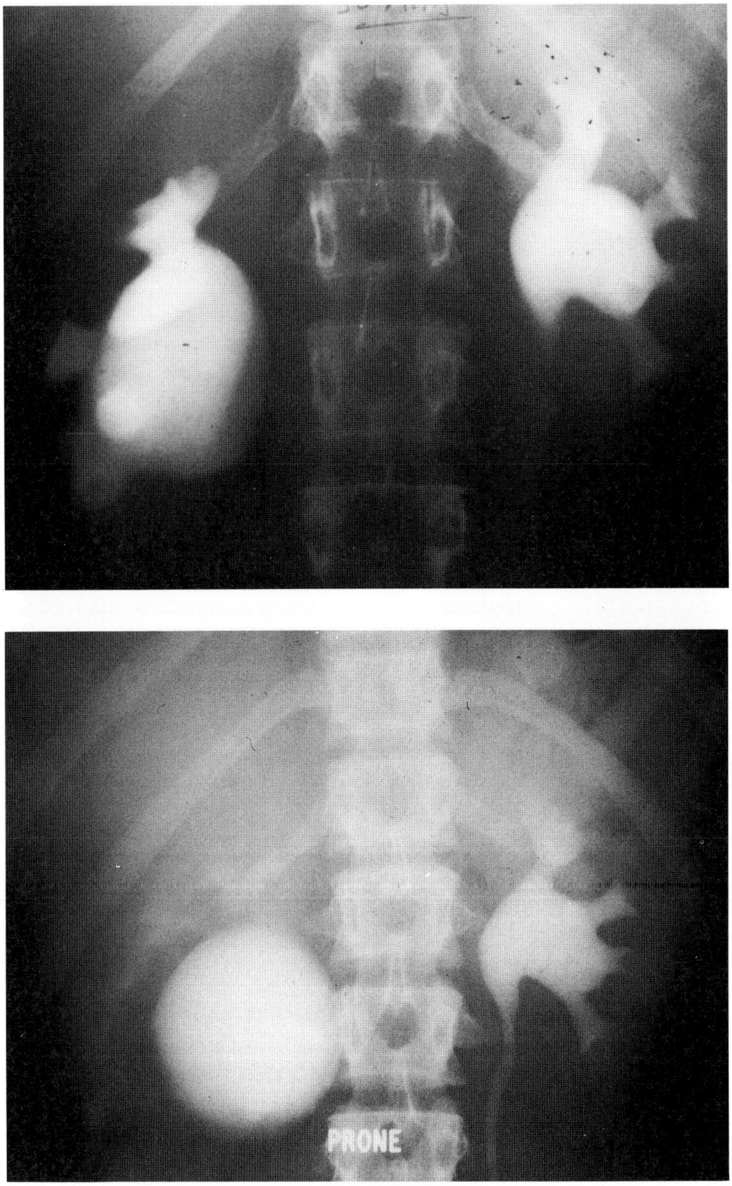


(a)

(b)

**Fig. 6.1** (a) IVU of a patient with occasional pain in the right flank. The dilatation of the right renal pelvis is suggestive of PUJ obstruction. (b) IVU during an episode of pain showing more significant dilatation of the renal pelvis.

amongst the elderly, have dilated and symptomless kidneys which appear to function normally. Although the IVU suggests PUJ obstruction, isotope scans are normal.

There are tantalising references in the literature to groups of the relevant patients: children with dilated kidneys proven not to be obstructed and followed without operation. Whitfield reported 15 of unknown ages followed for unknown periods, all doing well and remaining stable on isotope renography (Whitfield *et al.* 1979). Whitaker reported six similar cases with obstruction excluded by antegrade perfusion (Whitaker test). Follow-up for an unknown period showed the kidneys remaining stable (Whitaker 1975). The best series is probably that of O'Reilly. Twenty-five of 28 patients were followed for up to 5 years and their kidneys remained stable on isotope renography. Of the other three, two formed renal stones and one became obstructed and had a pyeloplasty (O'Reilly *et al.* 1981).

Unfortunately almost all of these cases were in adults. It is not known whether the same observations would apply to children. Koff strikes a cautious note. In a series of 82 patients of varying ages investigated by renography and Whitaker test, he found that children with a dilated renal pelvis were nearly always obstructed. In his subgroup of 20 patients who were found not to be obstructed, only one was a child. Follow-up of the 20 patients showed no deterioration in renal function. He comments that experimental and clinical evidence shows that the child's kidney is more easily damaged by distension than that of an adult (Koff 1982).

A practical problem remains. If a child is asymptomatic and has a non-obstructed hydronephrosis, for how long should follow-up continue and by what means? The answer can only be a guess. I suggest an isotope renogram every 3 years until 25 years old.

The answer to the second question is easier to come by. Successful pyeloplasty improves obstructed kidneys. Most large series in children record symptomatic cure in more than 90%. Although most of the children were treated on the basis of IVU appearances alone, few of them were discovered by chance and all had symptoms; it is likely that almost all were truly obstructed. I have not encountered a single patient with late relapse unless a complication such as stone had supervened.

The IVU appearances are another matter. It is unrealistic to expect the grossly dilated kidney to return to a normal shape. Kelalis claimed that 40% of his 109 children had normal IVUs postoperatively but Hendren reported that few IVUs were normal although 89% were improved (Kelalis *et al.* 1971, Hendren *et al.* 1980). The result appears to be maintained as the proportion of improved IVUs was the same at 3 months and at 1 to 5 years in a series of 44 children (Ahmed *et al.* 1986).

When assessed by isotope renography the results may be less impressive. In a group of all ages who had diuresis renography before and after pyeloplasty only 33% had better function in spite of a symptomatic improvement (Lupton *et al.* 1979). The outcome in children may be even worse: in one series it was found that there was no significant difference in the scintigraphy counts before and after pyeloplasty though the trend was better in patients under 2 years old (Dowling *et al.* 1988). However, it may be that the functional results take longer to become apparent. In Ahmed's series 67% of kidneys showed some renographic improvement at 3 months. On late follow-up (time unspecified) it had risen to 90%, with 77% showing moderate or great improvement. There was no late deterioration (Ahmed *et al.* 1986).

Improvement in renal function may follow pyeloplasty in adults but not always. If the preoperative GFR is low, it improves after successful reconstruction as does the concentrating ability when assessed at 8–10 years. If the function is near normal there is no change (Bratt *et al.* 1988). The effect of pyeloplasty on GFR in children is unknown. If it is true that the young kidney is more susceptible to damage from obstruction, the results may be similar.

Pyeloplasty in children does allow the kidney to grow but seldom to catch up with its expected size. The growth was more impressive after dismembered rather than non-dismembered in one series, though this may have reflected case selection (Rikalainen *et al.* 1986).

There is no information about the longer term. There is sometimes anxiety, in a unilateral case, that the other side will develop obstruction. The risk is only about 2% (Thomas *et al.* 1982) and there is usually some dilatation of the renal pelvis to give a warning at the time of original presentation. Otherwise long-term problems are uncommon. Some series have reported hypertension at presentation, 3% in Ahmed's series, but not at follow-up. I have not found any patient to have developed hypertension in adolescence.

In general, children operated for PUJ obstruction do well. The result achieved in the first few months is maintained. Late complications are rare.

## RENAL STONES

The aetiology of renal stones in children varies in different countries. In the UK the majority are due to infection in an otherwise normal urinary tract. At Great Ormond Street, UK between 1965 and 1974 only 12 cases of renal stone were of proven metabolic origin and one was in an exstrophy patient. Of the remaining 150 cases, 85% were associated with proven infection; 64% of the infections were with *Proteus* species (Androulakalis *et al.* 1982). These proportions are similar throughout the British Isles (Ghazali 1975).

In Jordan renal stones in children are common accounting for 2.9 per 1000 paediatric admissions in one series. Although half the children had urinary infection, 69% had a major urological malformation. In the infected cases, the most common organism was *Escherichia coli* (41%) and only three of 24 cases had *Proteus* (Dajani *et al.* 1988). Although some strains of coliform can produce urease the majority cannot and it therefore seems likely that the majority of stones were not, primarily, of infective origin.

In less developed parts of the world renal stones in childhood are frequently composed of ammonium acid urate and/or calcium oxalate. This suggests that malnutrition is an important aetiological factor. Dietary factors are also associated with a high incidence of bladder stones in childhood. This leads to two observations: firstly, that renal stones are becoming more common and bladder stones less common as countries become richer; and secondly, that the causes of renal stones are changing in many countries.

In a largely historical review Sutor found that 89% of renal stones from developing countries were composed of ammonium acid urate and/or calcium oxalate (Sutor *et al.* 1974). More recently, in Iran, the proportion of these stones had fallen to 48% (Cifuentes & Pourmand 1983).

In South Africa it is interesting to see that the incidence of renal stones in Blacks is increasing and their composition is changing. In the early 1980s those few renal stones that occurred were mainly of the phosphate type found in developing countries like the Sudan. By the end of the 1980s the incidence was higher and the majority were oxalate, identical to those found in white South Africans (Buekes *et al.* 1987). These findings were from adults. However, it seems probable that similar changes will be found later in children, though at present renal stones remain rare in Black children.

At the richest end of the spectrum, the renal stones in American children are found to be largely calcium oxalate in composition. In one series of 54 children, all of whom were white, the cause of stones was thought to be infection in 12, metabolic in 14, idiopathic in 15 and due to congenital anomalies in 13 (Sinno *et al.* 1979). In another series 81% of children were found to have hypercalciuria (Stapleton *et al.* 1982). There is a strong familial incidence of calcium oxalate stones, especially in those with hypercalciuria. In first degree relatives it may be as high as 45% in absorptive hypercalciuria and 20% overall. When a child presents with these diagnoses it is prudent to screen any siblings (Favus 1989).

In the very poorest countries renal stones in children are rare while bladder stones are still endemic. In the Institute of Child Health in Kabul 132 of 733 operations in 1 year were for bladder stone (95% in boys). Of the 30 stones that were analysed 78% were of calcium oxalate and uric acid. None of the children showed evidence of malnutrition or vitamin deficiency though the diet was high in cereals and low in animal protein. It was also commented that, at least in Afghanistan, severely malnourished children, including those with kwashiorkor, seldom developed bladder stones. Bladder stones rarely recur after removal (Srivastava *et al.* 1986).

### Results of treatment

When considering the results of treatment it is important to remember the aetiology of the stones. Metabolic abnormalities can be treated; structural or functional abnormalities of the urinary tract may be corrected; infections may be controlled. Just removing the stone may, in some cases, be a cure, but not always.

The treatment of the stones themselves has changed dramatically in the last decade. Open operations for stones are now rare. Percutaneous removal of renal stones is difficult because the renal pelvis is commonly too small to accommodate standard instruments. With special instruments such surgery is satisfactory and we have cleared stones from four children between 5 and 10 years old. Extracorporeal shock wave lithotripsy is accepted as first-line treatment in many centres including our own where 20 of 25 children were cleared of renal stones (T.A. McNicholas, personal communication 1989). Long-term results available now are based on conventional open surgery.

In the case of metabolic stones there is no good long-term follow-up study. The chance of recurrence would, probably, be related to the success in treatment of the metabolic problem. In the small number of cystine stones in St Peter's Hospitals we have seen a trend towards recurrence in teenagers as they rebel against intensive medical management.

In the 'stone belt' of the USA a rather high recurrence rate of 44% has been recorded (Sinno *et al.* 1979).

There have been two UK series that have followed up children for long enough to draw conclusions about the relapse rates: one from Great Ormond Street, London and the other from Glasgow (Androulakakis *et al.* 1982, MacDonald & Azmy 1988). The conclusions are similar for the 250 patients with urinary tract stones followed for 3 to 17 years (means 8.9 and 8.2 respectively). A few of the stones were located in the ureters, bladder or urethra at presentation but are thought to have originated in the kidneys and were, therefore, included in the analysis.

In 215 patients there was complete clearance of all stones at operation. Of these, 28 recurred (13%). The recurrence rate was significantly different in the two series. In Glasgow it was 20.4%, perhaps reflecting the fact that over half the children had a congenital anomaly of the urinary tract. The incidence of congenital anomalies in the London series is not recorded but was much lower and the recurrence rate was 8.3%. Recurrence was almost invariably associated with persistent *Proteus* infection. Only three recurrences were seen in 99 patients with a sterile urine 3 months postoperatively. Twenty-four of 28 recurrences occurred within 5 years; there were only two late recurrences at 14 and 16 years.

In 35 patients there were residual fragments. It is surprising what little trouble they caused. Only ten patients required re-operation for stone growth or infection. The main cause of trouble in this group was fragments left in the renal pelvis: all of four patients had to have a further operation.

In the long term it seems safe to discharge patients with no infection after 5 years. If there is infection or a persistent stone fragment, follow-up should be continued.

## REFERENCES

Ahmed S., Sparnon A.L., Savage J.P., Boucaut H.A. & Smith A.J. (1986) Surgery of pelviureteric obstruction in 101 children over 1 year of age. *Aust. N.Z. Surg.* **56**, 675–80.

Androulakakis P.A., Barratt T.M., Ransley P.G. & Williams D.I. (1982) Urinary calculi in children. *Br. J. Urol.* **54**, 176–80.

Avni E.F., Thoua Y., Lalmand B. *et al.* (1986) Multicystic dysplastic kidney: evolving concepts. *Ann. Rad.* **29**, 663–7.

Blackard C.E. & Mellinger G.T. (1968) Cancer in a horseshoe kidney: a report of 2 cases. *Arch. Surg.* **97**, 616–27.

Bratt C-G., Aurell M., Jonsson O., Nilsson S. (1988) Long term follow-up of maximum concentrating ability and glomerular filtration rate in adult obstructed kidneys after pyeloplasty. *J. Urol.* **140**, 273–6.

Buekes G.J., de Bruiyn H. & Vermaark W.J.H. (1987) Effect of changes in epidemiological factors on the composition and racial distribution of renal calculi. *Br. J. Urol.* **60**, 387–92.

Churchill D.N., Bear J.C., Morgan J. *et al.* (1984) Prognosis of adult onset polycystic kidney disease re-evaluated. *Kidney Int.* **26**, 190–3.

Cifuentes J.M. & Pourmand G. (1983) Mineral composition of 103 stones from Iran. *Br. J. Urol.* **55**, 465–8.

Cook D.J. & Takiff H. (1986) Original disease of the recipient. In: Terasaki P.I. (ed) *Clinical Transplants*. UCLA Tissue Typing Laboratory, Los Angeles, pp. 311–19.

Daalgard O.Z. (1957) Bilateral polycystic kidneys: a follow-up of 284 patients and their families. *Acta Med. Scand.* **328**, 1–251.

Dajani A.M., Abu Khadra A.L. & Bagdadi F.M. (1988) Urolithiasis in Jordanian children. A report of 52 cases. *Br. J. Urol.* **61**, 482–6.

Dowling K.J., Harmon E.P., Ortenberg J., Polanco E. & Evans B.B. (1988) Ureteropelvic junction obstruction: the effect of pyeloplasty on renal function. *J. Urol.* **140**, 1227–30.

Editorial (1987) Pain relief in polycystic kidney disease. *Lancet* **ii**, 1066.

Emanuel B., Nachman R., Aronson N. & Weiss H. (1974) Congenital solitary kidney: a review of 74 cases. *Am. J. Dis. Child.* **127**, 17–19.

Favus M.J. (1989) Familial forms of hypercalciuria. *J. Urol.* **141**, 719–22.

Frang D., Czvalinga I. & Polyak L. (1988) A new approach to the treatment of polycystic kidneys. *Int. Urol. Nephrol.* **20**, 13–21.

Ghazali S. (1975) Childhood urolithiasis in the United Kingdom and Eire. *Br. J. Urol.* **47**, 739–43.

Glassberg K.I., Stephens F.D., Lebowitz R.L. *et al.* (1987) Renal dysgenesis and cystic disease of the kidney. *J. Urol.* **138**, 1085–92.

Gordon A.C., Thomas D.F.M., Arthur R.J. & Irving H.C. (1988) Multicystic dysplastic kidney: is nephrectomy still appropriate? *J. Urol.* **140**, 1231–4.

Granberg P.O., Lagergren C. & Theve N.O. (1971) Renal function studies in medullary sponge kidney. *Scand. J. Urol. Nephrol.* **5**, 177–80.

Harrison A.R. & Williams J.P. (1971) Medullary sponge kidney and congenital hemihypertrophy. *Br. J. Urol.* **43**, 552–61.

Hendren W.H., Radhakrishnan J. & Middleton A.W. (1980) Pediatric pyeloplasty. *J. Ped. Surg.* **15**, 133–44.

Ho-Hsieh H., Novick A.C., Steinmuller D. *et al.* (1987) Renal transplantation for end stage polycystic kidney disease. *Urology* **30**, 322–6.

Kelalis P.P., Culp O.S., Stickler G.B. & Burke E.C. (1971) Ureteropelvic obstruction in children: experiences in 109 cases. *J. Urol.* **106**, 418–24.

Koff S.A. (1982) Ureteropelvic junction obstruction: the role of newer diagnostic methods. *J. Urol.* **127**, 898–901.

Lupton E.W., Testa H.J., Lawson R.S. *et al.* (1979) Diuresis renography and the results of pyeloplasty for idiopathic hydronephrosis. *Br. J. Urol.* **51**, 441–53.

MacDonald I. & Azmy A.F. (1988) Recurrent and residual renal calculi in children. *Br. J. Urol.* **61**, 395–8.

Mendelssohn D.C., Harding M.E., Cardella C.J., Cook G.T. & Uldall P.R. (1988) Management of end stage autosomal dominant polycystic disease with haemodialysis and transplantation. *Clin. Nephrol.* **30**, 315–19.

Murphy D.M. & Zincke H. (1982) Transitional cell carcinoma in the horseshoe kidney: report of 3 cases and review of the literature. *Br. J. Urol.* **54**, 484–5.

O'Reilly P.H., Lupton E.W., Testa H.J. *et al.* (1981) The dilated non-obstructed renal pelvis. *Br. J. Urol.* **53**, 205–9.

Osther P.J., Hansen A.B. & Rohl H.F. (1988) Renal acidification defects in medullary sponge kidney. *Br. J. Urol.* **61**, 392–4.

Pathak I.G. & Williams D.I. (1964) Multicystic and cystic dysplastic kidneys. *Br. J. Urol.* **36**, 318–31.

Patoir M.G. (1959) Les tumeurs du rein en fer a cheval. *J. d'Urologie* **65**, 799–803.

Pitts W.R. & Muecke E.C. (1975) Horseshoe kidneys: a 40 year experience. *J. Urol.* **113**, 743–9.

Reeders S.T., Breuning M.H., Corney G. *et al.* (1986a) Two genetic markers closely linked to adult polycystic disease on chromosome 16. *Br. Med. J.* **292**, 851–3.

Reeders S.T., Zeeres K., Gal A. *et al.* (1986b) Prenatal diagnosis of autosomal dominant polycystic kidney disease with a DNA probe. *Lancet* **ii**, 6–8.

Rikalainen H., Reunanen M. & Kekomaki M. (1986) Kidney growth after pyeloplasty. *J. Urol.* **135**, 1219–22.

Sahney S., Weiss L. & Levin N.W. (1981) Genetic counselling in adult polycystic kidney disease. *Am. J. Med. Genet.* **11**, 461–8.

Segura J.W., Kelalis P.P. & Burke E.C. (1972) Horseshoe kidney in children. *J. Urol.* **108**, 333–6.

Sinno K., Boyce W.H. & Resnick M.I. (1979) Childhood urolithiasis. *J. Urol.* **121**, 662–4.

Srivastava R.N., Hussainy M.A.A., Goel R.G. & Rose G.A. (1986) Bladder stone disease in children in Afghanistan. *Br. J. Urol.* **58**, 374–7.

Stapleton F.B., Noe H., Roy S. *et al.* (1982) Hypercalciuria in children with urolithiasis. *Am. J. Dis. Child.* **136**, 675–8.

Steyn J. & Logie J. (1964) Medullary sponge kidney. *Br. J. Urol.* **36**, 482–6.

Sutor D.J., Wooley S.E. & Illingworth J.J. (1974) A geographical and historical survey of the composition of urinary stones. *Br. J. Urol.* **46**, 393–407.

Thomas D.F.M., Agrawal M., Laidin A.Z. & Eckstein H.B. (1982) Pelviureteric obstruction in infancy and childhood. A review of 117 patients. *Br. J. Urol.* **54**, 204–8.

Watson M.L., MacNicol A.M. & Wright A.F. (1990) Adult polycystic kidney disease. *Br. J. Urol.* **300**, 62–3.

Whitaker R.H. (1975) Equivocal pelvi-ureteric obstruction. *Br. J. Urol.* **47**, 771–9.

Whitfield H.N., Britton K.E., Hendry W.F. & Wickham J.E.A. (1979) Frusemide intravenous urography in the diagnosis of pelvi-ureteric obstruction. *Br. J. Urol.* **51**, 445–8.

Woodhouse C.R.J., Hendry W.F. & Bloom H.J.G. (1985) Renal carcinoma. In: Whitfield H.N. & Hendry W.F. (eds) *Textbook of Genito-Urinary Surgery*. Churchill Livingstone, Edinburgh, Vol 2, pp. 945–61.

Zeier M., Geberth S., Ritz E., Jaeger T. & Waldherr R. (1988) Adult dominant polycystic kidney disease — clinical problems. *Nephron* **49**, 177–83.

# 7 *Ureteric anomalies*

## DUPLICATION

Duplication is the most common congenital anomaly of the ureters. In most cases it causes no problems in the short- or long-term and could be regarded as a variation of normal. Associated anomalies such as ureteroceles or ectopia may cause symptoms in childhood but they will usually have been dealt with before adult life.

The presence of duplication may complicate the management of incidental upper tract disease, especially if one moiety is completely obstructed and therefore unrecognised. Occasionally duplication may be an asset, for example in cases of renal pelvic neoplasm.

Amar has suggested that calculous disease may be more common in duplicated systems especially when there is previously unrecognised obstruction, reflux or ureterocele. In any event, surgery for the duplication may be needed to prevent recurrence of the stone (Amar 1972).

## MEGAURETERS

### Definition

It is only recently that urologists have come to realise that dilatation of the urinary tract does not always imply obstruction. It may indicate past and resolved obstruction or be a radiological observation of no significance. Dilatation of the ureter is only important if it causes deterioration of renal function or if it allows sufficient stagnation of urine to cause recurrent infection or stones.

Paediatric urologists are well aware of these distinctions and now are able to investigate the big ureter, only operating on appropriate cases. When a child presents with a megaureter four situations, recognised by an international classification, may be found:

**1** Obstructed megaureter.
**2** Refluxing megaureter.
**3** Non-refluxing, non-obstructed megaureter.
**4** Refluxing and obstructed megaureter.

### Obstructed and non-obstructed megaureters

It is the first and third ureters in this classification which give the most confusion. Until the advent of the Whitaker test and isotope renograms it was not possible to distinguish between the two. A megaureter which did not reflux was called 'congenital obstructive megaureter'.

#### *Follow-up*

The condition classified in most British paediatric units 20 or so years ago as 'congenital obstructive megaureter' is rare. Big series include around 50 cases collected over many years. Some were bilateral and unilateral cases had a high incidence of a different congenital abnormality on the other side. Most cases presented with recurrent infection, often severe and complicated by septicaemia. The presentation and the alarming appearance of the IVU were grounds enough for re-implantation with or without tailoring.

Considering the very gross dilatation of the ureter and kidney it is surprising how good the long-term outcome is. This diagnosis was made in 148 in-patients (108 male and 40 female) at Great Ormond Street, UK between 1950 and

1967. It is not known how many more were seen as out-patients and not admitted, but probably few. It proved difficult to achieve long-term follow-up. It is always dangerous to conclude that patients lost to follow-up are well, but in this instance I believe it to be so: it would be most unusual for a whole group of patients with severe renal damage or continuing urological problems to escape.

Some of these patients were the subject of an early report by Innes Williams. Although obstruction could not be excluded by the investigations of that time 27 of 88 ureters were treated conservatively with good outcome at 6 months to 2 years. Excellent early results were reported in the operated cases (Williams & Hulme-Moir 1970).

In 1987, a minimum of 20 years after presentation, only 78 patients could be traced and 47 responded to a postal questionnaire. Twenty-one of 47 agreed to attend for personal follow-up.

In the fully investigated group the 21 patients had 29 obstructive megaureters. At follow-up six patients had a solitary kidney which had originally been drained by a megaureter. The GFR of these kidneys ranged from 77 to 122 ml/min/1.73 $m^2$ surface area. When both sides had had a megaureter re-implanted, the GFR ranged from 76 to 139 with approximately equal distribution between sides. The least good results were seen in eight patients who had one normal ureter and one megaureter: four megaureter kidneys had normal function and four were atrophied, contributing less than 30% of overall function.

The one patient who had gross bilateral megaureters but was not operated had a GFR of 161 ml/min.

No patients were hypertensive and none had urinary infections. Taken overall only four of 29 megaureter kidneys would have any difficulty in supporting normal life on their own.

In the 26 patients followed by questionnaire alone, four were found to have died but only one of renal disease. One patient was on dialysis. None were hypertensive or had urinary infections (Cox *et al.* 1989).

The obvious flaws in this review are that we do not know the proper diagnosis of the patients originally and only one-third of the group had any follow-up. Nonetheless, it can be concluded that re-implantation of a megaureter, whether or not it is obstructed, is effective in eliminating infection. In spite of the frightening appearance on IVU, the outcome for the kidneys is good and hypertension must be rare.

### *Megaureters in adults*

It is rare for congenital megaureters to present in adult life. Minor degrees of fusiform dilatation of the lower ureter are sometimes seen by chance in routine IVUs (Fig. 7.1).

Full-blown cases that are seen are usually in sexually active girls with recurrent cystitis. As the infections are predominantly lower tract it is important not to promise that they will be cured by any upper tract surgery.

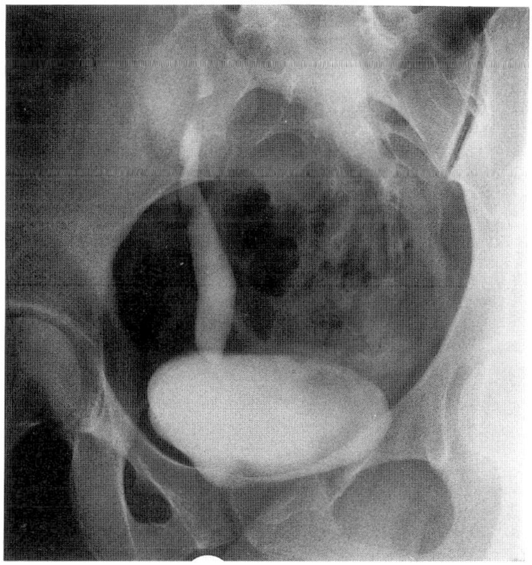

**Fig. 7.1** IVU showing a minor degree of megaureter affecting the lower ureter only.

Investigations should exclude reflux and establish whether or not there is obstruction. Many cases, for example that in Fig. 7.2, are not obstructed. If there is no obstruction and no disturbance of renal function, re-implantation of the ureter is not necessary. Nineteen megaureters in 15 adults have been followed for up to 40 years in two series with no change in the GFR (Heal 1973, Pagano & Passerini 1977). Surgical intervention was only recommended for clear-cut symptoms such as stones or recurrent upper tract infection. One patient in Heal's series who presented with haematuria was found to have a transitional cell carcinoma of the megaureter and he quoted three others from the literature, all in the middle third. This may indicate an increased risk of malignancy but as the neoplasms have been low grade and associated with haematuria, they are unlikely to be missed on conventional urological investigation.

If surgery is needed I have followed the principles suggested for children by Johnston (1967). The ureter is straightened as much possible, the redundant lower end is resected, the remaining ureter is tailored if necessary and re-implanted in a submucosal tunnel.

Although I have had no complications related to tailoring of the ureter, there is a potential for

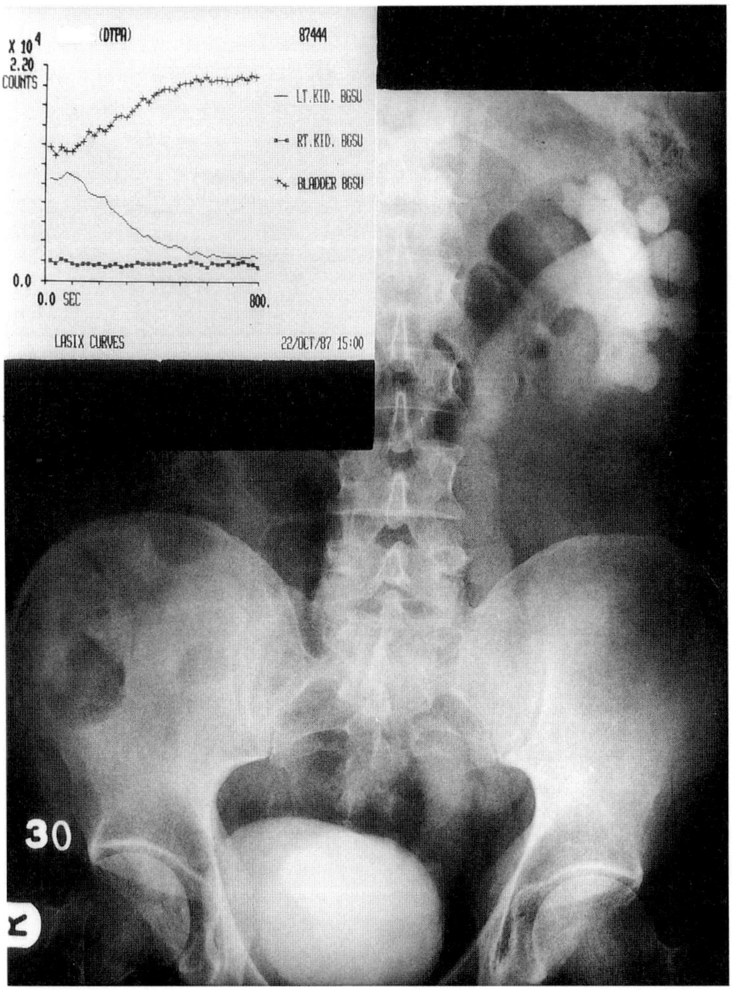


**Fig. 7.2** IVU in an adult showing gross left megaureter. The inset DTPA renogram shows good wash-out following injection of frusemide indicating absence of obstruction.

fistula formation and stenting for 7 to 10 days is essential. The surplus ureter does not have to be removed but may be folded in on itself to achieve tapering. This avoids the risk of fistula and may preserve the rather tenuous blood supply of the lower ureter; the bulky ureter left by the plication does not prevent re-implantation. A success rate of 95% has been reported in 74 megaureters. The patients were almost all children, but there were adults and the procedure worked as well in them as in the younger patients (Ehrlich 1985).

Turner-Warwick advocates re-implantation of the ureter without any form of tailoring. He makes a long enough sub-mucosal tunnel to give a lumen diameter:tunnel length ratio of 1:7 or 1:10. If necessary the available length of bladder is increased by a Boari flap or psoas hitch (Turner-Warwick 1989).

If the megaureter has been present from childhood, regardless of cause or treatment, effective follow-up is only possible if the kidney's GFR is known. Isotope scans and serial ultrasound are not able to pick up obstruction in the chronically dilated urinary tract (see Chapter 2).

### *The future*

The management of this condition will, I think, become more difficult as asymptomatic cases are picked up by fetal ultrasound examinations. Work is underway at Great Ormond Street, UK (amongst other centres) prospectively to follow such infants without surgery.

It must be remembered that so far we have only considered GFR as a measure of function. Although this is a good test, it may not detect all functional abnormalities. Grossly dilated kidneys may lack concentrating ability and this aspect needs further investigation.

If the child has repeated urinary infections there is no doubt that the ureter requires surgery whether it is obstructed or not, just to reduce the residual urine. The earlier suggestion that such children should be treated conservatively was based on the poor results from a surgical procedure that allowed reflux (Nesbit & Withycombe 1954).

It is equally clear that cases can be managed conservatively with antibiotics if necessary. I have several cases which have been followed for many years, one of which is included in Cox's series detailed above. Pitts and Muecke followed 17 (of 80) patients without surgery, all of whom did well.

It is also important to note that the re-implantation is not nearly so uncomplicated as that done for simple reflux. In Cox's series 24 megaureters had 31 re-implantations. In the 26 operated patients in Pitts and Muecke's series eight developed reflux or obstruction. It is clear from several series that reflux, whether or not there is obstruction, carries a poor prognosis in this condition (Nesbit & Withycombe 1954, Johnston 1967, Pitts and Muecke 1974).

There must be a flexible approach to the megaureter. Providing a kidney is not irreversibly damaged at presentation, the prognosis for renal function and hypertension is good. Surgery should be reserved for symptomatic patients or those with significant obstruction. Although most cases are cured by surgery, it must be recognised that re-implantation has a 20–25% complication rate.

## Refluxing and obstructed megaureters

The last type of megaureter is rare and carries a particularly poor prognosis for the function of the kidney drained by that ureter. Six patients with eight such ureters were reported by Whitaker & Flower (1979). Although all were shown to be obstructed, the renal function was only assessed by radiographic contrast excretion: the worse the obstruction, the worse the excretion. The ureteric orifice had a characteristic 'nipple-like' projection into the bladder.

It is a situation that may also be found in a ureter re-implanted (for whatever reason) at long-term follow-up. It is important to recognise because of its damaging effect even on an adult kidney but may be difficult because of our general view that the presence of reflux means the absence of obstruction.

## URETEROCELES

In the majority of children with ureteroceles diagnosis and treatment will have been completed long before adolescence. Some cases may be complicated and there may be anomalies of, or secondary damage to renal moieties not involved with the ureterocele. However, in a series of 31 patients with ectopic ureteroceles only one infant died of renal failure and the remainder were successfully reconstructed (Johnston & Johnson 1969). I have not encountered long-term problems in these patients. There may be a few patients who have lost so much parenchyma that they will suffer late renal failure due to hyperperfusion of the remaining nephrons. Obviously such patients must be carefully followed.

Problems specifically related to the ureterocele will only arise if a part of the system has been left behind. When the ureterocele is on a ureter draining a poor kidney or moiety, a child may well be treated by removal of the upper tract, leaving behind all or part of the ureter. This ureter then becomes a partly obstructed and stagnant diverticulum of the bladder. If the ureterocele has been incised, it may also reflux.

Many patients will have no problems from the residual ureter. The short-term results of partial nephrectomy and partial ureterectomy for duplex systems with ureteroceles are good. Ten of 22 patients investigated by pre-operative micturating cystogram had lower moiety vesico-ureteric reflux (VUR); in six it resolved after upper pole partial nephrectomy and partial ureterectomy (Caldemone *et al.* 1984). Thus the problems of both moieties were resolved by one simple operation.

However, with longer follow-up, nearly 50% of patients were found to have acquired reflux in the lower pole ureter, though not all were symptomatic (Caldemone *et al.* 1984). The redundant ureters are prone to infection and to stone formation.

More worrying is the malignant potential of the ureter left behind. As the number of ureters at risk is not known, the incidence of carcinoma cannot be calculated. Four of 42 symptomatic ureteric stumps (of all diagnoses) reported from the Mayo Clinic, USA had carcinomas. Eighteen cases had been reported in the literature review and other cases have been reported since, including one from a redundant ureterocele (Malek 1973, Heyman & Kalkt 1984). All the patients were in the normal age group for transitional cell carcinoma. One case of leiomyoma in a redundant ureterocele has also been reported (Sekar *et al.* 1980). These rarities may not influence the paediatric urologist. Nonetheless, since non-functioning parts of the urinary tract left behind are going to be a source of anxiety for 70 years or more, it should not take much prompting to remove them.

### Ureteroceles in adults

Small orthotopic ureteroceles may be a chance finding in adults and of no consequence because they are not causing obstruction.

It is commonly said that presentation in adults is with stones. Indeed Sir Peter Freyer is said to have thought that the stones caused the ureterocele (attributed by Gutierrez 1939). It would be expected that an anomaly that had been silent for many years would only present when some complication occurred. The reported incidence of stones in adult ureteroceles is four to 39%. Rodriguez reported that 6.3% of all patients with lower ureteric stones had a ureterocele, while 71% of adults with ureterocele presented with a stone (1984). Pain is the most common symptom, with or without symptoms of infection. Eleven percent present with bladder outflow obstruction (Thompson & Kelalis 1964, Wines & O'Flynn 1972).

Standard urological investigations will identify a significant ureterocele. They may be difficult to see on cystoscopy even when recognised on IVU (Fig. 7.3). I have found it helpful to do the cystocopy with carbon dioxide instead of water and to give the patient a fluid load and lasix. The urine can then be seen to fill the ureterocele and squirt into the gas-filled bladder like a fountain.

When a stone is present, especially with infection and overlying oedema, the appearance may be of a solid tumour (Nash & Knight 1973).

If the ureteric tone appears good and function of the renal moiety is preserved, endoscopic treatment is indicated. Although both incision and resection have been used, it is important to try to prevent subsequent reflux. In an uncontrolled series treated with incision or resection, the incision group fared better. Persistent or progressive hydronephrosis or parenchymal scarring followed in 44% of resected cases against 36% of incised cases (Wines & O'Flynn 1972). Better results have been reported with an endoscopic incision to produce a 'smiling mouth': 22 of 25 patients being cured and only one patient having reflux on follow-up (Rodriguez 1984).

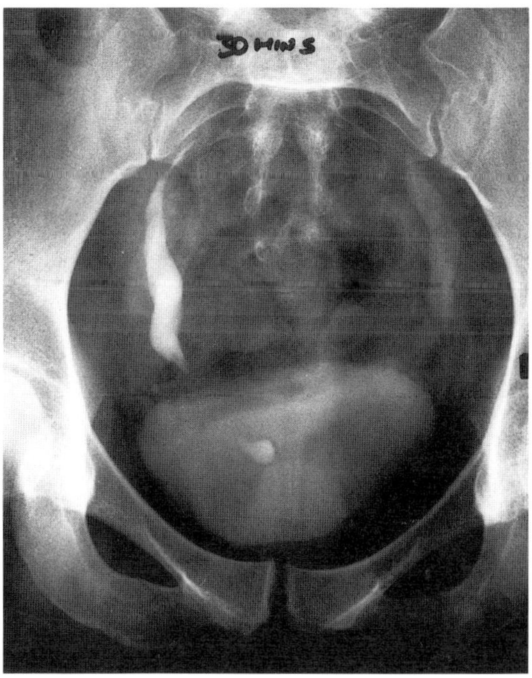


**Fig. 7.3** IVU in an adult showing the right ureter with an orthotopic ureterocele.

## ECTOPIC URETERS

Ectopic ureters, especially single ones, may open into the urethra between the internal and external sphincters. There will, therefore, be no symptoms until some damage occurs to the external sphincter when the classical incontinence of the ectopic ureter will occur. This may occur in women after delivery. Although reports in the literature are rare (Zimmern *et al.* 1986), I think it may be unrecognised in some women, the incontinence being attributed to prolapse alone: I have seen two cases and may have missed others.

The upper part of the ureter should be reimplanted in the bladder (assuming the kidney is worth saving). The debate concerns the treatment of the lower ureter which passes through, or close to, the bladder neck. In Zimmern's case, the stump was left at the first operation but subsequently acted as a urethral diverticulum and had to be removed. In my own cases I have removed the lower end of the ureter and successfully repaired the bladder neck.

Ectopic ureters in males are even rarer than in females. Most are single and drain dysplastic kidneys. They may present in adult life, especially if they drain into the genital tract. MacDonald has described a characteristic syndrome of urinary infection (especially epididymitis) with a boggy mass just above the prostate. On urography, the affected dysplastic kidney may not be visualised (MacDonald 1986).

This will be a rare cause of urinary infection. However, infections in men are worthy of investigation and the presence of a dysplastic or apparently absent kidney should alert the urologist to the possibility of a rare congenital anomaly. The affected kidney, ureter and seminal vesicle should be removed.

## BILHARZIA

It might be thought that discussion of bilharzia was out of place in a book on the long-term consequences of congenital anomalies. It must, though, be included as a reminder that it is one of the world's most common diseases, is very prevalent in children from some parts of the world and causes urinary tract damage that has important consequences in later life.

### Aetiology and epidemiology

Urinary bilharziasis is caused by infestation with *Schistosoma haematobium* through most of Africa and *S. japonicum* in the Far East. Other members of the *Schistosoma* family may be pathogenic in humans. Male and female worms, the female living in the gynaecophoric canal of the male, copulate in the veins of the lower urinary tract. The eggs are deposited in the wall of the bladder and excreted in the urine. It is the urinary tract's reaction to the presence of the eggs that causes the long-term damage. The prevalence of infection increases with age from early childhood, reaching a peak at 15 years old.

The distribution of the disease is controlled by the habitats of the snails which are primary hosts. The traditional areas are along the great tropical rivers of Africa, the Nile, Zambesi, Congo, Niger, Senegal and Gambia and in Arabia, the Tigris and Euphrates. However, migration of workers has carried the disease to other parts of Africa and the Middle East. The habitat of the snail has been widened by irrigation schemes which create areas of stagnant water. Countries which have (or have had until recently) endemic areas of bilharzia are shown in Table 7.1. With so wide a distribution and an estimated 200 million people infested, bilharzia is a disease that can never be forgotten.

**Table 7.1** Countries which have (or have recently had) endemic areas of bilharzia.

| High prevalence | | |
|---|---|---|
| China | Mali | South East Asia |
| Formosa | Mozambique | Sudan |
| Ghana | Nigeria | Volta |
| Ivory Coast | Saudi Arabia | Yemen |
| Japan | Senegal | Zimbabwe |
| Madagascar | South Africa | |
| **Medium prevalence** | | |
| Algeria | Iran | Philippines |
| Angola | Iraq | Sierra Leone |
| Botswana | Kenya | Somalia |
| Brazil | Lebanon | Syria |
| Cameroon | Libya | Tanzania |
| Chad | Mauretania | Turkey |
| Egypt | Morocco | Venezuela |
| Gambia | Niger | Zaire |
| Guinea | | Zambia |
| **Low prevalence** | | |
| Australia | India | Portugal |
| Cyprus | Mauritius | South Yemen |
| Ethiopia | Reunion | Uganda |
| Greece | Oman | Windward Islands |

### Adult consequences of childhood infestation

The clinical manifestations of bilharzia vary greatly in different groups. In endemic areas the rate of infestation of children is high and increases with age. Radiological changes occur in about a quarter of children and are more common and more severe in boys than girls.

The primary changes of the disease are due to the reaction to the presence of eggs. The reaction may take three forms: cicatrisation, calcification and polyp formation.

An adult who was infested as a child may have

been treated early in the disease and before irreversible changes had occurred; there are unlikely to be any long-term consequences. Even if radiological changes had occurred, successful treatment leads to radiological improvement in about two-thirds of patients.

Untreated patients may live in symbiosis with their ova for many years, especially if they are well-nourished and removed from possible reinfestation. They may present with haematuria or may be picked up on routine urine microscopy as young adults.

The principal late lesion is fibrosis leading to ureteric stenosis. Thin layers of calcification further worsen the problem by limiting peristalsis. The end result is obstruction and loss of renal function. The same changes occur in the bladder causing diminished volume and irritation, and in the vasa causing sterility. However, the variability of the reaction to infestation causes a very wide range of clinical manifestations and almost anything is possible.

### Investigation

In western culture it is most likely that the diagnosis will be suspected following a urogram. The urine should be microscoped to look for ova. The best specimen is collected after exercise in the middle of the day. Ova may also be found in rectal mucosal biopsies, bladder biopsies and bladder washings. Few urologists seem able to resist the temptation to cystoscope suspected cases, and, although it is understandable when the diagnosis is uncertain, great pains must be taken to avoid causing urinary infection.

Standard urological radiology is applicable to bilharzia. Antegrade pyelography and cystogram are particularly useful. Retrograde pyelography is usually unhelpful and may well cause infection of an obstructed upper tract. DTPA isotope scanning is the best method for the diagnosis of obstruction and there is a characteristic appearance of the bilharzial ureter caused by the patchy nature of obstruction in the ureter.

### Cancer

Cancer in the bilharzial bladder (it is very rare in the ureters) has a number of curious features. It occurs four times more often in men than women. It is much more common in some endemic areas such as Egypt than in others. It usually presents in an advanced stage in adults in their 30s and 40s. Although clinically aggressive, most cases seem histologically of low grade malignancy. About two-thirds are squamous cell carcinomas, adenocarcinomas and, occasionally, transitional cell carcinomas are seen.

Some of these features have tentative answers and others do not. Oestrogens are thought to inhibit copulation in the parasites and hence lessen the egg load in female patients. Thus all the manifestations of bilharzia are less in females.

The incidence of secondary urinary infection is closely related to the incidence of carcinoma. It has been shown that in Egypt, where the rate of bacterial infection is high, several carcinogens, especially nitrosamines, are found in the urine. The rate of bacterial infection is particularly high in adolescent boys.

The resulting cancers are often inoperable at presentation. They are resistant to radiation therapy and there have been few responses to chemotherapy. Radical cystectomy and diversion offer the best hope of cure.

### Treatment of bilharzia

An acutely obstructed kidney may, occasionally, require decompression by percutaneous nephrostomy. Otherwise, the first line of treatment is with drugs to eliminate the infestation. Several are available, the choice depending on the *Schistosoma* concerned; double infestation is common. The latest drug, praziquantel, is said to be effective in a single dose against the three main species and is probably the treatment of choice. The available drugs are shown in Table 7.2.

Surgery should wait for as long as possible as

effective medical treatment may allow slow resolution of radiological lesions. Early surgery is only indicated to save the function of a kidney that is seen to be deteriorating on serial renograms. Bladder outflow obstruction is treated by bladder neck incision, the small bladder by augmentation cystoplasty; the use of any of the techniques described in Chapter 11 should make cutaneous diversion unnecessary.

The biggest problem is in dealing with the obstructed and possibly refluxing ureter. If surgery is essential, there are obvious problems in operating on a fibrosed and calcified tube. Re-implantation into a bladder in the same state is also difficult.

Minor ureteric strictures at any level that are not associated with calcification may respond to one or more dilatations (Wishahi 1987). Another reasonably simple technique has been described from Kuwait. At open operation a complete ureterolysis is performed. All adhesive bands are divided and kinks are straightened out. A full length ureteric stent is then put into the ureter and left for 3 weeks. Resolution of obstruction was complete in all of 23 patients with follow-up to a maximum of three years (Rady & Rady 1987).

Although localised excision of parts of the ureter with direct anastomosis or re-implantation have been described, the results have not been good. If the ureter is extensively damaged, complete replacement is more satisfactory. Good results have been reported for complete replacement with ileum, especially if the kidney is protected by a nephrostomy before and for several weeks after surgery (Wallace 1979, Elem 1989).

## Further reading

This account of bilharzia is far from complete. It is intended to draw attention to the fact that one of the world's most common diseases may produce major urological problems in young adults. Aside from the current literature, the following books are helpful in practical management:

Husain I. (ed) (1984) *Tropical Urology and Renal Disease*, Churchill Livingstone, Edinburgh, Chapters 13–16.

Cowie A.G.A. (1981) Therapy for tropical urological diseases. In: Hendry W.F. (ed) *Recent Advances in Urology/Andrology 3*. Churchill Livingstone, Edinburgh, Chapter 8.

**Table 7.2** Therapy for schistosomiasis.

| Drug | Susceptible worms | Dose | Frequency |
|---|---|---|---|
| Praziquantel | *S. haematobium*<br>*S. mansoni* | 40 mg/kg | Once |
| | *S. japonicum* | 20 mg/kg | 8-hourly for 1 day |
| Metriphonate | *S. haematobium* | 7.5 mg/kg | 3 doses, 2 weeks apart |
| Oxamniquine | *S. mansoni* | 15 mg/kg | Once |
| Niridazole* | *S. haematobium*<br>*S. mansoni* | 7.5 mg/kg | 3 doses, 2 weeks apart |

* Niridazole is no longer used in the UK.

## REFERENCES


Amar A.D. (1972) The management of urinary calculous disease in patients with duplicated ureters. *Br. J. Urol.* **44**, 541–9.

Caldemone A.A., Snyder H.McC. & Duckett J.W. (1984) Ureteroceles in children: follow-up and management with an upper tract approach. *J. Urol.* **131**, 1130–2.

Cox R., Strachan J.R. & Woodhouse C.R.J. (1990) Twenty year follow-up of primary megaureter. *Eur. Urol.* **17**, 43–6.

Ehrlich R.M. (1985) The ureteral folding technique for megaureter surgery. *J. Urol.* **134**, 668–70.

Elem B. (1989) Preliminary nephrostomy and total ileal replacement of both ureters in advanced bilharzial obstructive uropathy. *Br. J. Urol.* **63**, 453–6.

Gutierriez R. (1939) The modern treatment of ureterocele. *Surg. Gynecol. Obstet.* **68**, 611–30.

Heal M.R. (1973) Primary obstructive megaureter in adults. *Br. J. Urol.* **45**, 490–6.

Heyman J. & Kalkt S. (1984) Transitional cell carcinoma ocurring in ureterocele. *Urology* **24**, 175–7.

Johnston J.H. (1967) Reconstructive surgery of megaureter in childhood. *Br. J. Urol.* **39**, 17–21.

Johnston J.H. & Johnson L.M. (1969) Experiences with ectopic ureteroceles. *Br. J. Urol.* **51**, 61–70.

MacDonald G.R. (1986) The ectopic ureter in men. *J. Urol.* **135**, 1269–71.

Malek R.S. (1973) Primary tumours of the ureteric stump. *Br. J. Urol.* **45**, 391–4.

Nash A.G. & Knight M. (1973) Ureterocele calculi. *Br. J. Urol.* **45**, 404–7.

Nesbit R.M. & Withycombe J.F. (1954) The problem of primary megalo-ureter. *J. Urol.* **72**, 162–71.

Pagano P. & Passerini G. (1977) Primary obstructed megaureter. *Br. J. Urol.* **49**, 469–75.

Pitts W.R. & Muecke E.C. (1974) Congenital megaloureter: a review of 80 patients. *J. Urol.* **111**, 468–73.

Rady M.Y.A. & Rady A.M.Y. (1987) Full length ureteric splintage in the management of bilharzial ureteric strictures. *Br. J. Urol.* **59**, 297–9.

Rodriguez J.V. (1984) Endoscopic surgery of calculi in ureteroceles. *Eur. Urol.* **10**, 36–9.

Sekar N., Nagrani B. & Yadav R.V.S. (1980) Ureterocele with leiomyoma of the ureter. *Br. J. Urol.* **52**, 400.

Thompson G.J. & Kelalis P.P. (1964) Ureterocele — clinical appraisal of 176 cases. *J. Urol.* **91**, 488–92.

Turner-Warwick R. (1989) The reflux preventing reimplantation of large ureters without 'reduction tailoring. In: Gingell J.C. & Abrams A. (eds) *Controversies and Innovations in Urological Surgery*. Springer Verlag, London, pp. 485–92.

Wallace D.M. (1979) Urinary schistosomiasis in Saudi Arabia. *Ann. Roy. Coll. Surg.* **61**, 265–70.

Whitaker R.H. & Flower C.D.R. (1979) Ureters that show both reflux and obstruction. *Br. J. Urol.* **51**, 471–4.

Wishahi M.M. (1987) The role of dilatation in bilharzial ureters. *Br. J. Urol.* **59**, 405–7.

Williams D.I. & Hulme-Moir I. (1970) Primary obstructive megaureter. *Br. J. Urol.* **42**, 140–9.

Wines R.D. & O'Flynn J.D. (1972) Transurethral treatment of ureteroceles. *Br. J. Urol.* **44**, 207–16.

Zimmern P.E., Cooper J. & Neustein P. (1986) Single ectopic ureter causing incontinence after childbirth. *J. Urol.* **136**, 92–3.

# 8 *Vesico-ureteric reflux*

It has been known for at least 300 years that urine should not reflux from the bladder to the ureters and that the tunnel of ureter through the bladder wall was able to prevent it (Snape 1683, Gibson 1697). The specialty of paediatric urology is presently busy with debate on the management of reflux in infants and children. The arguments will not be considered here. I am only concerned with the management of patients who have refluxed and have reached adult life. The adult urologist is interested in the condition of the kidneys, whether or not reflux persists and, if ureteric re-implantation has been done, whether there are any long-term complications thereof.

## SURGICAL COMPLICATIONS

Until the early 1970s ureteral re-implantation was done by intra- and/or extravesical dissection. The Leadbetter–Politano or Lich–Gregoir techniques were favourites. The Cohen transtrigonal advancement using intravesical dissection alone was first described in 1975 and was soon established as the method of choice (Cohen 1975).

Direct comparison, albeit retrospectively, between the Cohen and Leadbetter–Politano methods seems to confirm the technical superiority of the former. The last 100 Leadbetter–Politano cases were compared to the first 100 Cohens in one unit. Fortunately the child populations were well matched, though the distribution of reflux severity slightly favoured the Cohens. Reflux was cured in 88 of the Leadbetter cases and 97 of the Cohens. Of the 12 failures with the Leadbetter operation, three were obstructed and nine refluxed; all the Cohen failures were with reflux (Carpentier *et al.* 1982).

Late complications are rare. Reflux, obstruction or both occur in about equal numbers and the overall incidence is probably less than 5% (Arap *et al.* 1981, Mesrobian *et al.* 1985). Unfortunately it is not always clear from published reports which technique was used at the original operation. Obstruction may be caused by distal ureteric ischaemia (31%), paravesical scar tissue (30%) or a previously unrecognised neuropathic bladder (8%) and the type of original operation may be irrelevant. However, when obstruction is caused by kinking or angulation (12%), too cephalad an entry point to the bladder (10%) or an intraperitoneal course (9%), extravesical dissection must be to blame (percentages from Mesrobian *et al.* 1985).

Most complications are found soon after the initial surgery either because of symptoms or at routine postoperative imaging examinations. Late complications (beyond 4 years) are rare and 10 of 12 reported by Mesrobian had symptoms. The incidence of late, silent complications is unknown but it is doubtful if it is high enough to justify indefinite follow-up on its own. The need for further monitoring is likely to be determined by the condition of the kidneys. Our own experience has been that no child with a normal IVU 6 months postoperatively has developed a complication (Wallace *et al.* 1978).

Some patients have ureteric obstruction only when the bladder is full. This abnormality is due to extravesical dissection and re-implantation of the ureter in too lateral and cephalad a position. On IVU there may appear to be little ureteric dilatation but the lower end of the ureter has a rather pronounced 'J' shape as it enters the bladder (Hensle *et al.* 1982). When investigating, it is important to test upper tract emptying (e.g. by DTPA isotope scan) with the bladder full and empty. I have also encountered one patient whose implanted ureter passed through the broad ligament and obstructed as the uterus enlarged in pregnancy.

## SPONTANEOUS RESOLUTION OF REFLUX AND NO RENAL DAMAGE

Vesico-ureteric reflux (VUR) can resolve spontaneously. The proportion of patients in whom this occurs and the latest age at which it can happen are uncertain. With dilated ureters resolution has been reported in 40% with antibiotics alone, but with undilated ureters it may be as high as 80% (Edwards *et al.* 1977, Scholtmeijer & Griffiths 1988). There are no long-term studies on patients whose reflux has resolved spontaneously without renal damage. It is likely that such patients will have no problems.

Occasionally a young woman will present with bacterial cystitis which recurs frequently in spite of diligent preventitive measures. Investigation of such patients is commonly fruitless but it would be prudent, if she was known to have refluxed in childhood, to do a micturating cystogram. If the reflux had returned consideration could be given to ureteric re-implantation (see next section).

## UNRESOLVED REFLUX

Many patients with reflux are now treated without surgery. They may have urinary infections in childhood treated with antibiotics from time to time or they may remain symptom-free. In either case a problem will arise at puberty when they leave the care of their paediatrician and are still refluxing. The fate of these children is unknown.

Girls should not, I believe, be allowed to pass into adult life still refluxing. This view results from the belief that reflux predisposes to urinary tract infection. When girls become sexually active they are further predisposed to cystitis and are therefore likely to be taking antibiotics when at risk of pregnancy. In addition, pregnancy is the only time apart from early childhood when renal scars may occur from infected reflux.

Although it is true that re-implantation of the ureters may not prevent bacterial cystitis or renal scarring in pregnancy, the hazard is obvious enough and the surgical prevention is relatively easy. When antibiotics must be given to sexually active women only those that are thought to be safe in pregnancy should used (see Appendix II to this chapter).

In boys the problems of reflux are unlikely to arise until late in life when prostatic enlargement begins. Unless a boy is having repeated infections it would be difficult to justify re-implantation.

## REFLUX NEPHROPATHY

Much the most serious complication of reflux is nephropathy (see Chapter 3). It seems likely that most scars result from the first infection which occurs in early infancy. Scars are found in 12–20% of children presenting with urinary infection. Some apparently new scars seen on radiographs may, in fact, be old scars that become apparent as the kidney grows.

However, real new scars may occur at least up to 10 years old. In a collaborative series of 120 patients who had presented with infection new scars developed in 87 kidneys in 74 patients. In 58 children the kidneys were initially normal, 13 had unilateral and three bilateral scars. The new scars occurred in the presence of reflux of any degree, one patient developing global scarring with minimal reflux which did not reach the kidney or cause ureteric dilatation. One-third of the kidneys that developed scars were known to have been normal at 5 years old (Smellie *et al.* 1985).

Renal scarring may also result from infection in pregnancy. The sequence of radiographs in Fig. 8.1 illustrates a case associated with reflux, though reflux may not be necessary.

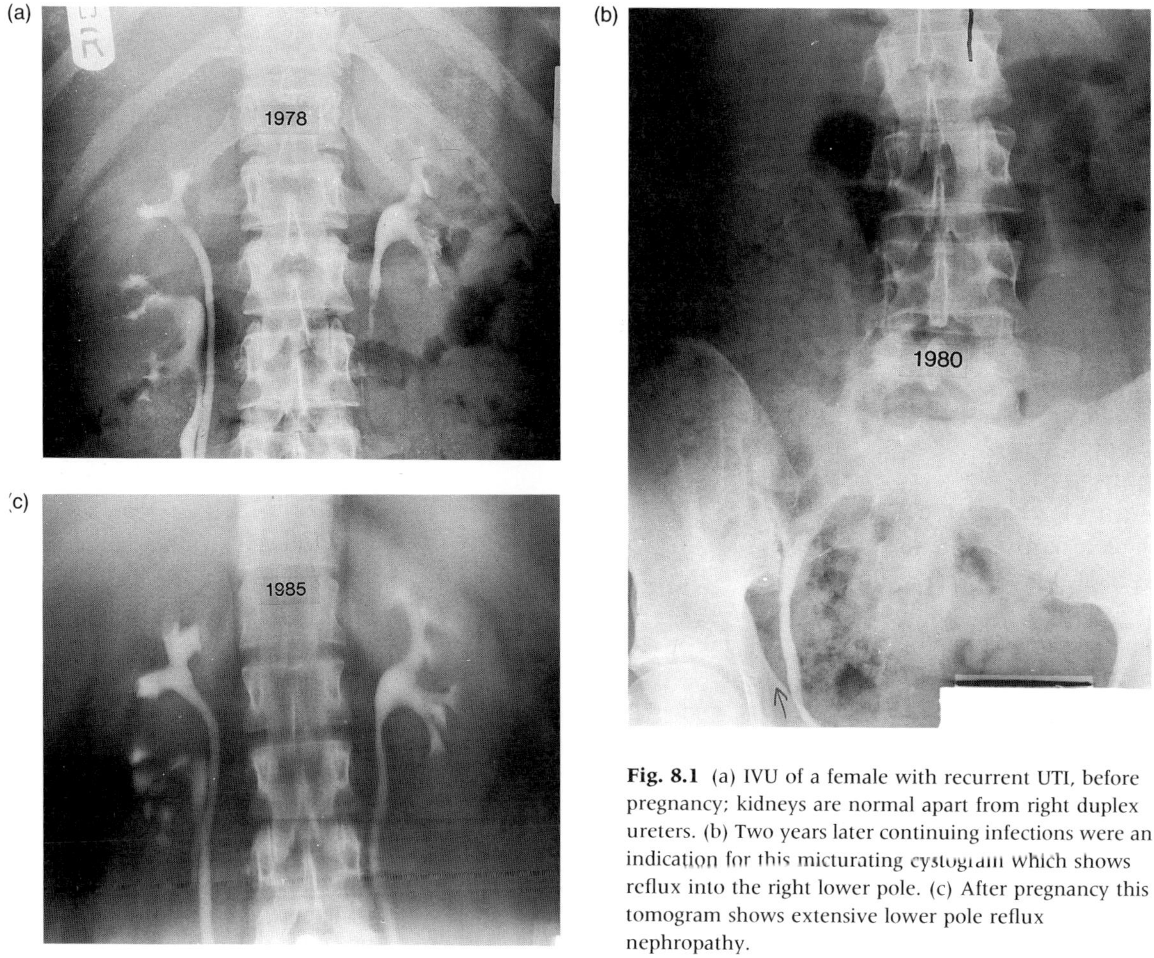


**Fig. 8.1** (a) IVU of a female with recurrent UTI, before pregnancy; kidneys are normal apart from right duplex ureters. (b) Two years later continuing infections were an indication for this micturating cystogram which shows reflux into the right lower pole. (c) After pregnancy this tomogram shows extensive lower pole reflux nephropathy.

Whatever the age at which the scars are acquired, the late consequences are considerable. Kincaid-Smith has stated that 'reflux nephropathy is not a benign disorder in adults' (Kincaid-Smith *et al.* 1984).

## Hypertension

Pyelonephritic scarring is the most common cause of hypertension in children and an important cause in young adults. Not only is there a high incidence of hypertension in young adults with abnormal kidneys, but also a rise in blood pressure may indicate the onset of a new problem in a previously quiescent, but damaged, urinary tract.

The mechanisms by which the damaged kidney raises the arterial blood pressure are the subject of some debate and are dealt with in more detail in Chapter 3. With the pyelonephritic kidney the most likely mechanism is increased renin production from relatively ischaemic tissue; in renal outflow obstruction, retention of sodium is more likely (Ledingham 1982).

Large groups of children with reflux nephropathy have been followed in the paediatric nephrology clinics of Great Ormond Street and University College Hospital in the UK. Although there are more data to come from prospective research projects, the most consistent finding has been raised peripheral plasma renin activity (PRA) in some groups. Of particular interest is a group of 35 young adults who were found to have significantly raised PRA, nine of whom had developed hypertension. Although some hypertensive patients do not have raised PRA, the levels may be inappropriately high considering the blood pressure: in other words the hypertension has not suppressed the production of renin (Dillon & Smellie 1984).

In adolescence normal blood pressure is lower than in adults. The systolic reaches adult levels in boys at about 19 and in girls at about 18 years old, the diastolic a year or so earlier. The centile charts for blood pressure are shown in Fig. 8.2. Although they are a good guide to normal levels, the working party that drew them up pointed out that they lack confirmatory evidence. The normal subjects examined to construct the charts were Negro and Caucasian up to 5 years old and there was no significant difference between them. From 5 onwards the subjects were almost exclusively Caucasian. A single abnormal reading in any individual does not constitute a diagnosis of hypertension but only a warning to make repeated measurements over several months. Unlike height and weight, blood pressure does not follow precisely the percentile tracks (Blumenthal *et al.* 1977). My experience has been that most patients with two high readings in the clinic do eventually go on to develop hypertension though it may be several years before they do so.

The incidence of hypertension in patients with reflux nephropathy has been investigated in our patients. Of patients with reflux, 166 had re-implantations between 1960 and 1967; 141 of them were reviewed especially for the study in

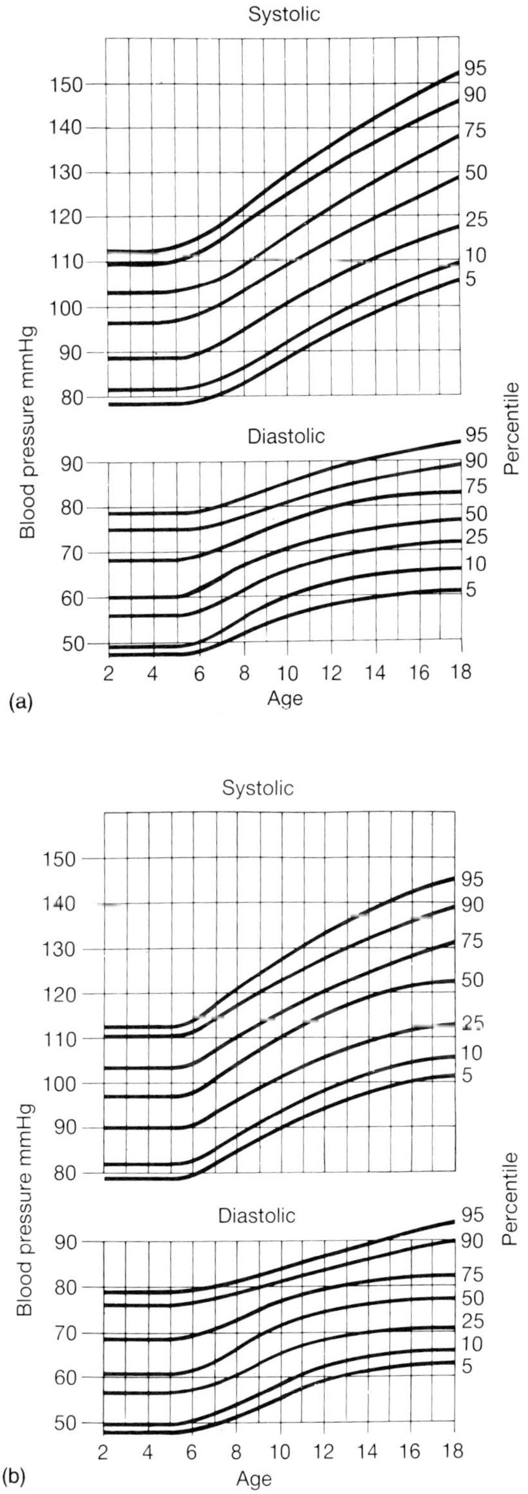


**Fig. 8.2** Percentile charts for normal blood pressure by age for girls (a) and boys (b) (from Blumenthal *et al.* 1977, reproduced with permission).

1977 so that the minimum follow-up was 10 years. The radiological findings in the study group are shown in Table 8.1. No child was hypertensive at presentation but 24 had one or both of the pressures above the 95th percentile for their age.

At follow-up, 11 patients (7.8%) were hypertensive and a further seven (5%) had at least one blood pressure reading of 140/90 mmHg or more. The incidence of true hypertension requiring treatment was 18.5% when both kidneys were scarred and 11.3% when only one was scarred. Hypertension was also found in three patients with normal pre-operative kidneys but who had acquired scars (two cases) or obstruction postoperatively. No patient with a normal IVU 6 months postoperatively developed hypertension.

The mean age at onset of hypertension was 19 (range: 12–23) and the mean time from operation was 12 years (range: 6 months to 15 years) (Wallace *et al.* 1978). Many of these patients remain under observation and new cases of hypertension are found each year.

In an older group with unilateral or bilateral scarring, reviewed at a mean age of 27 years, 23% had hypertension and the levels correlated with the PRA (Jacobson *et al.* 1989).

The risk of hypertension in patients with reflux nephropathy is such that they should never be discharged from follow-up and should have their blood pressure measured at least once a year. The severity of scarring cannot be used as a predictor of later hypertension although the risk is greater with more extensive scarring (Heale 1977, Braren *et al.* 1988).

The medical treatment is considered in Chapter 3. As a general rule surgical treatment should only be considered when medical treatment proves difficult. Nephrectomy or partial nephrectomy are the only options and so cases for surgical treatment must be very carefully selected especially if there is bilateral scarring. A small, scarred kidney that contributes less than 15% to overall function could be removed.

**Table 8.1** Radiological condition of the kidneys in 141 refluxers before surgery (Wallace *et al.* 1978).

| | Number (%) |
|---|---|
| Bilateral scarring | 38 (27%) |
| Unilateral scarring | 62 (44%) |
| Dilatation but normal kidneys | 12 (8.5%) |
| Normal | 26 (18.5%) |
| No information | 3 (2%) |

Cases can be selected on the basis of renal vein or even segmental vein renin. It has been established that the ratio of renin activity between the veins of normal kidneys is seldom more than 1.16:1 (95% confidence limit 1.4:1). In 22 hypertensive patients with a ratio of 1.5:1 or worse all were cured or significantly improved by surgery. In patients with asymmetrical or bilateral scarring it may be possible to select renal areas for resection on the basis of segmental vein renins (Dillon & Smellie 1984).

Unilateral nephrectomy in unselected cases, even when the other kidney is normal, is not always curative. A wide range has been quoted but so few of the patients are from a uniform group. Thirty percent is a generally accepted figure (Ledingham 1982) but recently 47% has been reported in a group of older children (Braren *et al.* 1988). In patients whose medical control is difficult, nephrectomy may led to improvement even if not a cure.

If the risk of hypertension is so great, should prophylactic surgery be considered? Further information from prospective studies on renin activity may help to select patients. In the meantime the results of a small prospective trial from New Zealand may be noted. Normotensive patients with one small kidney with a GFR of 10 or less and one normal kidney with a GFR of 62 or more were allocated to either observation or unilateral nephrectomy. Only one of six having nephrectomy have become hypertensive while three of eight controls have done so (Bailey *et al.* 1984a).

### Renal failure

Long-term follow-up consistently shows reduced GFR in patients with reflux nephropathy. In our 166 children at presentation 16 had a plasma urea above 7.0 mmol/l but in none was it higher than 11.0 mmol/l. At follow-up nine had a plasma creatinine above normal, three of whom were in renal failure. Twelve patients had a creatinine between 100 and 120 mmol/l (Wallace *et al.* 1978). In two other series seven of 145 and three of 30 patients developed end-stage renal failure. Thus the risk is 3.8% for all scarred kidneys. The higher figure of 10% in one series probably reflects an older group of patients. The risk is cumulative with age and patients with higher blood pressure and PRA have lower GFRs (Kincaid-Smith *et al.* 1984, Jacobson *et al.* 1989).

When the dialysis population is examined, between 12 and 20% appear to have reflux nephropathy, many of them previously undiagnosed. It is the most common cause of renal failure in children. In adults, especially men, it causes renal failure earlier than other diseases: mean of 22 years old for reflux nephropathy against 39 years old for all males. Hypertension or pregnancy accelerates the progress of renal failure (Kincaid-Smith *et al.* 1984).

It is becoming apparent in longer follow-up that even when the urinary tract is quite stable and there is no hypertension, progressive renal deterioration may occur (see Chapter 3). We do not yet know the incidence of this problem or the level of renal function at which it becomes a risk. Patients with severe renal damage should have the creatinine clearance measured. Those whose GFR is less than 40 ml/min corrected to 1.73 $m^2$ surface area should be watched closely. The onset of proteinuria is ominous.

## REFLUX IN ADULTS

### Incidence

The incidence of reflux in adults is uncertain: 5% has been quoted. Even when reflux has been found it is often unclear whether it is congenital or a consequence of another problem. A retrospective study of 1486 video cystometrograms in males is interesting because it showed that 5.4% of 174 patients with normal urodynamics had reflux. In those with abnormal urodynamics the highest incidence was found in men with bladder neck dyssynergia, 18.5% of whom had reflux. Both obstruction and detrusor instability were associated with reflux and the effects of the two were additive (Christmas *et al.* 1988).

The incidence of reflux in adult females is less clear. Theoretically it should be higher to reflect the higher incidence in female children. In adults presenting with established renal scarring there are four times as many women as men. This ratio falls to less than 2:1 in patients presenting with renal failure due to reflux nephropathy (Kincaid-Smith *et al.* 1984).

It is unclear how many women, especially in the older age groups, have uncomplicated reflux. It may even be the same 5% as is found in men. So low a figure might be explained by the higher rate of diagnosis in female children due to early infection (leaving fewer to be found as adults) and the higher rate of diagnosis in adult men with late complications from increasing bladder ouflow obstruction.

It is very important in adults to distinguish between primary congenital reflux and secondary reflux from bladder dysfunction or surgical damage to the ureteric orifices.

### Presentation

Great care must be taken in attributing symptoms to reflux in an adult. For example, reflux is not normally a painful condition. When symptoms, particularly recurrent urinary infection, have been present from childhood it is not unreasonable to blame reflux when it is found.

When cystitis begins in young, sexually active women, the causal relationship is more difficult.

Cystitis is so common in this group that investigation can only be justified in the most carefully selected patients. One percent of all new consultations in general practice are for symptoms of frequency and dysuria (Asscher 1980). I have found it helpful to give the patients written instructions on the avoidance of cystitis (see Appendix I to this chapter). Indications for the radiological investigation of adults with proven urinary infection are:

**1** Association with bacteraemia or pyelonephritis.

**2** Infection with uncommon organisms such as *Proteus* or *Pseudomonas* species.

**3** Frequent recurrence in spite of adequate preventive measures.

**4** Failure to clear infection in spite of appropriate antibiotic treatment.

**5** Association with other complications such as passage of stones.

**6** Family history of major congenital anomalies of the urinary tract.

**7** Infection beginning in older women who have not previously had urinary problems in spite of sexual activity and pregnancy.

**8** Males with cystitis and negative cultures of expressed prostatic secretion.

Reflux in adults is most commonly found during investigation of urinary infection — 61% of cases in one series (Hawtrey *et al.* 1983). Nevertheless, reflux is a rare cause of recurrent cystitis in adults. Even when it is found and thought to be worthy of surgical correction, the female patient should be warned that she may continue to have cystitis.

Other symptoms attributed to reflux in adults have included frequency and dysuria with sterile urine, enuresis, loin pain (especially during micturition), double micturition and intractable pyelonephritis in pregnancy. With all such symptoms it is possible that the reflux is a chance finding and quite unrelated. When pain is the main symptom, it can be easily tested by comparing the onset of pain with the beginning of reflux during the micturating cystogram. Most of the other symptoms may be co-incidental to the reflux.

The presentation of adults with established reflux nephropathy shows that half the women and two-thirds of the men do not have localised symptoms (Table 8.2, and see Kincaid-Smith 1984).

When reflux complicates other conditions, the situation may be more serious. About 6% of men with reflux and bladder outflow obstruction have pyelonephritis or septicaemia at presentation (Morillo *et al.* 1963, Amar & Das 1985a). It also seems that reflux can carry malignant cells to the upper tracts: in patients with bladder carcinoma and reflux the incidence of renal or ureteric carcinoma is 15-fold greater than in non-refluxers (Amar & Das 1985b).

## Treatment

The first step in the management of patients with outflow obstruction is to relieve the obstruction. Thereafter the reflux may resolve spontaneously in up to three-quarters of patients. In the few patients with persistent, gross, reflux and infection adequate control of infection may not be possible with antibiotics. Occasionally nephrectomy or antireflux surgery may be necessary (Amar & Das 1985a).

For primary congenital reflux it is important to select cases carefully and not to promise too much about the relief of symptoms, especially the relief of recurrent cystitis, though one series reported nine of 11 adults symptomatically cured (Weston *et al.* 1982). It has been suggested that persistent gross reflux accelerates renal failure (Bailey & Lynn 1984), but, conversely, there is little evidence that successful re-implantation prevents it, though it may help to maintain the status quo (Kincaid-Smith *et al.* 1984).

In patients who already have reflux nephropathy, the renal function and the degree of proteinuria at the time of surgery are more predictive of the outcome for renal function than the degree of reflux. In adults with normal renal

**Table 8.2** Presentation of 145 adults with reflux nephropathy. Patients often had more than one feature (Kincaid-Smith *et al.* 1984).

| | Female (123) | | Male (22) | |
|---|---|---|---|---|
| | *n* | (%) | *n* | (%) |
| UTI | 62 | 50.4 | 4 | 18.1 |
| Hypertension | 26 | 21.1 | 5 | 22.7 |
| Problems in pregnancy | 23 | 18.6 | — | — |
| Proteinuria | 4 | 3.2 | 11 | 50.0 |
| Impaired renal function | 5 | 4.0 | 2 | 9.0 |
| Loin or abdominal pain | 3 | 2.4 | 3 | 13.6 |
| Microscopic haematuria | 2 | 1.6 | 1 | 4.5 |
| Family history alone | 1 | 0.8 | — | — |

function, re-implantation of the ureters may prevent recurrent infection. In those with impaired function or who are already in renal failure successful re-implantation does not prevent further renal deterioration when proteinuria is already present. When there is no significant proteinuria, function may be stabilised (Weston *et al.* 1982).

As with children, the Cohen transverse advancement can be used in adults who have a normal bladder, near normal ureter and who have not had pelvic surgery. For other patients the Leadbetter–Politano technique is better. A psoas hitch will prevent kinking of the ureter at the re-implant site.

If surgery is needed for secondary reflux, the surgeon is usually faced with re-implantation into a very thick-walled and trabeculated bladder. A poorly functioning kidney with a grossly dilated and tortuous ureter may not survive and is best removed. A ureter with better function can be re-implanted. It is essential to prepare a flat muscle bed by division of trabeculations and closure of the defects of diverticula. In doing this the ureter is mobilised by intra- and sometimes extravesical dissection and can be re-implanted in a submucosal tunnel. Amar and Das (1985a) have pointed out that the whole procedure can be done intravesically and the re-implant is similar to the Cohen.

When a nephrectomy is indicated it is important to remove the lower stump of ureter. If the ureter is still refluxing it will act as a diverticulum. If previous surgery has abolished reflux, the stump will remain as a partly obstructed appendage of the bladder waiting to become infected and so form a pelvic abscess. All of 10 refluxing ureteric stumps were associated with recurrent infection in a series reported by Lipsky and Chisholm: five required excision of the stump and four were controlled with antibiotics (1971).

## PREGNANCY AND REFLUX

It has already been shown that pregnancy may unmask previously undiagnosed reflux and even predispose to reflux nephropathy. For this reason, among others, I have suggested that girls should not be allowed to pass into adult life while still refluxing. In patients with established reflux nephropathy, pregnancy may accelerate renal deterioration. Thus it is clear that reflux and pregnancy may not be happy bedfellows.

Women should be carefully advised. If they have uncorrected reflux the risk is in acquiring nephropathy. Meticulous monitoring of urine cultures and prompt treatment of bacteriuria is essential.

With established reflux nephropathy, pregnancy may cause deterioration in renal function which may not be reversible. Five patients have been reported who produced five live births. One had normal plasma urea and the others had a urea between 10 and 15 mmol/litre before pregnancy. All had rapid deterioration of renal function during pregnancy. Four, including one treated aggressively with heparin and plasma exchange, developed end-stage renal failure within a few months of delivery. The fifth patient, who was treated with heparin during pregnancy, recovered some function after delivery and had a plasma urea only slightly above her original level 1 year later (Kincaid-Smith *et al.* 1984). These poor results are not typical and many patients with scarred kidneys have gone through pregnancy with no difficulty. Jacobson, for example, found no difference in renal function or blood pressure control before and after 26 pregnancies in 16 women (Jacobson *et al.* 1989).

Women with extensive nephropathy must be told of the risks of pregnancy. At the very least pregnancy may bring forward the necessity for dialysis. In some it may be responsible for that need.

Even after successful re-implantation there may be complications in pregnancy. A postal and telephone survey of 67 women at least 15 years after surgery gave some worrying and unexpected results. Re-implantation had been by the Leadbetter–Politano method and the effect of nephropathy was not considered. Thirty women had had 64 pregnancies. Fifty-seven percent of pregnancies were complicated by urinary infections and 17% by pyelonephritis. One patient developed ureteric obstruction at 30 weeks requiring nephrostomy drainage. Thirteen percent of pregnancies ended in spontaneous abortions between nine and 21 weeks (mean 15.5), mostly in the group with recurrent infections. The usual spontaneous abortion rate at that time was considered to be 3.3%. All but one baby were delivered at term (Austenfield & Snow 1988).

We have not reviewed our own pregnancies in any detail. However, I have had three patients who developed ureteric obstruction in pregnancy following re-implantation be the Leadbetter–Politano technique. Curiously, one of the patients, with a solitary kidney, developed the obstruction in the second pregnancy, the first having been uncomplicated. Theoretically the risk of obstruction should be less after a Cohen re-implant.

Reflux is a common condition. Presumably many patients will go through pregnancy without problems and we should not raise unnecessary difficulties for them. On the early data we have available, the protocols shown in Table 8.3 seem reasonable. A guide to antibiotic prescribing in pregnancy is shown in Appendix II to this chapter.

## INHERITANCE OF REFLUX

Eighty-eight families have been investigated by Bailey and the literature reviewed. There seems no doubt that reflux has a genetic mechanism, is an autosomal dominant and has incomplete penetrance. There may be symptomless carriers of the gene. Thirty of the 88 families were found to have more than one affected member, adding up to 36 first-degree relatives of the index cases. The ratio of affected to non-affected relatives was 36:54. About one-third of the offspring of an affected parent will have reflux. A genetic marker has not been identified with certainty, but HLA-A9 occurs significantly more frequently in refluxers with renal failure than in the rest of the renal failure population (Bailey *et al.* 1984b).

The inherited risk is so high that all offspring of refluxers must be investigated at birth. Bailey suggests that a micturating cystogram should be done. Others might feel that a radionuclide cystogram or even an ultrasound might suffice. Abbeele found reflux by radionuclide cystography in 45% of the symptomless siblings of refluxers. Although no direct comparison was made in this series, the authors firmly recommended this investigation in preference to radiographic cystography or renal ultrasound. It is more sensitive and involves less radiation,

**Table 8.3** Suggested protocols for the management of the special risks of pregnancy in vesico-ureteric reflux.

| Problem | Special risks | Protocol |
|---|---|---|
| Corrected reflux: little or no nephropathy | UTI. Mid trimester abortion | Weekly MSU to 24 weeks |
| Corrected reflux: moderate nephropathy | Hypertension | Normal antenatal care |
| Uncorrected reflux | UTI. Nephropathy | Weekly MSU to term |
| Corrected reflux: major nephropathy | Accelerated renal failure | Nephrology supervision ?heparin ?plasma ex-change |
| Corrected reflux by extravesical approach | Ureteric obstruction | Ultrasound 2-monthly |
| Corrected reflux by extravesical approach: single kidney | Ureteric obstruction | Ultrasound monthly |

though it does not remove the need for a catheter (Abbeele *et al.* 1987).

## APPENDIX I: Notes given to young women with recurrent bacterial cystitis

The advice is sometimes helpful for those whose symptoms of cystitis are not due to bacterial infection. There is little scientific evidence to back up any of this advice but the majority of patients who follow it appear to have fewer episodes of cystitis.

All of the advice should be followed from the outset. If it becomes apparent that the patient is better as a result, she can start to experiment to find which items are of most value to her.

### Prevention

**1** High fluid intake: at least 2.5 litres of water should be drunk per day, more in hot weather or when travelling long distances. As a guide, you should pass at least 1.8 litres of urine a day.

**2** Do not allow your bladder to get over-full. Empty the bladder at least every 3–4 hours.

**3** Personal hygiene: the vulva (area around the entrance to the vagina) should be washed at least twice a day, after a bowel action and before sexual intercourse. For this and all other washing use simple soap (baby soap).

**4** Do not use perfumed soaps, detergents, antiseptics, bath oils, bath salts or vaginal deodorants. Do not wash your hair in the bath or shower: wash it over the sink to prevent contact with shampoo which may be irritant.

**5** Sexual intercourse: whether or not cystitis follows intercourse, the following points should be observed:

**a** Have a wash, bath or shower first.

**b** Ensure that intercourse is not uncomfortable or painful to avoid bruising.

**c** Always use a lubricant such as KY jelly or baby oil.

**d** Empty your bladder within 20–30 minutes of finishing intercourse.

**6** Use cotton underwear or tights with a cotton gusset. Wash your underwear in simple soap and do not use detergents or biological powders.

### Treatment

**1** Immediately start to drink extra fluid: half a litre as often as possible (e.g. every half hour) until you have drunk 2 litres.
**2** Take two tablets that you keep for headaches, etc. (e.g. aspirin or paracetamol).
**3** Keep warm. You may find a hot water bottle on your lower tummy or between your legs helpful.
**4** Pass a midstream specimen of urine into the specimen bottle with which you have been provided. Keep it in the ordinary fridge (not the deep freeze).
**5** Start the antibiotic with which you have been provided and continue for 3 days.
**6** Visit your doctor within 36 hours to deliver the urine specimen and to collect an antibiotic for next time.

## REFERENCES


Abbeele A.D. Van den, Treves S.T., Lebowitz R.L. *et al.* (1987) Vesicoureteral reflux in asymptomatic symptoms with known reflux: radionuclide cystography. *Pediatrics* **79**, 147–53.

Amar A.D. & Das S. (1985a) Vesicoureteral reflux in patients with obstructive prostatic disease. *J. Urol.* **133**, 194–7.

Amar A.D. & Das S. (1985b) Upper urinary tract transitional cell carcinoma in patients with bladder carcinoma and associated reflux. *J. Urol.* **133**, 468–71.

Arap S., Abrao E.G. & Menezes de Goes G. (1981) Treatment and prevention of complications after extra vesical anti reflux technique. *Eur. Urol.* **7**, 263–7.

Asscher A.W. (1980) *The Challenge of Urinary Tract Infections.* Academic Press, London, Chapter 3.

Austenfield M.S. & Snow B.W. (1988) Complications of pregnancy in women after reimplantation for vesicoureteric reflux. *J. Urol.* **140**, 1103–6.

Bailey R.R. & Lynn K.L. (1984) End-stage reflux nephropathy. In: Hodson, C.J., Heptinstall, R.H. & Winberg, J. (eds) *Reflux Nephropathy Update, 1983.* S. Karger, Basel, pp. 102–10.


## APPENDIX II: Antibiotics in pregnancy

No drugs can be considered entirely safe in pregnancy. The following list of antibiotics that might be used to treat urinary infections is a guide to the safer ones (Wise 1987).

| Antibiotic | Use | Notes |
|---|---|---|
| Penicillin<br>Ampicillin*<br>Amoxycillin*<br>Cloxacillins | Probably safe | |
| Augmentin<br>Pivampicillin | Inadequate data | |
| Carbenicillin<br>Mezlocillin<br>Azlocillin<br>Ticaricillin<br>Piperacillin<br>Mecillinam | Inadequate data | Reserve for severe infection with susceptible organisms |
| Cephalosporins | Inadequate data | Probably safe: injectable forms (except latamoxef and cefamandole) first choice in severe infections |
| Sulphonamides* | Probably safe | |
| Trimethoprim† | Probably safe | ?Teratogenic |
| Co-trimoxazole | Probably safe | |
| Tetracyclines | Not safe | |
| Erythromycin | Not safe | |
| Aminoglycosides | Not safe | |
| Nalidixic acid | Caution | Theoretical risks |
| Ciprofloxacin | Not safe | Theoretical risks |
| Nitrofurantoin† | Probably safe | Not with 6PD deficiency |
| Metronidazole | Caution | Theoretical risks |

* First choice
† Second choice

Bailey R.R., Lynn K.L. & McRae C.U. (1984a) Unilateral reflux nephropathy and hypertension. In: Hodson, C.J., Heptinstall, R.H. & Winberg, J. (eds) *Reflux Nephropathy Update, 1983*. S. Karger, Basel, pp. 116–25.

Bailey R.R., Janus E., McLoughlin K., Lynn K.L. & Abbott G.D. (1984b) Familial and genetic data in reflux nephropathy. In: Hodson, C.J., Heptinstall, R.H. & Winberg, J. (eds) *Reflux Nephropathy Update, 1983*. S. Karger, Basel, pp. 40–51.

Blumental S., Epps R.P., Heavenrich R. *et al.* (1977) Report of the task force on blood pressure control in children. Standards for blood pressure. *Pediatrics* **58** (Supplement), 802–3.

Braren V., West J.C., Boerth R.C. & Harmon C.McW. (1988) Management of children with hypertension from reflux or obstructive nephropathy. *Urology* **32**, 228–34.

Carpentier P.J., Bettink P.J., Hop W.C.J. & Schroder F.H. (1982) Reflux — a retrospective study of 100 ureteric reimplantations by the Politano–Leadbetter method and 100 by the Cohen technique. *Br. J. Urol.* **54**, 230–3.

Christmas T.J., Chapple C.R., Milroy E.J.G., Turner-Warwick R.T. & Rickards D. (1988) Vesico-ureteric reflux in the adult male. *Br. J. Radiol.* **61**, 776–7.

Cohen S.J. (1975) Ureterozystoneostomie. Eine rene antirefluxtechnik. *Akt. Urol.* **6**, 1–8.

Dillon M.J. & Smellie J.M. (1984) Peripheral plasma renin activity, hypertension and renal scarring in children. In: Hodson, C.J., Heptinstall, R.H. & Winberg, J. (eds) *Reflux Nephropathy Update, 1983*. S. Karger, Basel, pp. 68–80.

Edwards D., Normand I.C.S., Precod N. & Smellie J.M. (1977) Disappearance of vesicoureteric reflux during long-term prophylaxis of urinary tract infection in children. *Br. Med. J.* **ii**, 285–8.

Gibson T. (1697) *The Anatomy of Humane Bodies Epitomized*. Awnsham & Churchill, London, pp. 133–7.

Hawtrey C.E., Culp D.A., Loening S., Fallon B. & Maynard M. (1983) Ureterovesical reflux in an adolescent and adult population. *J. Urol.* **130**, 1067–9.

Heale W.F. (1977) Hypertension and reflux nephropathy. *Aust. Paed. J.* **13**, 56.

Hensle T.W., Berdon W.E., Baker D.H. & Goldstein H.R. (1982) The ureteral 'J' sign: radiographic demonstration of iatrogenic distal ureteral obstruction after ureteral reimplantation. *J. Urol.* **127**, 766–8.

Jacobson S.H., Eklof O., Eriksson C.G. *et al.* (1989) Development of hypertension and uraemia after pyelonephritis in childhood: 27 year follow-up. *Br. J. Med.* **299**, 703–6.

Kincaid-Smith P.S., Bastos M.G. & Becker G.J. (1984) Reflux nephropathy in the adult. In: Hodson C.J., Heptinstall R.H. & Winberg J. (eds) *Reflux Nephropathy Update, 1983*. Karger & Co, Basel, Chapter 8.

Ledingham J.G.G. (1982) Renal disease and hypertension. In: Williams D.I. & Chisholm G.D. (eds) *Scientific Foundations of Urology*. William Heinemann Medical Books, London, Chapter 16.

Lipsky H. & Chisholm G.D. (1971) Primary vesico-ureteric reflux in adults. *Br. J. Urol.* **43**, 277–83.

Mesrobian H-G.J., Kramer S.A. & Kelalis P.P. (1985) Re-operative ureteroneocystostomy: review of 69 patients. *J. Urol.* **133**, 388–90.

Morillo M.M., Orandi A., Fernandes M. & Draper J.W. (1963) Vesicoureteral reflux in male adults with bladder neck obstruction. *J. Urol.* **89**, 389–94.

Scholtmeijer R.J. & Griffiths D.J. (1988) Treatment of vesicoureteric reflux: preliminary report of a prospective study. *Br. J. Urol.* **61**, 205–9.

Smellie J.M., Ransley P.G., Normand I.S.C., Prescod N. & Edwards D. (1985) Development of new renal scars: a collaborative study. *Br. Med. J.* **290**, 1957–60.

Snape A. (1683) *The Anatomy of an Horse*. M. Flesher, London, p. 39.

Weston P.M.T., Stone A.R., Bary P.R., Leopold D. & Stephenson T.P. (1982) The results of reflux prevention in adults wth reflux nephropathy. *Br. J. Urol.* **54**, 677–81.

Wallace D.M.A., Rothwell D.L. & Williams D.I. (1978) The long term follow-up of surgically treated vesicoureteric reflux. *Br. J. Urol.* **50**, 479–84.

Wise R. (1987) Prescribing in pregnancy. *Br. Med. J.* **294**, 42–6.

# 9 *Neuropathic bladder*

## MYELOMENINGOCELE

The neuropathic bladder of childhood is almost always due to disorders of the spinal cord, principally myelomeningocele. A few patients are seen with bladders that behave in a neuropathic manner without overt neurological disease: the so-called non-neurogenic neurogenic bladder (or occult neuropathic bladder). Children with enuresis may have a neuropathic bladder but more often the symptom occurs in otherwise normal individuals.

It is difficult to consider the urinary tract of the myelomeningocele patient in isolation from the other disabilities. The neurological deficit ranges from the very minor to dense paraplegia with intellectual impairment. The urological requirements vary with the function of the other organs and the long-term prognosis depends on both.

The mortality of myelomeningocele has lessened considerably with aggressive neurosurgical management. The result is a larger number of the more severely affected children and adults, 97% of whom have urological problems (Durham Smith 1972). Renal morbidity is high without active urological help, but deaths in early adulthood are uncommon. In a series of 215 patients only eight died between 16 and 24 years old, three of the deaths being from chronic renal failure (Rickwood *et al.* 1984).

Better understanding of the pathophysiology of the neuropathic urinary tract in the last 20 years has led to more satisfactory management. This is not relevant to the children of 20 or more years ago, many of whom were diverted, permanently catheterised or left to drip into nappies. It is of value, however, to review current opinions to help decide what form of undiversion would be appropriate for an older patient.

### Current views of neuropathic bladder

The neuropathic bladder and sphincters may exhibit three types of behaviour: contractile, intermediate and acontractile (Rickwood 1984, Mundy *et al.* 1985). About one-third of patients have a contractile bladder in that the detrusor has sufficient contraction to produce some bladder emptying. Unfortunately, 95% of such patients have sphincter dyssynergia so that there is no relaxation during detrusor activity and emptying is incomplete. Patients with incomplete cord lesions may have some voluntary control over the distal sphincter and the same patients usually have normal anal tone and positive sacral reflexes.

About 40% of patients have an intermediate bladder. The detrusor does contract but lacks the force to produce bladder emptying. Although the external sphincter has some tone it shows little activity in response to detrusor contractions and incontinence occurs solely because of the pressure rise in the bladder. There is no voluntary control of the sphincters. If the bladder outflow resistance is increased by, for example, the implantation of an artificial urinary sphincter, an intermediate bladder may develop more forceful detrusor contractions and become a contractile one (Murray *et al.* 1988).

An acontractile bladder is seen in about 25% of patients. In this group there is little sphincter activity but incontinence occurs when the volume reaches a critical level even though the intravesical pressure is still low.

In about half the patients with contractile bladders the bladder neck is competent. In the other half and in all patients in the other two groups it is open. It is almost never obstructive.

The distal sphincter is nearly always dyssynergic in contractile bladders, contracting at the same time as the detrusor, so creating obstruction. The sphincter then relaxes ahead of the detrusor and incomplete bladder emptying occurs. Children with incomplete cord lesions have some voluntary control of the external sphincter. In intermediate and acontractile bladders the external sphincter shows little if any activity, remaining closed until opened passively by a detrusor contraction or an excessive volume of urine (Mundy *et al.* 1985).

Although it might be thought that the patients with the least neurological deficit would have best bladders, it is not so. The essential element in the bladder is the function of the detrusor and the sphincters in harmony. Dyssynergia between the two may occur with only minor neurological deficit elsewhere and will result in poor overall bladder function. The motor and sensory levels cannot be used to predict bladder function. But 70% of patients with a positive anocutaneous reflex have detrusor hyperreflexia, good sphincter tone and a competent bladder neck (Williams *et al.* 1988).

The long-term natural history of congenital neuropathic bladder is unknown. It is likely that there is no spontaneous change from one type of bladder to another, though there may be a quantitative change within a type. The sphincters worsen with time, the obstructive becoming more so and the weak becoming more incontinent.

The function of the bladder controls not only continence but also renal function. Bladder function is thus a major determinant of the overall prognosis in myelomeningocele. About 14% of myelomeningocele patients have renal complications at birth and subsequent risk is greatest in the first 5 years of life. Ultimately about 50% will develop upper tract complications but they may be delayed for up to 30 years. The incidence is equal between the sexes (Rickwood 1984). In some older patients renal damage has been so severe that remedial measures, although successful in the short-term, do not save the patient from late renal failure: this outcome was seen in seven of 42 patients in whom neither intermittent clean self-catheterisation (ICSC) nor cutaneous diversion prevented progressive deterioration (Brem *et al.* 1987).

Hydronephrosis and renal damage have been associated with several parameters of bladder function. The relative importance of each has been assessed in a prospective series of 215 patients on a programme of ICSC. The most significant determinants of hydronephrosis were increased thickness of bladder wall and grade of vesicoureteric reflux (VUR) assessed by radiography, urethral pressure above 70 cm $H_2O$ and bladder capacity below the mean for age (McLorie *et al.* 1988). Bladder pressures of 35 to 40 cm $H_2O$ have been shown to reduce glomerular filtration rate (Steinhardt *et al.* 1988).

Aside from dilatation, reflux probably has the same effect in these children as in others. It has been shown experimentally that reflux nephropathy occurs with intrarenal reflux plus infection at normal pressures and with vesicoureteric reflux alone at high pressures (Ransley & Risdon 1982). It can be inferred from this work and from some clinical observation that the high pressure bladders with reflux seen in many spina bifida patients will cause scarring even without infection.

The incidence of hypertension is high, presumably because of renal scars. At 16 years old it is said to be 11% overall and 29% in patients with damaged kidneys. During follow-up for 12 years 28 of 196 adult patients developed hypertension, six of them with normal kidneys on IVU (Rickwood *et al.* 1984).

Urodynamic assessment in children can be difficult. As far as renal impairment is concerned, the important factor is the level of storage pressure rather than the much higher pressure that may be associated with transient detrusor contractions.

## Results of management of neuropathic bladder

These relatively recent reports of urinary tract function have provided some new information and confirmed a good deal of that which was already known. Obviously they come too late to affect the management of patients who are now adults. They make a considerable difference to plans for urinary undiversion (see Chapter 11), providing the bladder was not surgically altered before diversion. They also explain why some aspects of management from the past have been more successful than others.

Traditional management was based on spontaneous or induced bladder emptying, incontinence devices and pads and permanent catheters. Sphincterotomy was used to aid bladder expression and, sometimes, in an attempt to improve the kidneys. Renal deterioration and repeated infections were sometimes (but not always) treated by ileal conduit diversion. Once diversion had been made, and often it was a life-saving procedure, the prognosis became dependent on the function of the conduit (see Chapter 10).

### *Bladder expression*

Treatment by bladder expression was successful in many cases, presumably because the patient had an acontractile bladder and a low urethral pressure (Pekarovic *et al.* 1970). Those with contractile and most with intermediate bladders would fare badly. External sphincterotomy lowered the outflow resistance and made expression easier in 80% of patients but did little to reduce residual volumes (Thomas *et al.* 1973). The effect on hydronephrosis was unpredictable, with some patients, mainly with high bladder pressures and external sphincter dyssynergia, improved and others remaining dilated (Thomas *et al.* 1973, Rickwood 1982). Bladder emptying by manual expression remains an important method of treatment when there is no upper tract dilatation (Rickwood *et al.* 1982, Borzyskowski *et al.* 1982).

The danger to the kidneys of residual urine and vesico-ureteric reflux has been known for many years. Johnston initially regarded reflux as an indication for diversion. Later he advised increased efforts to achieve emptying and re-implantation of the ureters. Although the technique was difficult, using a modified Leadbetter–Politano reflux was corrected in 95% of patients and 79% of kidneys were improved or stabilised (Johnston *et al.* 1976).

### *Intermittent clean self-catheterisation (ICSC)*

The introduction of ICSC by Lapides produced a revolution in the management of this and many other conditions (Lapides *et al.* 1972). Its apparently obvious value may explain why there is little recorded long-term follow-up! When his own series of 60 patients was reviewed at a minimum of 10 years' follow-up it was surprising to find that less than a half were still performing ICSC. However, this apparently poor result was largely accounted for by 25% who were lost to follow-up and specific reasons for giving up in most of the others (such as death and change in neurological status); one patient stopped because of a false passage and the mother of one child disliked the procedure. Of the original 60, 46 were children or adolescents, 10 having myelomeningocele. It is not possible to distinguish the outcome of these from the whole group, but it appears that they formed the majority of those still catheterising after 10 years. 'Several' patients had persistent bacteriuria without coming to harm and there was no recorded renal deterioration (Diokno *et al.* 1983). In another review from the same unit it was confirmed that bacteriuria was not harmful except in patients with high grade reflux, 60% of whom suffered intermittent pyelonephritis (Kass *et al.* 1981).

Although ICSC remains the single most useful means of managing the congenital neuropathic bladder, it is not the answer for all. It has been estimated that only 30% of patients are suitable (Enrile & Crooks 1980). However, in suitable patients up to 84% may become dry though many only with drug supplements (Mulcahy *et al.* 1977).

It does not always allow improvement of renal dilatation: in a cross-over controlled trial comparing ICSC and manual expression (with supplementary drugs as required), ICSC was shown to produce significantly better continence but there was no difference between the two in improving renal function. It is important to note that ICSC appeared to produce better renal function at 18-month follow-up but this advantage was lost at later review up to 4 years later. Renal function in patients with reflux and external sphincter dyssynergia does not improve with either management alone. CISC is only suitable for this group after surgical treatment for reflux and/or a sphincterotomy (Borzyskowski *et al.* 1982).

ICSC is unhelpful for those who lack motivation or the ability actually to perform the catheterisation. Those with incomplete sacral lesions may have sufficient urethral sensation to make ICSC too painful for regular use. Finally, mobility can present problems: the wheelchair-bound patient, especially female, may find the frequent transfers on and off the lavatory unacceptable.

### *Bladder outflow surgery*

If the sphincters are too weak to maintain continence, one of two possible paths may be followed. The goal may be either for 'normal' voiding or to establish fixed outflow resistance and empty by ICSC. 'Normal' voiding can be achieved by destroying the natural sphincters and implanting an artificial urinary sphincter (AUS). Although Brantley Scott himself reported that 90% of his patients were continent and had unchanged upper tracts (Brantley Scott *et al.* 1986), the AUS has a poor reputation in the congenital neuropathic bladder. Insufficient attention has been paid to the likely function of the bladder when continence has been established. In a series of 40 young patients good results were achieved for continence at 3 to 5 years' follow-up. However, nine patients had a deterioration in detrusor function. The group most at-risk had intermediate-type bladders. The authors pointed out that any detrusor contraction seen in an otherwise flat trace preoperatively indicated that a change to a contractile bladder was possible postoperatively. Close urodynamic follow-up or elective bladder augmentation at the time of AUS implant are essential (Murray *et al.* 1988).

The alternative to AUS, particularly in females, is to increase the outflow resistance by bladder neck reconstruction or colposuspension and accept that ICSC is likely to be necessary. Raz has reported an excellent result in 79% of 42 young females managed with a combination of denervation (for hyperreflexia), augmentation and colposuspension. All patients used ICSC and all kidneys remained stable or improved at 3 to 9 years' follow-up (Raz *et al.* 1988).

In a comparison of similar patients (though not randomly allocated) both Young–Dees reconstruction and AUS had similar results for continence. The AUS patients had a mean of 1.5 re-operations each and the reconstruction patients had 0.8 re-operations each. Admittedly most patients had the older model AUS and the results with the AS800, on much shorter follow-up, were better at 0.375 re-operations per patient. Ten of 11 reconstructed patients and seven of 16 AUS patients had to self-catheterise (Sidi *et al.* 1987).

### *Other managements*

There remains a group of patients for whom

none of these managements is suitable. There are usually many factors involved: difficult bladders, difficult patients, difficult parents and difficult social circumstances. For these, the possibilities are sphincterotomy and a penile appliance (for boys), permanent catheter (for either sex but especially females) or incontinence pads. These unsatisfactory forms of management may compound the difficulties that made them necessary in the first place.

### Undiversion in neuropathic bladder

The current management of congenital neuropathic bladder does not commonly include cutaneous diversion. In a recent series only seven of 174 patients were diverted (Brereton *et al.* 1987). Current management has been considered here because it is relevant to ideas about undiversion (and alternatives to a bag) for adults who were diverted in the past. It should go without saying that undiversion should not result in an incontinent urinary reservoir or a lower tract that is a danger to the kidneys.

Before deciding on undiversion for an adult with a neuropathic bladder it is essential to consider the type of bladder that will result, the likely effects on the kidneys and the advantages for the patient as a whole. The first two of these follow from the foregoing description. The techniques and results of undiversion are covered in Chapter 11.

The overall advantages of undiversion are less certain. In a patient with a cutaneous diversion that works well and has no complications, undiversion involves a major operation for a cosmetic reason. It should only be done if the patient is able to take advantage of the improved appearance. This implies that the patient is sufficiently well motivated to advance in life, either in work or in social relationships. In those who have only minor disabilities getting rid of the bag usually confers a great improvement in self-confidence. Such patients should be considered in the same way as any others who are candidates for undiversion (see Chapter 11).

It might be thought that patients who are severely crippled or confined to a wheelchair should not be undiverted. I do not believe that this is the case. In carefully selected patients I have seen considerable improvements following removal of the bag. A second benefit is that, in some patients, changing a bag may be impossible without help, whereas ICSC may be possible independently. In these patients careful consideration must be given to the orifice that is to be catheterised: a suprapubic or even an upper abdominal stoma may be more satisfactory than the external urinary meatus.

## MINOR DEGREES OF NEUROPATHIC BLADDER

About 20% of patients with spina bifida have such minor neurological deficits that the bladder functions normally. They may be recognised in childhood and, if so, should be carefully followed because of the known tendency of sphincter function to deteriorate. Occasionally, because of the neurological deterioration, patients with spina bifida occulta, especially those with a tethered cord, may present in adolescence. Early diagnosis is important as the bladder dysfunction may be curable by neurosurgery in up to 67% of patients (Kondo *et al.* 1986).

There is a small sub-group that gives me particular cause for concern. I have seen one male with a good bladder and minor incontinence in childhood who became continent spontaneously in puberty. He defaulted from follow-up for 6 years and represented with bilateral hydronephrosis and advanced renal failure. Presumably the extra outflow resistance provided by the developing prostate unmasked detrusor hyperreflexia. I have now identified 18 other patients in a similar situation who are being followed prospectively, one of whom has started to develop hydronephrosis.

Bearing in mind the known outcome on the detrusor of increasing bladder outflow resistance and the potential for late renal damage, we must beware of the incontinent child who becomes dry.

## SEXUAL FUNCTION WITH A NEUROPATHIC BLADDER

Even the most crippled spina bifida patient has sexual desires. Very often it is beyond the training of the urologist to help when there are emotional difficulties. The very least that can be done is to give an opportunity for the subject to be discussed, to give 'medical permission' for sexual acts, and to arrange appropriate counselling when necessary. Normal sexual intercourse, pregnancy and delivery are quite possible even when life is spent largely in a wheelchair. It is very disappointing to find that, in spite of the openness of the 'swinging sixties', 23% of adolescents in one series did not know how babies were conceived and many more had no knowledge of contraception (Dorner 1976).

Pubertal development is normal. It has been said that the menarche is early in myelomeningocele girls, especially the severely affected. In a group of English patients it occurred at a mean of 12 years and 4 months which is not particularly early. The boys' voices broke at a mean age of 12 years and 6 months which is early (Dorner 1976).

In a series of 52 postpubertal males, including some of my own patients, 70% claimed to have erections, in most cases supported by parental observation. Erections occurred in all patients with a positive anocutaneous reflex and in 64% of those with a negative reflex and a sensory level at or below the sympathetic outflow (D10 to L2). Only 14% of males with higher lesions and absent reflex had erections (Diamond *et al.* 1986). It is not known whether these erections were in response to appropriate sexual stimuli; in the most severely affected patients it seems more likely that they were reflex actions. Likewise, it is not known how many were able to ejaculate or to have intercourse. It is reasonable to think that the 20% of myelomeningocele patients who have normal bladder function will also have normal sexual function (Diamond *et al.* 1986).

In a smaller series of men ejaculation and orgasm were recorded in two of three with lesions at L2 and above, three of five with intermediate lesions and all of four with lesions at S1 or below. Six were having intercourse; one of them was the father of three normal children. Amongst 35 females no patient with a lesion at L2 or above was having intercourse though one had orgasms with masturbation. With lower lesions 17 of 27 had intercourse, 12 having orgasms (Cass *et al.* 1986). Absence of genital sensation in females does not preclude physical enjoyment of sex: such girls have been shown to derive erotic pleasure from cuddling and kissing (Dorner 1976).

Translating theory into practice is altogether more difficult. In Dorner's series 80% of adolescents expressed interest in the opposite sex but only 28% had dated. In the males only those with minimal handicaps had dated, none had established a steady relationship and none had had intercourse. In the females the pattern was different. There was no relationship between handicap and dating. Four girls, three of whom were severely handicapped, were engaged to normal men, but there was little physical contact. Only one girl (not engaged) had had intercourse on one occasion. It is clear that adolescents with spina bifida are very different from others of their age (Dorner 1976).

The situation improves as the patients get older. In a review of 49 adults it was found that nine had steady partners and 22 were married. Of the others, 10 were under 20 years old, two were mentally handicapped and two had overprotective parents. It could, therefore, be said that 88% of those with realistic prospects were married or had a steady partner. Many of the patients were severely handicapped and incontinent which seemed no bar to their achievements (Laurence & Beresford 1975).

Patients who are impotent or do not ejaculate should be investigated along conventional lines. Although there have been no studies specifically on these patients, it is known that patients with spinal cord defects can be managed with intracorporeal injections of papaverine and other agents with appropriate dose reductions (Lue & Tanagho 1987). Electro-ejaculation may have a role in a few patients (Brindley 1981).

In Cass's series 12 women had 20 pregnancies resulting in 16 children, 11 by vaginal delivery apparently without difficulty (1986). An obstetrician, reporting his own cases and reviewing the literature has a different view of pregnancy. Complications in severely affected patients are almost invariable. Urinary tract infection in all and deterioration of bladder function in those who are not diverted are frequent. A deformed pelvis makes accommodation of the fetus difficult, leading to premature labour and a high rate of caesarean section. The patients are often themselves poor and have further social problems, as well as the obvious physical ones, in coping with the child (Richmond *et al.* 1987).

Combined series have shown an increased risk of neural tube defects as high as 4%. The risk is the same whether the affected parent is male or female, but daughters have a one in 13 incidence while the risk for sons is only one in 50 (Laurence & Beresford 1975). Diagnosis *in utero* by ultrasound and alpha-fetoprotein estimation is now routine.

## NON-NEUROGENIC NEUROGENIC BLADDER

It is well known that a bladder may behave in a manner identical to that seen in spina bifida without overt neurological disease and without abnormalities in other organs except the lower bowel. Many names have been given to this condition, usually reflecting different views of aetiology, but most accept that this is 'non-neurogenic neurogenic bladder'.

An extensive paediatric literature indicates the controversies of diagnosis, aetiology and classification that surround this mysterious condition.

In patients with normal kidneys, treatment is likely to have included antibiotics, anticholinergics, biofeedback techniques and a variety of psychological regimes. In reviewing 15 years of literature Hinman (after whom the syndrome is sometimes named) recorded good results for most of these techniques but was unable to give a long-term prognosis (1986).

In those with dilated upper tracts, regimes for the spina bifida patient will have been used. However, as virtually all of these patients have normal intelligence and manual dexterity, the overall results are likely to have been better. ICSC has been the most widely used treatment. Occasional patients have been diverted. The longer-term future is unknown and few centres have enough properly documented patients to find out.

I have patients who have presented in renal failure, have recovered on optimal bladder management, only to go into irreversible renal failure as adults. In these patients the renal damage was presumably so extensive that hyperperfusion of the surviving nephrons lead to nephrosclerosis (see Chapter 3). Transplantation is the logical treatment but care must be taken that the bladder which has already killed two native kidneys does not kill the transplant as well (see Chapter 5).

At the other end of the scale, I have patients who, after a period of diversion or ICSC, have developed normal bladder function. Their long-term prognosis depends on the degree of renal damage before diagnosis.

Other syndromes are recognised in which patients have unstable detrusor contractions and sphincter dysfunction but do not develop retention. These patients frequently have VUR and infection and may only be recognised when antireflux surgery has failed. In a prospective study of 53 such patients 58% were able to remain free of infection and have normal voiding with anticholinergics alone. This suggests that the bladder dysfunction (rather than the infection) is the primary problem. The long-term outcome was not known nor was it recorded whether any children were able to give up medication (Koff *et al.* 1979).

## SACRAL AGENESIS

This rare condition is usually diagnosed in early childhood because of a neuropathic bladder and the orthopaedic anomalies that are associated. The management is the same as that in myelomeningocele though, at least in adolescence, the bladders often prove very refractory to treatment and dangerous to the kidneys. Occasionally a patient presents in late childhood or even adolescence. In all such patients it is most important to obtain good X-rays of the sacrum or the diagnosis will be missed.

## ENURESIS

Bed-wetting is a common paediatric problem that usually gets better spontaneously in childhood. Treatment may speed up that which will happen naturally anyway. By the age of 15 years only about 2% of enuretic children are still wet (Forsyth & Redmond 1974). Most of this small group will have been treated intensively in childhood with little response. A few will seldom have been brought to a doctor by their parents and this pattern of non-attendance is often continued by the adolescent.

The adult bed-wetter should be completely reassessed. Even a history of normal day time voiding does not exclude detrusor dysfunction. Urodynamic studies are indicated in adults (though not in children) as up to 75% may have detrusor instability, through many of these patients do have diurnal symptoms on close questioning (Torrens & Collins 1975).

Others have reported sudden spikes of detrusor contraction during filling which provoke external sphincter contraction. The important observation was that the patients were unaware of any sensation of detrusor contraction and the sphincter action was dyssynergic allowing the patient to leak transiently. Most of the 55 patients in this report, aged 4 to 43, had severe and refractory symptoms and 13 had features of non-neurogenic neurogenic bladder. There may, therefore, be an overlap between enuresis and occult neuropathy (McGuire & Savastano 1984).

The treatment depends on the urodynamic findings. If the bladder is normal treatment is similar to that used in childhood. The choice must be tempered by a knowledge of regimes that have already been tried and failed. It is important to establish exactly what has been tried: many patients are treated with inadequate doses of drugs for an inadequate time. Buzzers and alarm clocks are more likely to work in well-motivated adults than in difficult teenagers, but still have an important role.

Two drugs may not have been used in childhood. Desmopressin, a synthetic analogue of antidiuretic hormone, has shown promising results. In one cross-over controlled trial patients had significantly fewer wet nights on desmopression than on placebo, but only eight of 21 patients became completely dry. Three patients followed for 2 years remained dry but became wet if they missed a dose (Ramsden *et al.* 1982).

In my own experience mazindol, a synthetic amphetamine, has proved the most successful drug. Unfortunately the side-effects limit its use, though they are lessened by increasing the dose slowly over 10 days from 1 mg to 3 mg. In a double-blind cross-over trial 10 of 16 patients became dry and five were improved. Five patients followed for a year were able to stop treatment and remained dry (Tiptaft *et al.* 1984).

With a stable bladder and a capacity over 400 ml good results may follow bladder transection. At follow-up of at least a year 53% of patients have been cured (Hindmarsh *et al.* 1977).

If the bladder is unstable, the usual anticholinergic regimes should be tried. Oxybutinine and terodiline are currently the most useful drugs. If drug treatment fails there may be a dilemma — if enuresis is truly the only symptom, aggressive surgical treatment may only change one unpleasant symptom for another. Although injection of the pelvic plexus with phenol may help in women, the cure rate at 1 year in those under 55 years old is only 14% (Blackford *et al.* 1984). Aside from this, only clam cystoplasty is likely to abolish instability and this is usually too drastic an operation for enuresis alone.

## REFERENCES


Blackford H., Murray K., Stephenson T.P. & Mundy A.R. (1984) Results of transvesical infiltration of the pelvic plexuses with phenol in 116 patients. *Br. J. Urol.* **56**, 647–9.

Borzyskowski M., Mundy A.R., Neville B.G.R. *et al.* (1982) Neuropathic vesicourethral dysfunction in children. *Br. J. Urol.* **54**, 641–4.

Brantley Scott F., Fishman I.J. & Shabsigh R. (1986) The impact of the artificial urinary sphincter in the neurogenic bladder on the upper urinary tracts. *J. Urol.* **136**, 636–42.

Brem A.S., Martin D., Callaghan J. & Maynard J. (1987) Long term renal risk factors in children with meningomyelocoele. *J. Pediatr.* **110**, 51–4.

Brereton R.J., Narayanan R. & Ratnatunga C. (1987) Ureteric reimplantation in the neuropathic bladder. *Br. J. Surg.* **74**, 1107–10.

Brindley G.S. (1981) Electro ejaculation: its technique, neurological implications and uses. *J. Neurol. Neurosurg. Psychiatr.* **44**, 9–18.

Cass A.S., Bloom B.A. & Luxenberg M. (1986) Sexual function in adults with myelomeningocoele. *J. Urol.* **136**, 425–6.

Diamond D.A., Rickwood A.M.K. & Thomas D.G. (1986) Penile erections in myelomeningocoele patients. *Br. J. Urol.* **58**, 434–5.

Diokno A.C., Sonda L.P., Hollander J.B. & Lapides J. (1983) Fate of patients started on clean intermittent self catheterisation therapy 10 years ago. *J. Urol.* **129**, 1120–2.

Dorner S. (1977) Sexual interest and activity in adolescents with spina bifida. *J. Child. Psychol. Psychiatr.* **18**. 229–37.

Durham Smith E. (1972) Urinary prognosis in spina bifida. *J. Urol.* **108**, 815–17.

Enrile B.G. & Crooks J.K. (1980) Clean intermittent catheterisation for home management in children with myelomeningocoele. *Clin. Pediatr.* **19**, 743–9.

Forsyth W.I. & Redmond A. (1974) Enuresis and spontaneous cure rate. A study of 1129 enuretics. *Arch. Dis. Child.* **49**, 259–63.

Hindmarsh J.R., Essenhigh D.M. & Yeates W.K. (1977) Bladder transection for adult enuresis. *Br. J. Urol.* **49**, 515–21.

Hinman F. (1986) Nonneurogenic neurogenic bladder (the Hinman syndrome) — 15 years later. *J. Urol.* **136**, 769–77.

Johnston J.H., Shapiro S.R. & Thomas G.G. (1976) Anti reflux surgery in the congenital neuropathic bladder. *Br. J. Urol.* **48**, 639–42.

Kass E.J., Koff S.A., Diokno A.C. & Lapides J. (1981) The significance of bacilluria in children on long-term intermittent catheterisation. *J. Urol.* **126**, 223–5.

Koff S.A., Lapides J. & Piazza D.H. (1979) Association of urinary tract infection and reflux with uninhibited bladder contractions and voluntary sphincteric obstruction. *J. Urol.* **122**, 373–6.

Kondo A., Kato K., Kanai S. & Sakakibara T. (1986) Bladder dysfunction secondary to tethered cord syndrome in adults: is it curable? *J. Urol.* **135**, 313–16.

Lapides J., Diokno A.C., Silber S.J. & Lowe B.S. (1972) Clean intermittent self catheterisation in the treatment of urinary tract disease. *J. Urol.* **107**, 458–61.

Laurence K.M. & Beresford A. (1975) Continence, friends, marriage and children in 51 adults with spina bifida. *Dev. Med. Child. Neurol.* **17** (Supplement 35), 123–8.

Lue T.F. & Tanagho E.A. (1987) Physiology of erection and pharmacological management of impotence. *J. Urol.* **137**, 829–36.

McGuire E.J. & Savastano J.A. (1984) Urodynamic studies in enuresis and the nonneurogenic neurogenic bladder. *J. Urol.* **132**, 299–302.

McLorie G.A., Perez-Marero R., Csima A. & Churchill B.M. (1988) Determinants of hydronephrosis and renal injury in patients with myelomeningocoele. *J. Urol.* **140**, 1289–92.

Mulcahy J.J., James H.E. & McRoberts J.W. (1977) Oxybutinin chloride combined with intermittent catheterisation in the treatment of myelomeningocoele patients. *J. Urol.* **118**, 95–7.

Mundy A.R., Shah P.J.R., Borzyskowski M. & Saxton H.M. (1985) Sphincter behaviour in myelomeningocoele. *Br. J. Urol.* **57**, 647–51.

Murray K.H.A., Nurse D.E. & Mundy A.R. (1988) Detrusor behaviour following implantation of the Brantley Scott artificial urinary sphincter for neuropathic incontinence. *Br. J. Urol.* **61**, 122–8.

Pekarovic E., Robinson A., Zachary R.B. & Lister J. (1970) Indications for manual expression of the neurogenic bladder in children. *Br. J. Urol.* **42**, 191–6.

Ramsden P.D., Hindmarsh J.R., Price D.A., Yeates W.K. & Bowditch J.D.P. (1982) DDAVP for adult enuresis — preliminary report. *Br. J. Urol.* **54**, 256–8.

Ransley P.G. & Risdon R.A. (1982) Pathophysiology of chronic pyelonephritis (reflux nephropathy). In: Chisholm G.D. & Williams D.I. (eds) *Scientific Foundations of Urology*, 2nd edn. William Heinemann, London, pp. 98–106.

Raz S., Ehrlich R.M., Zeidman E.J., Alarcon A. & McLaughlin S. (1988) Surgical treatment of the incontinent female patients with myelomeningocoele. *J. Urol.* **139**, 524–7.

Richmond D., Zaharievski I. & Bond A. (1987) Management of pregnancy in mothers with spina bifida. *Eur. J. Obstet. Reprod. Biol.* **25**, 341–5.

Rickwood A.M.K. (1982) Use of internal urethrotomy to reverse upper renal tract dilatation in children with neurogenic bladder dysfunction. *Br. J. Urol.* **54**, 292–4.

Rickwood A.M.K. (1984) The neuropathic bladder in children. In: Mundy A.R., Stephenson T.P. & Wein A.J. (eds) *Urodynamics: Principles, Practice and Application.* Churchill Livingstone, Edinburgh, pp. 326–47.

Rickwood A.M.K., Hodgson J., Lonton A.P. & Thomas D.G. (1984) Medical and surgical complications in adolescent and young adult patients with spina bifida. *Health Trends* **16**, 91–5.

Rickwood A.M.K., Thomas D.G., Philp N.H. & Spicer R.D. (1982) System of management of the congenital neuropathic bladder based upon combined urodynamic and radiological assessment. *Br. J. Urol.* **54**, 507–11.

Sidi A.A., Reinberg Y. & Gonzalez R. (1987) Comparison of artificial sphincter implantation and bladder neck reconstruction in patients with neurogenic urinary incontinence. *J. Urol.* **138**, 1120–2.

Steinhardt G.F., Goodgold H.M. & Samuels L.D. (1988) The effect of intravesical pressure on glomerular filtration rate in patients with myelomeningocoele. *J. Urol.* **140**, 1293–5.

Thomas G., Zachary R.B. & Lister J. (1973) 'Closed' external sphincterotomy for bladder outlet obstruction in myelomeningocoele. *Br. J. Urol.* **45**, 515–19.

Tiptaft R.C., Woodhouse C.R.J. & Badenoch D.F. (1984) Mazindol for nocturnal enuresis. *Br. J. Urol.* **56**, 641–3.

Torrens M.J. & Collins C.D. (1975) The urodynamic assessment of adult enuresis. *Br. J. Urol.* **47**, 433–40.

Williams M.P.L., Katz Z., Escala J.M. & Rickwood A.M.K. (1988) Peripheral neurology as a predictor of bladder dysfunction in congenital neuropathic bladder. *Br. J. Urol.* **62**, 51–3.

# 10 *Urinary diversion*

## INTRODUCTION

Great ingenuity has gone to devise systems for urinary diversion. The historical pattern is shown in Fig. 10.1. Traditionally, systems using the anal sphincter were preferred, until the suggestion of an ileal conduit was made by Bricker (1950). It is ironic that the Bricker conduit was introduced and thought to be so wonderful at just the time when the complications of the ureterosigmoidostomy were beginning to be understood and treated.

The consequences of diversions may be considered as: psychosocial, renal, 'histological' and biochemical. We tend to think, today, that all the consequences are bad. It must be remembered, however, that the alternatives were continuous incontinence, renal failure or both. Although in children there are now almost no indications for permanent cutaneous diversion, in adults with pelvic cancer a diversion is often essential and sometimes welcomed.

It may well be that the reconstructions and continent diversions done today will have just as many problems in 20 or 30 years' time (see Chapter 11). It is reasonable to consider the problems of earlier diversions, especially ureterosigmoidostomy, in some detail to show what the future might hold in store.

## URETEROSIGMOIDOSTOMY AND VARIATIONS

The use of the anal sphincter to maintain urinary and, if possible, faecal continence has a long history. The classical ureterosigmoidostomy is shown in Fig. 10.2, but there are many variations on the theme (Fig. 10.3). Only a very small number of patients with the variations remain: no general figures are available, but the choice of first diversion for benign disease in a 28 year period at Great Ormond Street and St Peter's hospitals in the UK is shown in Table 10.1. Seventeen of the 25 with the variations are thought to have the diversion intact.

Systems that have retained the bladder and drained it into the colon with the faecal stream have proved very unsatisfactory (Fig. 10.3c and d). The inevitable stagnant mixture of urine and faeces in the bladder has caused chronic infection and stones. When they are encountered in follow-up, they should be converted to another system.

Good results have been reported for an isolated vesicorectal diversion with an end colostomy for the faecal stream (Fig. 10.3b, the Mauclaire or Boyce–Vest procedure). Eighteen of 24 patients from Boyce's own unit have reached adulthood and it is claimed that none are 'handicapped by urinary incontinence' at work, though a few have occasional incontinence and one is enuretic

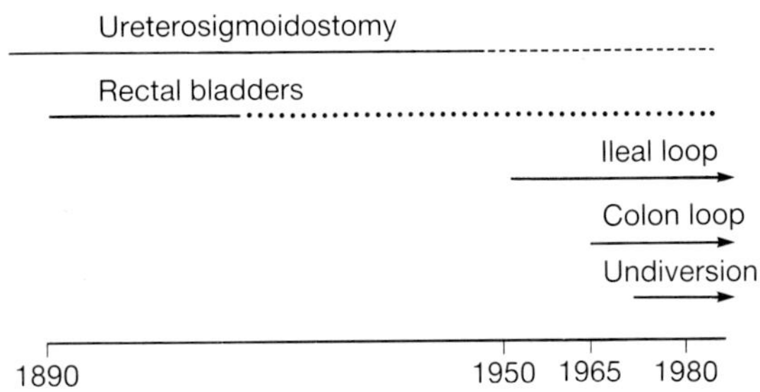


**Fig. 10.1** Diagram of the history of types of urinary diversion. Broken line indicates: declining popularity; dotted line indicates: rare.

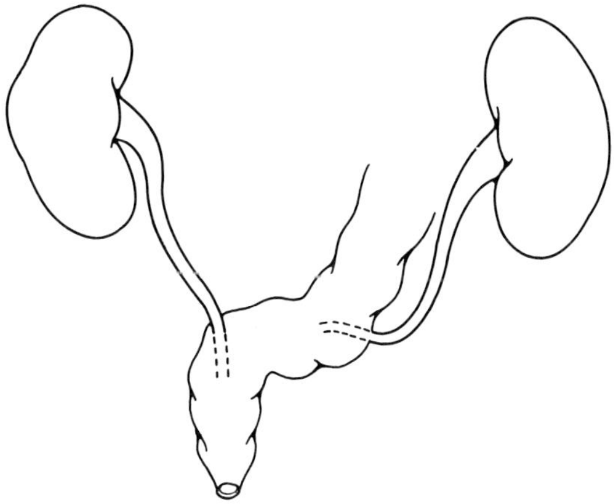

**Fig. 10.2** Diagram of classical ureterosigmoidostomy.

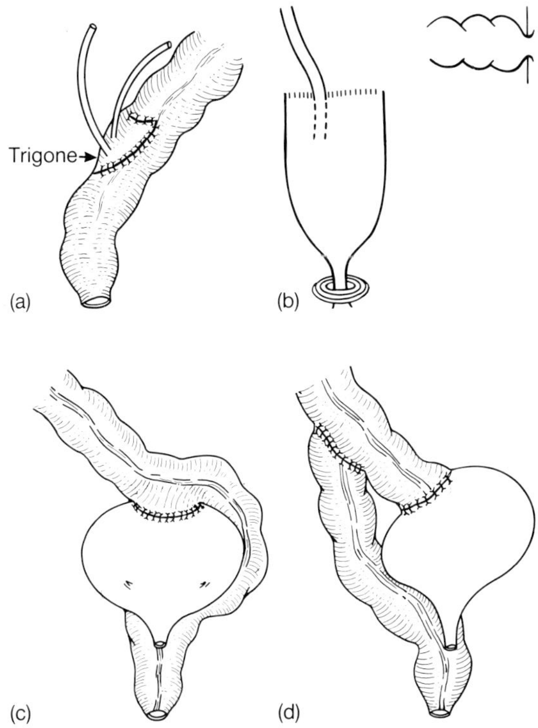


**Fig. 10.3** Diagrams of variations on ureterosigmoidostomy, all using the anal sphincter to maintain urinary continence. (a) Trigonal-colonic anastomosis (Maydl's operation). (b) Ureterorectal anastomosis and end colostomy for stools (Mauclaire or Boyce–Vest procedure). (c and d) Types of colovesicostomy. (From Silverman *et al.* 1986, reproduced with permission.)

periodically. None have suffered renal deterioration. Judging from their occupations they have grown up well and only one is unemployed (but two have been in prison). Sixteen of 18 adults have been married, two later getting divorced (Kroovand & Boyce 1988).

The Gersuny operation (Fig. 10.4a) is a lovely idea that seldom works in practice. I have encountered one or two patients in whom the system works well. On direct questioning most patients admit that the effluent is runny and very smelly, suggesting that urine and faeces are mixed in the colon/rectum. On rectal examination it is rare to find two openings (rectum and colon) presenting at the anal margin as they should. In the worst cases the common wall between rectum and colon has retracted, leaving a large cavity containing faeces and urine (Fig. 10.4b and c). Such patients are usually incontinent.

Patients with these variations will not be considered in detail any further. It is assumed that

**Table 10.1** Distribution of forms of primary urinary diversions in 303 patients with benign disease performed at The Hospital for Sick Children, Great Ormond Street and St Peter's Hospitals, UK, 1954–1981 (Stewart 1986).

| Type | Number | Diagram in figure |
|---|---|---|
| Ureterosigmoidostomy | 106 | 10.2 |
| Vesicocolic anastomosis | 9 | 10.3c and d |
| Gersuny | 15 | 10.4a |
| Maydl's | 2 | 10.3a |
| Colon conduit (up to 1975) | 56 | |
| Ileal conduit (up to 1975) | 115 | |

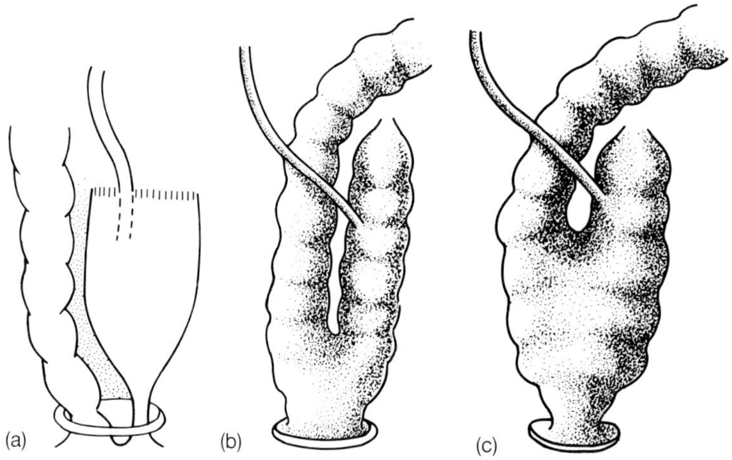


**Fig. 10.4** Diagrams of the Gersuny bladder and its deterioration. (a) Normal Gersuny bladder: the colon has been brought down behind the rectum and through the anal sphincter. The ureters have been anastomosed to the isolated rectum. Note that the common wall between the two ends is at or below the anus. (b) With time the common wall retracts allowing communication between colon and rectum distally. (c) Further retraction of the common wall to form a single large cavity containing urine and stool.

they have the same long-term risks for cancer and for hyperchloraemic acidosis as other patients with urine and faeces stored together, although it must be said that I have not seen such complications nor was either reported for the Boyce–Vest procedure (Kroovand & Boyce 1988).

## URETEROSIGMOIDOSTOMY

### Psychosocial problems

Patients who have had ureterosigmoidostomies since early childhood are satisfied with their lot. I have never encountered one who would volunteer to change the diversion. Even in five patients operated for neoplasm of the ureteric anastomosis, all wished to have a new uretero-sigmoid anastomosis rather than a different diversion (Silverman *et al.* 1986).

The effluent of mixed urine and faeces has a very offensive smell. It is not a suitable diversion for children from socially deprived families where no private lavatory is available. Likewise, the misery of incontinence is worsened by the ostracism due to the smell.

Incontinence has been reported in older patients. When the diversion is made in child-hood, continence is more reliable. Those who fail to become dry are usually given a different diversion; thus incontinence is rare in long-term follow-up. In my own series of 28 patients followed for a mean of 20 years, five have minor leakage (Silverman *et al.* 1986). Late onset of incontinence has only been seen once.

When reviewed as adults, all our patients have been content with their form of diversion. However, they are a selected group since those who were unhappy or had unacceptable complications, about 39%, had their diversion changed earlier (Aaronson & Morgan 1979). Those who survive the first 5 years rarely require a change.

This happy experience has not been shared by all and the more searching the questions asked of patients, the more worrying is the information obtained. In a series of nine exstrophy patients diverted between two and 16 years old, Macfarlane found all patients had leakage at some time, three only at night. In addition, eight had to empty the bowel one- to two-hourly by day and one to five times at night with urgency. None were able to pass gas without some urine/faeces as well. Two of the patients had their diversion changed to an ileal conduit because of such problems. The authors attributed the unwillingness of others to change to the excessive number of operations that they had already had (Macfarlane *et al.* 1979), though this is not an argument that I can accept as much-operated ileal conduit patients are happy enough to change.

Patients given ureterosigmoidostomies as adults commonly have poor results. McConnell and Stewart condemn this form of diversion because of the 'bizarre life-style' that is forced on the patients. However, the majority of their 13 living patients were able to undertake normal social activities providing they did not have to travel by bus (Table 10.2).

My patients have normal educational and social achievements. For example, 19 of 28 young adults with long-standing ureterosigmoidostomies have regular sexual intercourse (Table 10.3). The poor paternity record is probably because most of the patients had exstrophy with its associated penile problems (see Chapter 13).

The employment record of a group of 34 patients is shown in Table 10.4. Forty per cent were in professional or skilled occupations and only three were unemployed. Even in older patients McConnell and Stewart report that only two of 13 patients were unemployed because of their ureterosigmoidostomy.

It is difficult to reconcile the conflicting opinions about ureterosigmoidostomy. It is probable that there are severe and partly hidden social problems, but the system certainly works well for some patients. Prospective patients and their parents must be carefully and honestly counselled. Existing patients must be very closely followed to be sure they are not sinking into a life almost entirely revolving around the lavatory.

**Table 10.2** Ability of 13 patients with uretero-sigmoidostomy (formed at mean age of 66 years) to undertake social functions (McConnell and Stewart 1975).

| | No problem | Difficult | Impossible |
|---|---|---|---|
| Shopping | 10 | 3 | 0 |
| Theatre | 10 | 3 | 0 |
| Church | 6 | 1 | 6 |
| Visiting | 10 | 3 | 0 |
| Bus travel | 4 | 0 | 9 |

## Renal problems

The renal and metabolic problems were the main causes of the poor reputation of this diversion. Although the metabolic problems are better understood and antibiotics have lessened the consequences of infection, the long-term effects on the kidneys are still very worrying.

Table 10.5 compares the fate of 151 kidneys in 76 patients with various forms of diversion. All the patients had exstrophy and were born with normal kidneys. Diversions were done in early childhood and follow-up was at least 18 years. After ureterosigmoidostomy about 50% of kidneys are damaged to some extent, in eight of 25 patients sufficiently badly for a change of diversion to be necessary (Woodhouse *et al.* 1983). It has been estimated that 15% of kidneys are damaged during or immediately after early reconstructive surgery in exstrophy (Turner *et al.* 1980). Thereafter, the renal damage is the consequence of the diversion.

Many of the patients had early complications with stones, infection and benign ureteric stric-

**Table 10.3** Sexual function and marital status in 28 patients with ureterosigmoidostomy. Diversions were all before 22 years of age (Silverman *et al.* 1986).

| | Regular sexual intercourse | | | | |
|---|---|---|---|---|---|
| | Yes | No | Married | Pregnancies | Children |
| Females | 6 | 2 | 5 | 6 | 5 |
| Males | 13 | 4 | 8 | 2 | 2 |

**Table 10.4** Employment in 34 patients with ureterosigmoidostomy and its variations (Silverman *et al.* 1986).

| | Number |
|---|---|
| Professional | 7 |
| Skilled | 7 |
| Semi-skilled | 7 |
| Manual | 1 |
| At college | 4 |
| Housewife | 3 |
| Unemployed | 3 |
| Retired | 2 |

tures. Such problems were unusual in late follow-up. Five of 28 patients in our series had had recent stones and two had recurrent infections (Silverman *et al.* 1986). Late ureteric obstruction was always due to neoplasm.

Although these figures are somewhat depressing, they may not reflect the true consequences for the adult. Patients who have a ureterosigmoidostomy formed in early childhood and are then followed for 18 years have had a long follow-up by conventional medical standards. But the patients have grown through the period of greatest vulnerability for the kidneys. The next 18 years may not be so difficult. In following adults from 20 years old onwards, I have not detected further deterioration in the renal function. It seems that a stable state is reached which may be maintained through adulthood. A policy of active follow-up may be useful to identify complications and start treatment before renal damage occurs (see Chapter 2).

## Histological changes

The presence of urine within the intact sigmoid colon does not cause major histological changes on conventional examination. At laparotomy,

**Table 10.5** Effects of diversion on the *kidneys*. This table includes 151 normal *kidneys* in 76 patients born with exstrophy (one patient had a solitary but normal kidney). Follow-up is at least 18 years (Woodhouse *et al.* 1983).

| | Norm | Renal damage: Mild/Mod | Renal damage: Sev | Change of diversion needed | Total with renal damage |
|---|---|---|---|---|---|
| Continent bladder | 18 | 6 | | | 6/24 |
| Incontinent bladder | 2 | 2 | | | 2/4 |
| Ureterosigmoidostomy | | | | | |
| Failed closure | 6 | | | 8 | 14/28 |
| Primary diversion | 3 | | 1 | 8 | 12/22 |
| Ileal conduit | | | | | |
| Failed closure | 5 | 14 | 9 | 2 | 25/30 |
| Primary diversion | 9 | 11 | 4 | | 15/24 |
| Rectal bladders | | | | | |
| Failed closure | | 2 | | 2 | 4/4 |
| Primary diversion | 3 | 1 | | | 1/4 |
| Colonic conduit | | | | | |
| Failed closure | 1 | 3 | | | 3/4 |
| Primary diversion | 6 | | | | 0/6 |
| Cutaneous ureterostomy | 2 | 3 | | | 3/5 |

Norm: normal
Mild/Mod: mild or moderate
Sev: severe

however, the bowel is seen to be dilated and the wall thin.

On colonoscopy the ureteric orifice usually looks like a small cherry 3 or 4 mm in diameter. Sometimes it is a flat opening that can be hard to see. On haematoxylin and eosin staining of biopsies normal colonic epithelium is seen abutting normal transitional cell epithelium with inflammatory cell infiltrate. The orifice may become sufficiently prominent and inflamed to earn the title of inflammatory polyp (Fig. 10.5). Even in long-standing anastomoses the junction between the two epithelial types is abrupt.

Histochemistry, however, does show differences from normal. For example, staining with high iron diamine alcian blue identifies areas of sialomucin production (Filipe 1975). Sialomucins are produced by cells in the bottom of normal colonic crypts. Production by other cells is a premalignant condition at least in some circumstances: it is seen as an intermediate change when carcinomas are induced in the rat colon and in areas adjacent to human colonic carcinomas where it is called transitional mucosa (Filipe & Branfoot 1976). Positive sialomucin staining has been found through the full depth of the crypts in colonic biopsies in 17 of 19 patients with ureterosigmoidostomies. The appearances were the same even when the urine had been through the colon for only a short time before conversion to a different diversion (Silverman *et al.* 1986). In a patient with adenocarcinoma of the ureterosigmoid anastomosis positive silaomucin staining was found in all areas of the colectomy specimen (Strachan *et al.* 1987a).

Colonic cellular activity is also increased both in the presence of urine alone and, more so, with urine and faeces. Strachan found increased crypt cell production rates and cellular diploid DNA in rats (Strachan *et al.* 1987b).

The significance of this type of change is unknown. It could be an innocent change in colonic mucosa caused by the presence of urine. Or it could indicate that urine produces, almost invariably, a premalignant change of long latency. It is not seen in colonic conduits.

## Ureterosigmoid cancer

The most important change that occurs in ureterosigmoidostomies is neoplastic. The first case of carcinoma of a ureterosigmoidostomy was reported in 1929 (Hammer 1929). However, little interest was taken of this complication until

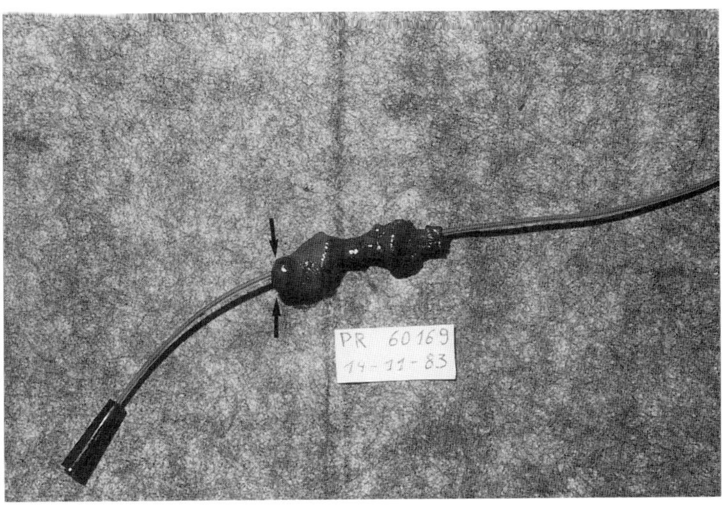


**Fig. 10.5** Resected specimen of ureterosigmoid anastomosis showing a small inflammatory polyp (arrowed).

about 20 years ago. Only 18 adenomas or adenocarcinomas were recorded in the literature up to 1970. Presumably few patients with ureterosigmoidostomies lived long enough to develop the tumours. It is interesting that the first recorded patient had exstrophy but did not have his diversion until the age of 50, developing the carcinoma 10 years later at a time of life when colonic carcinoma is common.

*Aetiology*

The tumour arises at the anastomosis or very close to it in 90% of cases (Fig. 10.6). In patients diverted for benign disease 95% are adenomatous (adenomas or adenocarcinomas) but one transitional cell and one lymphomatous tumour have been reported (Stewart 1986). The most important aetiological factor both experimentally and clinically, is the mixture of urine and faeces at the anastomotic site. Urine can be found throughout the colon but tumours do not occur as a result (Fig. 10.7).

In rats union of the urinary and faecal streams is as potent a carcinogen as dimethylhydrazine (DMH) or N-[4-(5-nitro-2-furyl)-2-thiazolyl] formamide (FANFT) which are themselves very potent urinary and bowel carcinogens respectively. Union of the urinary tract with colon but with the faecal stream excluded does not precipitate tumours (Crissey *et al.* 1980, Strachan *et al.* 1987b).

In humans, the same applies: neoplasms occur when the two streams are mixed. They are very rare in isolated colonic conduits where only two carcinomas have been reported (Chiang *et al.* 1982, Wilson & Morales 1982). No neoplasms have been found in 37 years of follow-up of the Boyce–Vest diversion (Kroovand & Boyce 1988).

The increased risk of carcinoma in patients with ureterosigmoidostomy has been variously estimated at 100 to 7000 times that in the normal population (Stewart *et al.* 1982). Stewart accepts the lower figure.

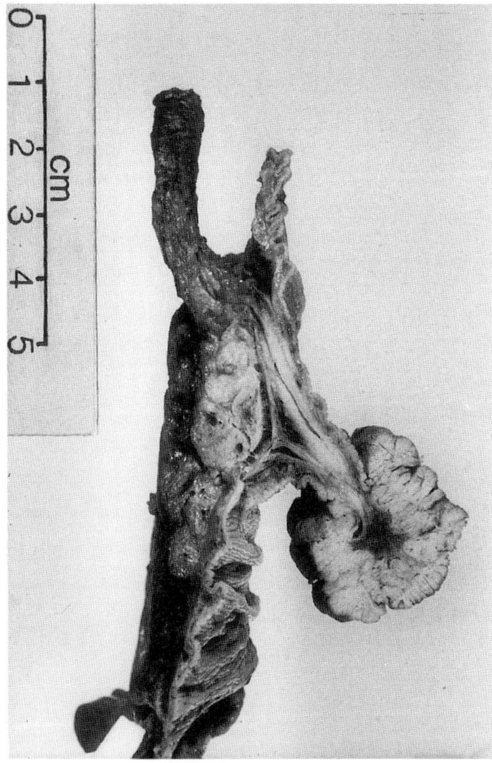


**Fig. 10.6** Resected specimen of ureterosigmoid anastomosis showing a carcinoma arising exactly at the mucosal anastomosis. The ureter can be seen forming the 'stalk' of the tumour.

Estimates of risk have been plagued by the lack of a uniform population at low risk of other neoplasms. It is, therefore, particularly interesting to look at the outcome of diversions in patients with exstrophy of the bladder. In my 103 adult exstrophy patients, Strachan has looked at the cancer incidence at a minimum follow-up of 20 years. He divided them into those who had ever had urinary and faecal streams mixed (at-risk group — 42 patients) and those who had had an early diversion by colonic or ileal loop (non-risk group — 61 patients). There were no cancers in the non-risk group. In the 'at-risk' group there were four cancers and four non-invasive neoplasms at the ureterosigmoidostomy. Two further patients in this group

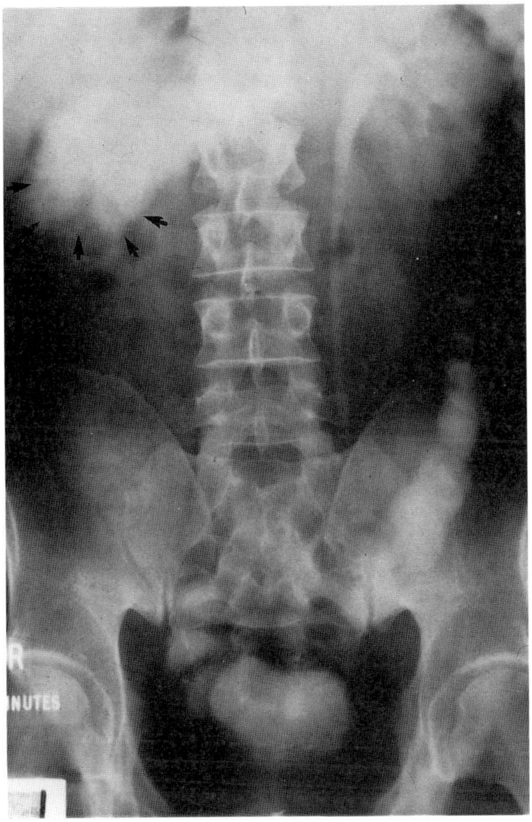

**Fig. 10.7** IVU of a patient with a ureterosigmoidostomy and a solitary left kidney. The contrast can be seen as far proximally as the middle of the ascending colon (arrowed).

died of adenocarcinomas said to have arisen in the bladder (but see Chapter 13 for discussion). The mean age of the 'at-risk' patients was 36.1 years and the cumulative risk of developing colonic cancer at that age is 6.1 per 100 000 for normal patients. In the ureterosigmoid patients the incidence was 10 526 per 100 000. Therefore, in this relatively pure group, the risk is 1726 times the expected incidence (J.R. Strachan & C.R.J. Woodhouse, unpublished data).

It is unfortunate that the urine is diverted into the sigmoid colon rather than any other part. When a colonic carcinoma occurs in a normal patient under 40 years old, the sigmoid is the site in over 60% of cases (Pitluk & Poticha 1983).

These clinical and experimental observations do not explain the cause of the tumours. Because they are adenomas and adenocarcinomas and because adenomatous metaplasia has not been reported in ureteric biopsies at colonoscopy, it has been assumed that they arise from the colon. Research has, perhaps, been biased in this direction. It is equally possible that the tumours arise from the ureter (that is the anatomical site at which they are found). In my patients biopsies from the ureteric orifice have nearly always shown inflammation and in one case, dysplasia. In five cases the transitional cell mucosa has formed an inflammatory polyp (Fig. 10.5).

Experimentally, no neoplasms are seen when a length of ileum is interposed between the urothelium and the colon (Gittes 1986). On the other hand, when a free graft of transitional urothelium is made to colon in a rat, the same neoplasms are seen at the graft edge but they are smaller and more delayed than with a ureterosigmoidostomy (Strachan *et al.* 1987b). A good experimental model with one ureter anastomosed to the colon by a microsurgical technique has been described; the other ureter is left in the bladder as a control (Miersch 1988). No results are available yet, but it should allow a distinction to be made between colonic and ureteric neoplasms.

The carcinogenic agent may be an N-nitroso compound. These potent carcinogens are present in ureterosigmoid effluent in a concentration ten times greater than in normal bladder urine. The concentrations found in isolated ileal and colonic conduits are variable between patients and in individual patients at different times of day: the only reasonably consistent finding is low concentrations when the diverted urine is sterile.

The relevant compounds are amines. They may be produced by the action of bacteria on urinary nitrates and faecal secondary amines (Stewart 1986). Whether any combination of mixed bacteria can do this is uncertain. Stewart has suggested this to be the case, and a consistently high carriage rate of *Peptostreptococcus* species has been found in ureterosigmoid effluent in my patients (Silverman *et al.* 1986). This interesting organism is a powerful ureolytic agent (the first step in producing nitrates from urea) and is also capable of performing many of the major biotransformations of bile which have been implicated in the formation of procarcinogens and tumour promotors involved in the pathogenesis of bowel carcinomas.

*Presentation*

Symptoms from adenocarcinoma of a ureterosigmoidostomy occur late in the disease. Half the patients have rectal bleeding and about one-quarter each abdominal pain or constipation (Stewart 1986). In patients with no bowel symptoms, some patients have been found with ureteric obstruction which may or may not have been painless.

Now that this condition has been found to be so common, all cases should be found early during colonoscopy. Any 'lump' at the ureteric orifice should be regarded with suspicion and biopsied. I have found a tumour of 6 mm in diameter which was a moderately differentiated adenocarcinoma with invasion (Fig. 10.8). In other words, such tumours do not behave as primary colonic neoplasms where a tumour under 1 cm in diameter would not be malignant.

The predisposing factor to neoplasia is that there has *ever* been an anastomosis between the urinary and faecal streams. Thus the anastomosis is at risk in patients whose diversion was changed to an ileal conduit leaving the original anastomosis between ureters and colon *in situ*. Another small group to beware of will have had a ureterosigmoidostomy converted to a colonic conduit maintaining the original ureterocolic anastomosis.

The shortest period of exposure to risk (that is the period with a ureterosigmoidostomy before conversion to an ileal conduit) is 9 months (Spence *et al.* 1979). The mean time from exposure to development of the tumour is 18 years for benign tumours and 25 years for malignant tumours (benign tumours probably becoming malignant in 5 to 10 years). The mean age at presentation is 35 years (Stewart 1986).

Bearing these figures in mind it would be prudent to begin annual colonoscopies on the tenth anniversary of the ureterosigmoid diversion and to continue indefinitely.

A surgeon who is converting a ureterosigmoidostomy to any other diversion should make

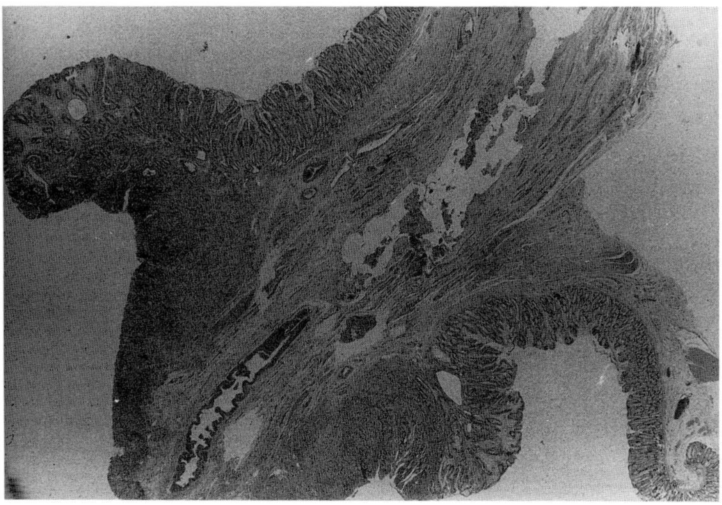

**Fig. 10.8** Haematoxylin and eosin stain of a ureterosigmoid anastomosis showing a 6 mm invasive carcinoma at the mucosal junction. The ureter is seen running through the middle of the tumour and there is normal colonic mucosa on either side (x6).

a point of resecting the original anastomosis. Similarly, if a laparotomy is required in a patient with the original anastomosis still intact, the opportunity should be taken to resect it.

*Treatment*

The rarity of this problem makes the development of a scientifically based protocol impossible. Patients presenting with symptoms usually have extensive local disease and many have metastases. There is a high early death rate whatever is done (Spence *et al.* 1979).

When the condition is found at colonoscopy, the tumour should be small, localised and often benign. My practice is to excise the lower 2 cm of ureter and an adjacent cuff of colon (Fig. 10.6). I also resect the other lower ureter and a smaller cuff of colon though in six specimens only inflammation has been found (Fig. 10.5).

The problem of diversion then arises. The patients are offered an alternative diversion or re-formation of a ureterosigmoidostomy with annual colonoscopies starting at one year. So far, all patients have opted for a new ureterosigmoidostomy (even knowing the risks) but I have had only one case since the advent of continent urinary diversions. This practice has an honourable tradition being the choice in 50% of the collected cases reviewed by Spence (Spence *et al.* 1979). Only one case of recurrence at the new anastomotic site has been reported (Urdanetta 1966).

## Biochemical abnormalities

*Hyperchloraemic acidosis*

The only clinically important biochemical abnormality is hyperchloraemic acidosis. There is some dispute about the exact mechanism that produces this condition. The plasma has an excess of chloride and a deficiency of bicarbonate ions, sometimes with potassium deficiency as well.

The urine secreted by the kidneys is probably acid and the more acidotic the plasma the lower is the pH of the urine. Certainly when ureterosigmoidostomy was done as a two-stage procedure (one ureter at a time), the bladder urine maintained a very low pH (4.8–5.5) and the bowel effluent a very high pH. Biochemical changes did not occur until the second ureter was implanted into the colon (Jacobs & Barr Stirling 1952, Parsons *et al.* 1952).

When the urine has been in the sigmoid colon, mixed with faeces, for only a short time, the mixture is highly alkaline. The alkalinity is due to high levels of ammonia and bicarbonate. It seems unlikely that renal tubular acidification defects have anything to do with these biochemical changes (Hayward *et al.* 1961a).

The changes must, therefore, be due to activity in the colon. In experimental animals the speed of development and the severity of acidosis is proportional to the surface area of colon in contact with urine (Hayward *et al.* 1961b). In humans the condition does not occur when the ureterosigmoidostomy is incontinent (Jacobs & Barr Stirling 1952).

The production of ammonia by the action of mixed faecal bacteria on urinary urea must be important at least in making the effluent alkaline and producing the full syndrome (Imler *et al.* 1979). When urine alone enters the colon (as in the Boyce–Vest diversion) patients have hyperchloraemia but are not acidotic according to the plasma bicarbonate estimation (Ghoneim 1970).

It is a moot point, probably clinically irrelevant, whether the main active pathway is absorption of ammonium chloride or secretion of bicarbonate. There is good evidence in humans to suggest that the normal response of the colon to the presence of an acid medium is secretion of bicarbonate and that this causes the acidosis (McConnell *et al.* 1979).

Although low plasma and total body potassium have been reported they are not consistent findings. When allowance is made for uncorrected metabolic acidosis it is probable that normal total body potassium is maintained.

Care must certainly be taken when prescribing potassium supplements just on the basis of a low plasma potassium (Boddy *et al.* 1975).

If potassium is lost, it is not by exchange but through the diarrhoea that occurs with ureterosigmoidostomy or by osmotic diuresis caused by excess urea resorption from the colon (Madsen 1964, Boddy *et al.* 1975).

Fortunately, there is some room for compensation in the system. As the bicarbonate concentration in the colon becomes excessively high diffusion occurs back into the blood stream of the colon. Many patients thus stabilise in mild acidosis (McConnell *et al.* 1979).

*Presentation.* The clinical features of hyperchloraemic acidosis were described in 1931 (Boyd 1931). Familiarity with the risk and ease of treatment have made symptomatic presentation rare. Persistent biochemical acidosis is, however, still common. The incidence ranges from 50 to 100%. A constant watch must be kept and new cases turn up even after many years of biochemical normality (Silverman *et al.* 1986). It may be that the problem is always present to some degree as a compensated metabolic acidosis is always found on arterial blood gas analysis when urine is stored in a reservoir which includes bowel (Nurse & Mundy 1989).

The importance of such sub-clinical abnormalities is unknown and sometimes it is difficult to distinguish problems arising from the diversion and those from the primary condition. In a combined series of 1673 patients followed for up to 10 years there is no mention of the long-term effects of the metabolic complications that were meticulously recorded (Jacobs & Barr Stirling 1952).

Bone demineralisation and osteomalacia are recognised complications of hyperchloraemic acidosis. All of the small number of cases reported in the literature have occurred in patients with severe and uncorrected acidosis. Patients present with bone pains, tenderness and weakness but the demineralisation must be far advanced before radiological changes are seen. Treatment is principally of the acidosis with alkalis and reduced dietary chloride. The calcium and phosphorus intake must be adequate. The role of vitamin D is unclear: patients have been shown to recover without supplements but it is likely to be faster if supplements are given early and in small doses such as 10 000 to 100 000 U of $D_2$ daily (Harrison 1958).

Experimental evidence suggests that minor degrees of hyperchloraemic acidosis can do the same (McDougal *et al.* 1988). It is not known whether it is clinically important but it seems likely that children would suffer some damage to growing bones. I have a clinical impression (the most notoriously inaccurate of all medical measurements) that children growing up with ureterosigmoidostomies are smaller than those with ileal loops. This impression was partly confirmed in a rat experiment where hyperchloraemic acidosis with ureterosigmoidostomy was corrected in half the animals. The animals receiving corrective supplements grew quicker and achieved a greater weight at the time of sacrifice after 8 weeks (Imler *et al.* 1979). However, a similar experiment but with all animals given antibiotics, produced equal growth in supplemented and non-supplemented animals (McDougal *et al.* 1988).

Surprisingly, osteomalacia is not accompanied by hypercalciuria either clinically or experimentally (Harrison 1958, McDougal *et al.* 1988). Patients do not have nephrocalcinosis. Renal stones occur as a relatively early complication in about 2% of patients surviving at least 6 months (Jacobs & Barr Stirling 1952). In my own series 7% of patients had stones at some time up to 10 years of follow-up but no new cases were seen thereafter.

Acute hyperchloraemic acidosis is rare except when there is a severe intercurrent illness and impairment of renal function. Presentation is, therefore, usually with that illness. The symptoms of acute hyperchloraemic acidosis are, most strikingly, extreme thirst in spite of nausea and vomiting and a salty taste in the mouth. Other symptoms include fatigue, weakness, weight loss, susceptibility to cold, anorexia, polyuria, rectal urgency and diarrhoea (Jacobs & Barr Stirling 1952). The accompanying hyperammonaemia causes coma and encephalopathy.

*Treatment.* The art of treating this condition has probably been lost. Even 40 years ago when the condition was poorly understood, treatment was quite easy (Jacobs & Barr Stirling 1952). The essential features were to drain the rectum with a large catheter, slowly to correct the acidosis with bicarbonate and to correct the dehydration but not with sodium chloride, of which the patient already has an excess.

By far the most important aspect is prophylaxis. The plasma bicarbonate and chloride should be measured at least annually. On the assumption that potassium deficiency is not a problem, I prescribe sodium bicarbonate tablets. Most patients require 90–150 mmol/day.

## ILEAL CONDUITS

### Psychosocial problems

The current general view is that all external urinary diversions are unacceptable and impose a severe burden on the child and adolescent. I agree with this view but with some reservations. Firstly, the ileal conduit undoubtedly saved the kidneys of many children whose lower tract disorders were untreatable or ill understood at the time. Secondly, many children, especially with exstrophy, have grown up to be well-adjusted and normal adults in spite of the bag. Thirdly, in considering 58 young adults for operations to remove the bag in one way or another, I have found six who claimed to be happy as they were. One woman even said that her two (normal) children would like to have bags too as it seemed better than going to the lavatory.

There have been several large reviews of the long-term results of ileal conduits. All testify to the high complication and re-operation rates, problems that must weigh heavily on the children and their parents. For example in a series with 75 children who could be reviewed between 10 and 16 years after diversion, only 12 had *not* had at least one complication (Shapiro *et al.* 1975).

With such poor operative results it would be difficult to identify psychosocial problems specifically related to the bag. Dunn found a 27% incidence of psychological problems in 55 children followed for a mean of 10 years. The children attended special schools for the handicapped. They had educational problems through lack of contact with teachers and ordinary children. Older children restricted their social lives and suffered sexual problems (Dunn *et al.* 1979).

Psychological problems have been found in adults with ileal conduits. In a group largely of cancer patients it was commented that many of the problems could be avoided by good pre-operative counselling and surgical techniques that gave an easily managed stoma. Twenty of 29 working patients returned to their previous jobs but nearly two-thirds of all the patients restricted their social lives because of the stoma (Jones *et al.* 1980). The lessons of these findings should not be lost on paediatric surgeons.

The quality of life with an ileal conduit or a Kock pouch have been compared. Surprisingly there was little difference between the two groups. Both felt happy in their social surroundings and there was no difference in the rate of return to work or the performance of daily tasks. Ileal conduit patients had lower expectations, poor self-image and less physical contact. Of ileal conduit patients 22% were sexually active against 48% of Kock patients. The most satisfied patients were a small subgroup who had had an ileal conduit converted to a continent Kock pouch (Boyd *et al.* 1987). Although this survey was done largely on cancer patients, it does have some important lessons for other groups. It emphasises the value of proper counselling. It may indicate that even continent diversions are not a perfect answer though patients who have experienced both types certainly prefer to be without a bag.

### Renal aspects

The short-term follow-up of patients with ileal conduits was very encouraging. Although it was recognised that some normal kidneys were damaged by the diversion, the most common situation was improvement of grossly distended kidneys or stabilisation of moderately distended ones. For example 83% of 62 children undergoing ileal conduit diversion because of renal deterioration were improved or stable according to the first postoperative urogram (Stevens & Eckstein 1977). Even at 10 to 16 year follow-up Shapiro found that 70% of previously normal kidneys had remained so (Shapiro *et al.* 1975).

With longer follow-up the rate of renal deterioration was frightening. The figures in Table 10.5 show the fate of kidneys that were normal at the time of diversion. They are slightly unfair to the ileal conduit as patients who had been diverted by ureterosigmoidostomy but failed were then converted to a cutaneous diversion, in some cases with kidneys that were already damaged. Nonetheless, damage of some kind to 75% of kidneys is worrying.

There are insufficient data from other centres to check whether these figures are representative. It is likely that the kidneys are more vulnerable in childhood, especially up to 8 years old. Therefore it is only in adulthood that the full effect of the diversion can be assessed: the 30% renal damage rate found by Shapiro at 10 to 16 years' follow-up must have included many patients who were still children. A similar incidence of renal damage was found by Frank at 'up to 25 years' but only nine of 80 patients were children and the mean follow-up was only 7 years (Shapiro *et al.* 1975, Frank *et al.* 1985). Efforts to protect the kidneys by anastomosing the trigone with the ureters to the ileal conduit have not been successful either in preventing reflux or renal damage (Lowe & Jeffs 1983).

Presumably the ileal conduit is not inherently bad for the kidneys. So the question arises of the causes and whether they are preventable. Three types of renal damage are seen: dilated kidneys, small and scarred kidneys and stones.

New dilatation in this context is due to obstruction which may be anatomical or functional. There are some circumstances where the ureteric peristalsis is inadequate to overcome the resistance of the uretero-ileal junction so that dilatation ensues without overt obstruction. When this happens, the dilated ureter becomes even less efficient and there is a vicious circle. Whether this leads to renal damage is unknown. The critical flow rate of urine may be as low as 1 ml/min. The clinical importance of this is that where there is dilatation without frank obstruction, increased fluid intake may worsen the problem (R.O. Witherow, personal communication).

The most common site of obstruction is in the stoma, secondly in the uretero-ileal junction, and thirdly where a ureter passes behind the root of the intestinal mesentery to reach the conduit lying on the other side.

Stomal stenosis is reported in 5 to 75% of patients. It is important to put a finger in the stoma at routine follow-up to search for this complication as the obstruction is commonly at fascial level. The stoma itself may look normal.

The stenosis may also provoke vigorous peristaltic waves which are of high amplitude and are associated with raised resting pressure (type III/IV activity). Kidneys draining into conduits with this activity almost invariably are dilated. True anatomical, or a functional obstruction of the stoma appears to be the cause and the dilatation will be improved by stomal revision (Neal *et al.* 1985).

Uretero-ileal stenosis may occur at any time. It is much less common than stomal stenosis, being reported in 5 to 10% of patients. It may be the cause of up to 25% of episodes of renal dilatation (Shapiro *et al.* 1975). If the Wallace system of anastomosing the ureters side to side and then joining them to the ileum is used, it is likely that both will stenose together.

The residual urine on catheterisation of the conduit should be small: 3 to 15 ml have been quoted (Shapiro *et al.* 1975, Frank *et al.* 1985). I am inclined to take 15 ml as the upper limit of normal. However, too much importance should not be attached to a single high residual, especially if the urine is sterile on culture. A repeatedly high residual of infected urine, not cleared by appropriate antibiotic therapy, is an indication for further investigation.

The search for obstruction must be relentless and the surgical treatment aggressive. There has been a tendency to think that urinary diversion is the end of a child's urological problems: really it is the beginning of a new set of problems.

Small scarred kidneys are caused by infection with or without obstruction. An ileal conduit should not be infected. The urine in the bag and swabs of the stoma are invariably positive on culture. Urine collected from the depths of the conduit by catheter should not be. Ideally, specimens should be collected with a catheter passed down the lumen of an outer catheter to avoid contamination (Bishop *et al.* 1971). In practice a pure culture of a typical organism is acceptable.

A statistically significant association has been shown between the urographic finding of small kidneys and the antibody titre to *Escherichia coli* or *Proteus mirabilis*. In 26 patients with raised antibodies only four had normal kidneys, whereas 89% of patients with normal urograms had normal antibody titres (Bergman *et al.* 1979). Although this does not prove a cause and effect, others have noted the association between bacteriuria, urinary tract dilatation and renal damage and it certainly supports the clinical impression.

Stones are seen in 5 to 30% of patients. They most often occur in the kidneys but have been seen in the ureters and even, occasionally, in the conduit. In patients who are not stone formers before diversion, 90% of stones are associated with *Proteus* infection. Other precipitating factors are ureteral dilatation, recurrent pyelonephritis, conduit residuals above 10 ml and minor degrees of hyperchloraemic acidosis (Dretler 1973). Although this information comes from a study of adults, there is no reason to suppose that it does not apply to children.

Renal deterioration with ileal conduits has a recognisable cause in most patients. Most causes are preventable, or at least identifiable at an early stage. Many of the complications are symptomless. Conduit patients should be carefully and actively followed (see Chapter 2). The same mistakes should not be made with patients having continent diversions or reconstructions using intestine.

## Histological changes

The histological changes seen when urine is passed through a length of ileum are quite characteristic and of no great importance. They do, however, explain why there are so few metabolic problems. Partial and sub-total villous atrophy of the epithelium are seen, increasing in severity with the age of the conduit.

In partial villous atrophy the overall thickness of the mucosa is unchanged but the villi are shorter and the basal layer (containing the crypts of Lieberkuhn) is thicker. Sub-total atrophy is a more severe change in which the villi all but disappear and the mucosa takes on an appearance similar to colon. Villous atrophy is seen at a mean conduit age of 4.9 years, a mixed pattern at 10.6 years and widespread sub-total change at 13 years. The range is very variable and different patterns of change may be seen in conduits of similar age. There is no relationship with obstruction or infection.

The bowel wall has a considerable infiltration of inflammatory cells. The sub-mucosa and muscularis layers are always thickened and splintered. The lymphatics are grossly dilated and the submucosa is oedematous. Transitional epithelium grows in from the ureters and displaces the ileal epithelium over a radius of 3 to 5 mm. The stomas show superficial ulceration (Deane *et al.* 1984). The distribution of changes is shown in Fig. 10.9.

These changes have been widely reported in biopsies from ileal conduits and in ileal patches grafted into dog bladders. They have no sinister implications and there is no evidence that they are premalignant. Ileal conduits have been widely used for 40 years and there are only two reports of primary neoplasms: one was a benign polyp and the other an adenocarcinoma in a patient with exstrophy (Shousa *et al.* 1978, Tomera *et al.* 1982).

### Metabolic problems

The literature has many papers on the ability of the ileum to absorb or secrete ions. In practice, the metabolic consequences of forming an ileal conduit are negligible. Experiments have usually been done on relatively fresh conduits that still maintain their normal villi. Well-established conduits with the villous atrophy described above have little metabolic function. Two cases of diabetics who did not have glycosuria soon after ileal conduit diversion have been reported (McGournan 1977). Investigation of glucose handling by long-established conduits in diabetics and non-diabetics showed that there was no absorption of glucose except in one diabetic (Sridhar *et al.* 1983).

Occasional metabolic problems may be seen. Hyperchloraemic acidosis, absorption of drugs secreted in urine and vitamin $B_{12}$ deficiency are important. They are so rare that routine screening is not indicated.

## COLON CONDUITS

The colon conduit is newer than the ileal conduit and large, long-term series are lacking. Its stoma is unlikely to be different in its psychological effects from that of the ileum. Table 10.5 suggests that its effects on the kidneys may be better than other diversions, but the follow-up was shorter.

In follow-up to 21 years colon conduits have been shown to have similar complication rates to ileal conduits: stomal stenosis up to 61%, ureterocolic stenosis up to 22%, stones up to 16% and renal deterioration in 48%. There has been some suggestion that the anti-reflux mechanism, when successful (about 50% of anastomoses) protects the kidneys from parenchymal scarring (Elder *et al.* 1979, Hill & Ransley 1983).

The histological changes are different to those seen in ileal conduits. The mucosal pattern is not greatly changed from normal colon except that the goblet cells are decreased in size. There is a dense inflammatory cell infiltrate with plasma cells and eosinophils. The severity of inflammation worsens with the age of the conduits and mitotic figures are seen with increasing frequency (Moorcraft *et al.* 1983). It has been sug-

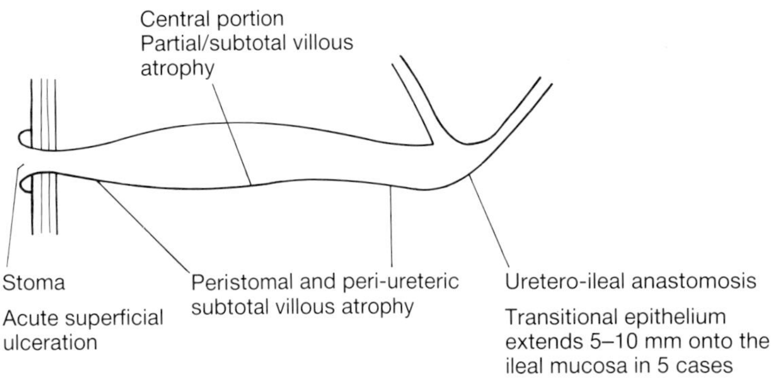


**Fig. 10.9** Diagram showing the distribution of histological changes in ileal conduits (from Deane *et al.* 1984, reproduced with permission).

gested that the changes are premalignant: this would be the case if they were seen in a patient with inflammatory bowel disease such as ulcerative colitis but whether they are in a colonic conduit remains to be seen. Only two colonic conduit tumours have been reported (Chiang *et al.* 1982, Wilson & Morales 1982).

The colon is not a very metabolically active part of the intestine. Although many experiments have documented theoretical metabolic problems with colonic conduits, very few are seen in practice. The theoretical risk of metabolic acidosis is greater than with ileal conduits but still rare enough to be ignored.

## REFERENCES


Aaronson I.A. & Morgan T.C. (1979) Ureterosigmoidostomy in childhood: the quality of life. *J. Ped. Surg.* **14**, 74–6.

Bergman B., Kaijser B. & Nilson A.E. (1979) Conduit urinary diversion and urinary tract infection. *Scand. J. Urol. Nephrol.* **13**, 65–70.

Bishop R.F., Smith E.D. & Gracey M. (1971) Bacterial flora of urine from ileal conduits. *J. Urol.* **105**, 452–9.

Boddy K., King P.C., Stewart W.K. & Flemming L.W. (1975) Whole body potassium in patients with ureterosigmoid anastomoses. *Br. J. Urol.* **47**, 277–82.

Boyd J.D. (1931) Chronic acidosis secondary to ureteral transplantation. *Am. J. Dis. Child.* **42**, 366–70.

Boyd S.D., Feinberg S.M., Skinner D.G., Leiskovsky G., Baron D. & Richardson J. (1987) Quality of life survey of urinary diversion patients: comparison of ileal conduits versus continent Kock ileal reservoirs. *J. Urol.* **138**, 1386–9.

Bricker F.M. (1950) Bladder substitution after pelvic exenteration. *Urol. Clin. North Am.* **30**, 1511–21.

Chiang K.S., Minton J.P., Clausen K., Clatworthy H.W. & Wise H.A. (1982) Carcinoma in a colon conduit urinary diversion. *J. Urol.* **127**, 1185–7.

Crissey M.M., Steele G.D. & Gittes R.F. (1980) Rat model for carcinogenesis in ureterosigmoidostomy. *Science* **207**, 1079–80.

Deane A.M., Woodhouse C.R.J. & Parkinson C.M. (1984) Histological changes in ileal conduits. *J. Urol.* **132**, 1108–11.

Dretler S.P. (1973) The pathogenesis of urinary tract calculi occurring after ileal conduit diversion. *J. Urol.* **109**, 204–9.

Dunn M., Roberts J.B.M., Smith P.J.B. & Slade N. (1979) The long-term results of ileal conduit diversion in children. *Br. J. Urol.* **51**, 458–61.

Elder D.D., Moisey C.U. & Rees R.W.M. (1979) A long-term follow-up of the colonic conduit operation in children. *Br. J. Urol.* **51**, 462–5.

Filipe M.I. (1975) Mucus secretion in rat colonic mucosa during carcinogenesis induced by dimethylhydrazine: a morphological and histochemical study. *Br. J. Cancer* **32**, 60–77.

Filipe M.I. & Branfoot A.C. (1976) Mucin histochemistry of the colon. In: Morson B.C. (ed) *Current Topics in Pathology*. Arnold & Co, London, pp. 149–62.

Frank P.P., Pernet M. & Jonas U. (1985) Ileal conduit diversion: early and late results of 132 cases in a 25 year period. *World J. Urol.* **3**, 140–4.

Ghoneim M.A. (1970). The rectosigmoid bladder for urinary diversion. *Br. J. Urol.* **42**, 429–33.

Gittes R.F. (1986) Carcinogenesis in ureterosigmoidostomy. *Urol. Clin. North Am* **13**, 201–5.

Hammer E. (1929) Cancer du colon sigmoide dix ans apres implantation des ureteres d'une vessie exstrophie. *J. Urol. (Paris)* **28**, 260–3.

Harrison A.R. (1958) Clinical and metabolic observations on osteomalacia following ureterosigmoidostomy. *Br. J. Urol.* **30**, 455–62.

Hayward R.H., Wakim K.G., Remine W.H. & Grindlay J.H. (1961a) An experimental study of the role of the kidney in hyperchloraemic acidosis. *Surg. Gynecol. Obstet.* **112**, 600–8.

Hayward R.H., Wakim K.G., Remine W.H. & Grindlay J.H. (1961b) An experimental study of the role of the colonic mucosa in hyperchloraemic acidosis. *Surg. Gynecol. Obstet.* **112**, 357–65.

Hill J.T. & Ransley P.G. (1983) The colonic conduit: a better method of urinary diversion? *Br. J. Urol.* **55**, 629–31.

Imler M., Schlienger J.L. & Batzenschlager A. (1979) Hyperammonemia following ureterocolostomy in the rat. *Surg. Gynecol. Obstet.* **149**, 183–8.

Jacobs A. & Barr Stirling W. (1952) The late results of ureterocolic anastomosis. *Br. J. Urol.* **24**, 259–316.

Jones M.A., Breckman B. & Hendry W.F. (1980) Life with an ileal conduit: results of questionnaire surveys of patients and urological surgeons. *Br. J. Urol.* **52**, 21–5.

Kroovand R.L. & Boyce H.H. (1988). Isolated vesicorectal internal urinary diversion: a 37 year review of the Boyce–Vest procedure. *J. Urol.* **140**, 572–3.

Lowe F.C. & Jeffs R.D. (1983) Ileal trigonal conduits: 10 year follow-up. *J. Urol.* **130**, 874–7.

McConnell J.B., Murison J. & Stewart W.K. (1979) The role of the colon in the pathogenesis of hyperchloraemic acidosis in ureterosigmoid anastomosis. *Clin. Science* **57**, 305–12.

McConnell J.B. & Stewart W.K. (1975) The long-term management and social consequences of ureterosigmoid anastomosis. *Br. J. Urol.* **47**, 607–12.

McDougal W.S., Koch M.O., Shands C. & Price R.R. (1988) Boney demineralisation following urinary intestinal diversion. *J. Urol.* **140**, 853–5.

Macfarlane M.T., Lattimer J.K. & Hensle T.W. (1979) The unheralded hazard of ureterosigmoidostomy. *Pediatrics* **64**, 668–71.

McGournan R.C.M. (1977) Glucose reabsorption from ileal loops. *Br. Med. J.* **ii**, 932.

Madsen P.O. (1964) The etiology of hyperchloraemic acidosis following urointestinal anastomosis: an experimental study. *J. Urol.* **92**, 448–54.

Miersch W-D. (1988) A new microsurgical model for the study of carcinogenesis in colonic urinary diversion in rats. *Urol. Int.* **43**, 269–71.

Moorcraft J., DuBoulay C.E.H., Isaacson P. & Atwell J.D. (1983) Changes in the mucosa of colon conduits with particular reference to the risk of malignant change. *Br. J. Urol.* **55**, 185–8.

Neal D.E., Hawkins T., Gallaugher A.S., Essenhigh D.M. & Hall R.R. (1985) The role of the ileal conduit in the development of upper tract dilatation. *Br. J. Urol.* **57**, 520–4.

Nurse D.E. & Mundy A.R. (1989) The metabolic complications of cystoplasty. *Br. J. Urol.* **63**, 165–70.

Parsons F.M., Pyrah L.N., Powell F.J.N., Reed G.W. & Spiers F.W. (1952) Chemical imbalance following ureterocolic anastomosis. *Br. J. Urol.* **24**, 317–22.

Pitluk H. & Poticha M. (1983) Carcinoma of the colon and rectum in patients less than 40 years of age. *Surg.Gynecol.Obstet.* **157**, 335–7.

Shapiro S.R., Lebowitz R. & Colodny A.H. (1975) Fate of 90 children with ileal conduit urinary diversion a decade later. *J. Urol.* **114**, 289–95.

Shousa S., Scott J. & Polak J. (1978) Ileal loop carcinoma after cystectomy for bladder exstrophy. *Br. Med. J.* **ii**, 397–8.

Silverman S.H., Woodhouse C.R.J., Strachan J.R., Cumming J. & Keighley M.R.B. (1986) Long term management of patients who have had urinary diversions into colon. *Br. J. Urol.* **58**, 634–9.

Spence H.M., Hoffman W.W. & Fosmire G.P. (1979) Tumour of the colon as a late complication of ureterosigmoidostomy for exstrophy of the bladder. *Br. J. Urol.* **51**, 466–70.

Sridhar K.N., Samuell C.T. & Woodhouse C.R.J. (1983) Absorption of glucose from urinary conduits in diabetics and non-diabetics. *Br. Med. J.* **287**, 1327–9.

Stevens P.S. & Eckstein H.B. (1977) Ileal conduit urinary diversion in children. *Br. J. Urol.* **49**, 379–83.

Stewart M. (1986). Urinary diversion and bowel cancer. *Ann. Roy. Coll. Surg. (England)* **68**, 98–102.

Stewart M., Macrae F.A. & Williams C.B. (1982) Neoplasia and ureterosigmoidostomy: a colonoscopy review. *Br. J. Surg.* **69**, 414–16.

Strachan J.R., Rees H.C. Cox R. & Woodhouse C.R.J. (1987a) Mucin changes adjacent to carcinoma following ureterosigmoidostomy. *Eur. Urol.* **13**, 419.

Strachan J.R., Matthews J., Rees H.C. & Cooke T. (1987b) Kinetic changes in experimental colonic urinary diversion. *Br. J. Surg.* **74**, 1046–8.

Tomera K.M., Unni K.K. & Utz D.C. (1982) Adenomatous polyp in an ileal conduit. *J. Urol.* **128**, 1025–6.

Turner W.R., Ransley P.G. & Williams D.I. (1980) Patterns of renal damage in the management of vesical exstrophy. *J. Urol.* **124**, 412–16.

Urdanetta L.P., Duffell D., Creevy C.D. & Aust J.B. (1966) Late development of primary carcinoma of the colon following ureterosigmoidostomy; report of 3 cases and literature review. *Ann. Surg.* **164**, 503–13.

Wilson J.W. & Morales A. (1982) Development of adenocarcinoma in transverse colon conduit. *Urology* **20**, 182–3.

Woodhouse C.R.J., Ransley P.G. & Williams D.I. (1983) The patient with exstrophy in adult life. *Br. J. Urol.* **55**, 632–5.

# 11 Undiversion and alternatives to a cutaneous urinary diversion

## INTRODUCTION

There are now very few indications for a permanent cutaneous urinary diversion in a child. In the past, however, diversion was sometimes a life-saving procedure and in other patients the only practical method of managing incontinence or recurrent urinary infection. In adolescents, the reconstructive techniques that are used in children can be applied to get rid of the bag. Almost anyone can have a reconstruction, but as the original surgery may have included resection of some of the urinary tract, more extensive and imaginative techniques may be needed.

Before doing such surgery it is important to establish the benefits that will result. The only certain improvement is cosmetic: the patient will not have an external appliance. If the bladder is, in fact, normal the long-term results of undiversion should be good. Some patients will be able to void normally but others may have to empty the bladder by intermittent clean self-catheterisation (ICSC).

The long-term results of more complex reconstructions, especially those using bowel, are unknown. The long-term results of cutaneous diversion are poor (see Chapter 10). It is reasonable to expect that a closed urine drainage system would be better for the kidneys than one that drains into a bag. The other long-term results of such reconstructions are unknown and unpredictable. It is salutary to remember that ureterosigmoidostomy had been used for nearly 100 years before the real risk of neoplasia was appreciated.

Those who undertake such surgery must be sure that the patients know of the uncertain future. Both surgeon and patient must be prepared for careful follow-up.

## PRINCIPLES OF UNDIVERSION

When a patient is seen for consideration for undiversion, three questions arise:

**1** Was the original diversion appropriate?

**2** Would modern methods allow use of the abnormal bladder?

**3** Could the bladder abnormality have got better?

In some patients, gross upper tract dilatation was an indication for diversion. The real diagnosis might never have been sought or might have been considered untreatable. Most undiversion series include patients whose original diagnosis was vesico-ureteric reflux (VUR) or 'congenital obstructive megaureter'. Our own first series included six such patients (Frank *et al.* 1982).

Most of these patients have a normal bladder. Undiversion can be done with the minimum of preliminary investigation. After surgery the bladder develops a normal pattern of micturition within a day or two. Even patients who have never consciously experienced micturition understand their new sensations and do not require 'potty training'. The duration of the diversion is irrelevant: restoration of normal function has been reported after 16 and 32 years (Pawar & Davenport 1986).

When the bladder is abnormal it may still be usable. The most common circumstance is the neuropathic bladder of myelomeningocele which, before diversion, was in chronic retention with overflow. Such bladders would now be managed with ICSC and the same technique can be used after undiversion.

Detrusor instability is another condition that is more easily managed nowadays. Drugs such as oxybutinine allow continence and may keep the intravesical pressure low enough to protect the kidneys. As life-long medication may not be very appealing to the adolescent, the 'clam cystoplasty' can also be used to reduce the intravesical pressure.

Spontaneous recovery of an abnormal bladder is unusual. It has been noted occasionally in the 'non-neurogenic (or occult) neurogenic bladder'. The aetiology of this condition remains an enigma (see Chapter 9). Spontaneous recovery is seen sufficiently often that all patients should be re-investigated with a view to undiversion.

## SELECTION AND INVESTIGATION

Selection of adolescents for undiversion is not as straightforward as it might seem. When the problems of the unknown long-term effects and the extent of the surgery have been explained, some patients may prefer to continue with their cutaneous diversion. In my own series six of 24 patients declined. All were either married or in a stable sexual relationship, some had children and some were trying to establish their careers. Those whose ileal conduit needed revision were more likely to accept (Cumming *et al.* 1988).

When undiversion was first practised on a large scale purely 'social' indications were uncommon. In one unit only one of 25 patients was considered for this indication in 1982 and two of 30 in its 1987 report; all the others had a specific 'medical' indication such as renal failure or a conduit complication (Stone *et al.* 1982, Galloway *et al.* 1987). With more experience undiversion is offered much more freely and I discuss the possibility with all adolescents with a cutaneous stoma. Nonetheless, it is important to establish what 'social' improvement will follow from undiversion. Those who feel that all their adolescent problems will fall away with the disappearance of the bag are usually (but not always) disappointed. Even with the very strict criteria used in Stone's series, one patient was not pleased with her technically successful operation (Stone *et al.* 1982).

There is some dispute about the extent of investigation that is necessary before undiversion. My own protocol includes a wide assessment of urinary tract anatomy and function, at least a part of which can only be justified as the establishment of a base line for long-term follow-up (Table 11.1). The essential investigations are those that establish the bladder function.

The patients should be examined under anaesthetic (EUA). Urethroscopy is performed to check that there are no strictures or false passages which might prevent voiding or self-catheterisation. The bladder is inspected and its capacity measured. Two small suprapubic catheters are inserted; an 8 FG catheter and an epidural catheter are convenient.

The EUA may provide other useful information particularly in patients who are wheelchair-bound with severe spina bifida. It gives the anaesthetist the opportunity to assess the reaction to anaesthesia. Some adolescent spina bifida patients have little respiratory reserve and have greater difficulty with anaesthesia than has been predicted by pre-operative testing. We have rejected two patients for reconstruction on the basis of these findings.

The EUA also gives the whole surgical team a view of how the patient will lie on the operating table. Some patients have such fixed flexion deformities that positioning is difficult and access to the pelvis is restricted.

On return to the ward the patient begins to 'cycle' the bladder. It is filled with saline through the larger catheter; when the bladder is full the continence is tested; an attempt is made to void and the residual, if any, is measured. If the bladder emptying is incomplete, the patient is taught ICSC. The cycle is repeated as often as possible until a steady state is reached. Video cystometrogram (VCMG) is then done.

**Table 11.1** Investigations before urinary undiversion.

| | |
|---|---|
| Urine: | Microscopy<br>Culture<br>Test for protein |
| Blood: | Full blood count<br>Electrolytes, urea and creatinine<br>Alkaline phosphatase<br>Calcium |
| Imaging: | Chest X-ray<br>Intravenous urogram |
| Isotopes: | Glomerular filtration rate |
| EUA: | Cystourethroscopy<br>Measurement of bladder capacity<br>Insertion of suprapubic lines<br>Anaesthetic assessment<br>Assessment of positioning for surgery |
| Cycling: | Filling of bladder<br>Attempts at voiding<br>Measurement of residuals<br>Assessment of sphincter function<br>Teaching of self-catheterisation<br>Video cystometrogram |

## CRITERIA FOR SIMPLE UNDIVERSION

In this context simple undiversion means that the kidneys are re-attached to the bladder by one means or another. The natural bladder, without enhancement, stores the urine. The bladder is emptied through the urethra either naturally or by ICSC. The original diagnosis in suitable cases is likely to have been reflux, megaureter, acontractrile neuropathic bladder, prune belly syndrome or, occasionally, posterior urethral valves. Particular care must be taken in valve patients because of the long-term bladder problems described in Chapter 14.

The criteria that are acceptable for simple undiversion are seldom stated in the literature. Most agree that the urinary tract function should be assessed and abnormalities are an indication for more elaborate reconstruction.

Poor renal function or renal failure is not a contraindication to undiversion. In fact undiversion may improve renal function or at least stabilise it. In one series 16 of 50 patients were undiverted specifically because of renal failure; in none did unexpected renal deterioration occur (Gonzalez *et al.* 1986). Occasionally renal function is markedly improved afterwards, as in three of nine children reported from Dublin (Sheehan *et al.* 1984).

The function of the ureters must be considered but investigation when they are not in use is virtually impossible. Ureteric failure contributes significantly to renal deterioration. The best guides to lower ureteric function are knowledge of the original diagnosis and function of the upper ureter. It has been suggested that the lower ureter should not be used in undiversion (Stone *et al.* 1982), however in seven children and adolescents we have used the lower (previously defunctioned) ureter without problems at up to 10 years' follow-up (Frank *et al.* 1982, Cumming *et al.* 1988).

Assessment of bladder and urethral function is critical. After cycling, the bladder must exhibit nearly normal urodynamic criteria. It does not have to be perfect as we have noted a uniform tendency for continued improvement after undiversion. I accept good compliance, capacity of 350 ml, stable detrusor and an end-filling pressure below 40 cm water.

The urethral sphincters must be synergic with the detrusor and continent. With a neuropathic urethra that has clearly demonstrated its competence with cycling, the patient will self-catheterise after undiversion. It is more difficult to predict continence with the apparently normally innervated sphincters. Cycling gives the best guide and fine needle electromyography may be helpful in difficult cases.

### Results of simple undiversion

In the literature on undiversion it is difficult to identify the cases that had a simple undiversion, for how long they were followed and what were the results. In the five series already quoted there were 29 patients who appear to fill the criteria. All have done well in the short follow-up that has been possible. There has been no incontinence and no unexpected renal deterioration.

Lack of proper data makes it impossible to conclude with certainty that this type of undiversion is acceptable. But logic suggests that it should be successful in the long-term. In the 12 years that St Peter's, UK has been doing such operations in any numbers, we have had no cause for regret.

## COMPLEX UNDIVERSION

When one or more components of the lower urinary tract are unusable, the surgeon must use his imagination to devise a system that avoids the dreaded bag. Lower urinary tract reconstruction should be tailored to the situation of each patient. There are three components to be considered and they are largely independent of each other: a reservoir for the urine, an outlet to the surface and a continence mechanism. The structures that have been used for each of these are shown in Table 11.2.

**Table 11.2** Tissues that may be used in the reconstruction of the lower urinary tract.

| Reservoir | Conduit | Control system |
|---|---|---|
| Bladder | Urethra | Urethral sphincters |
| Stomach | Appendix | Mitrofanoff |
| Ileum | Fallopian tube | Kock |
| Caecum | Ureter | Ileocaecal valve |
| Colon | Skin tube | Artificial sphincter |
| | Umbilical vein | Anal sphincter |
| | Ileum | |

The reservoir may be made of one or more of the items in the first column; the outlet from an item in the second column (lengthened by a skin tube if necessary); the continence mechanism comes from column three. The whole may be emptied by clean intermittent self-catheterisation or by spontaneous voiding.

My preference is to include in the reservoir as much normal bladder as possible. The urethra, if it is easily catheterisable and accessible to the patient, is the best outlet. The natural sphincters, if they can retain urine, are the best control mechanism.

Otherwise the choice of reconstruction depends on the material available, the needs of the patient, the possibilities for follow-up and the skills of the surgeon. It is a mistake to confine one's skills to one system, such as a particular type of pouch: if they extend to only one system, they should not be used in this field at all.

There seems to be little to choose between the different segments of intestine. The entire bladder capacity can be replaced by 20 cm of large bowel or 40 cm small bowel. There seems to be general agreement that jejunum should not be used. In a very extensive experience Mitchell has found ileum, caecum and sigmoid colon equally able to produce a compliant bladder substitute of good volume. Detubularisation in one form or another reduced the mass peristaltic contractions which were the most common cause of incontinence (Mitchell & Piser 1987).

In patients with acidosis from chronic renal failure there is a theoretical advantage in using stomach (Adams *et al.* 1988). It must be remembered that patients in chronic renal failure are likely to have a renal transplant and so lose their acidosis. Although the stomach may have other advantages as a bladder substitute, they remain just as unproven in the long-term as those of the other bowel segments.

### Choice of reservoir: augmentation cystoplasty

The reservoir may be made of any of the tissues in the first column of Table 11.2, either alone or in combination. The bowel is detubularised to disrupt the circular muscle and is generally used as a patch. To reduce the amount of bowel to be sacrificed from the intestinal tract, I incorporate as much normal bladder as possible. If there is an existing diverting conduit, it is incorporated in the reservoir.

Thus the first 'complex technique' that may be involved in undiversion is the augmentation of an unstable or poorly compliant bladder. Other techniques for the surgical treatment of an unstable bladder, such as detrusor transection or sub-trigonal phenol, have not stood the test of time and have not found favour with surgeons doing undiversions.

Augmentation cystoplasty has been used for many years in the treatment of the shrunken bladder of tuberculosis or bilharzia. It would be difficult to name a single 'inventor'. Dounis and Gow attribute the scientific work to Tizzoni and Foggi in 1888, while the clinical use is attributed to Von Mikulicz in 1899 (Dounis & Gow 1979). Under these circumstances the bowel was really being used as a substitution.

In detrusor instability, the 'clam' ileocystoplasty is the simplest augmentation and was popularised, if not invented, by Bramble (Bramble 1982). Particularly in the young and in the male, clam cystoplasty is the best long-term management of severe, refractory, detrusor instability (Mundy 1988a). It does lead to poor bladder emptying which may require ICSC, though this is less of a problem in congenital neuropathies. In practice any type of intestine can be used; for undiversion, the detubularised conduit is the most appropriate.

### *Results of undiversion with clam cystoplasty*

Clam cystoplasty became a treatment for congenital neuropathic bladder before it was used in undiversion. Children with high pressure and incontinent bladders were thus given a 'safe' bladder and a bag was avoided. Even so the length of experience is short. Undiversion plus clam experience is even shorter.

There seem to be about 120 patients in the literature who would fit into this category but many have not been followed even for 5 years. Again, it is difficult to pick out their details from the mass of data about a variety of different patient types. There do not seem to have been any major problems. ICSC is commonly necessary but I have been more optimistic recently about the prospects for complete voiding: the most surprising patients seem to be able completely to empty their bladders. An overall success rate for a safe bladder, continence and complete emptying (including ICSC) is about 85%. The complication rate (excluding incontinence) is about 20%.

## Choice of reservoir: substitution cystoplasty

The distinction between augmentation and substitution may be a fine one. Augmentation, particularly the clam, is mainly indicated to reduce the pressure and improve the compliance of the bladder. The storage volume will be increased by augmentation, but that is a lesser benefit. Substitution is indicated where the bladder can contribute no worthwhile volume. A rim of bladder is retained as the best means of connecting the intestinal pouch to the urethra.

It is unlikely that so small a bladder could also be used for implantation of the ureters which will, therefore, have to be implanted into the pouch. If the patient has not been diverted but has urine running through such a small bladder which must, almost by definition, be incontinent, non-refluxing vesico-ureteric junctions may sometimes be retained. Although any bowel can be used for substitution, I find it easier to achieve a non-refluxing and non-obstructed ureteric anastomosis with large bowel.

Bearing in mind that the urethra is the ideal outlet from the bladder, it should be obvious that the substituted bladder will always be anastomosed to the residual bladder base or upper urethra if they are present. It is not always so straight forward. Grossly abnormal bladders are often associated with other major abnormalities.

Firstly, the substituted bladder cannot always be emptied to completion. There is high probability that ICSC will be necessary. Patients with a neuropathic bladder which is so poor that substitution is necessary are often severely affected by myelomeningoceles. They may lack the manual dexterity to self-catheterise the urethra. The problem is worse if they walk with crutches or are wheel-chair-bound. If the bladder is not neuropathic, for example has been damaged by cyclophosphamide or surgery, the urethra, especially in the male, may be too sensitive for ICSC.

Secondly, the urethral sphincters may be incontinent. Therefore, either an artificial urinary sphincter (AUS) or a bladder reconstruction will be necessary as well. The feasibility and desirability of these procedures must be taken into account when deciding to anastomose the pouch to the urethra.

Thirdly, if an adolescent boy has been diverted all his life his penis will only ever have been a sexual organ. If, after undiversion, he will have to self-catheterise, the philosophical question arises as to whether he should catheterise his sexual organ. It seems unlikely that there is a 'right' answer to this question.

As lower urinary tract reconstruction becomes more complex in its surgery, so the choice of technique becomes more difficult.

### *Results of undiversion with bladder substitution*

Many of the patients whose undiversions with bladder augmentation have been reported have in fact had substitutions. Undiversion with colocystoplasty was reported in two young adults in 1979. Maximum follow-up was about 3 years (Bruce *et al.* 1979).

Since then bladder substitution has become increasingly popular though the number of patients followed for more than a few years is small. There are 111 cases in the seven papers quoted before and two others (Mundy *et al.* 1986, Goldwasser *et al.* 1987). A great majority of the patients had other procedures as well, particularly implantation of an AUS.

It is impossible to determine anything more than the broadest outcome from these series as so much detail is omitted. In particular it cannot be said which components of the complex operations were responsible for the successes and failures. A few general conclusions can be drawn.

Almost any patient can be 'undiverted'. Cases are even quoted where reconstruction (including renal transplantation) has been performed on patients with no urinary tract at all (Mundy *et al.* 1988b). Selection is based mainly on the patient's motivation and manual skills.

The surgery required is technically taxing. The complication rate is around 25 to 30%. Most of the complications requiring re-operation have been related to the continence mechanism rather than to the cystoplasty. One 19-year-old patient died two days postoperatively from respiratory complications (Gonzales *et al.* 1986).

The intestine is a suitable container for the storage of urine. The intrinsic peristaltic contractions must be abolished by one means or another. In my view this is best achieved by longitudinal incision through the full thickness of the wall. The opened out conduit is then sutured into the cystoplasty as a patch. If there is no conduit, the bowel is sutured transversely to form a cup (Fig. 11.1). Gonzales used bowel without transection of the muscle. Anticholinergics were given to suppress peristalsis in the 50% of patients who had unacceptably high pressures.

It is not always possible to abolish peristalsis even by complete transection of the circular muscle. I have also had two patients who re-established high pressure peristalsis after a period of bowel inertia. I have not found anticholinergic drugs to be effective.

The problem of the inert (or absent) ureter remains unsolved. If there is one good ureter, every effort should be made to preserve it and to get a good tunnelled re-implantation; the other ureter is joined to it as a transuretero-

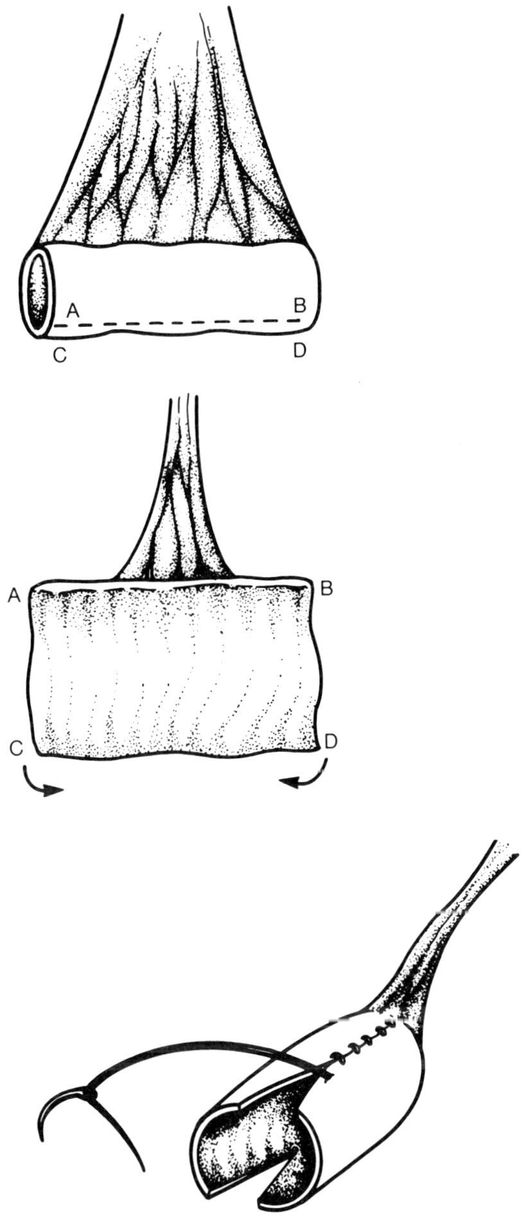


**Fig. 11.1** Detubularisation of bowel to form a pouch.

ureterostomy (TUU). Baggy, aperistaltic ureters should not be tunnelled into the new bladder as they will inevitably be obstructed: a simple end-to-side anastomosis should be done. The length of poor ureter that is used should be minimised by bringing the bladder implantation site as high as possible with a psoas hitch or Boari flap. Tailored ileum can be used as a substitute for ureter. In the long term, ureteric failure may be the greatest threat to renal function.

## CONTINENCE AND THE BLADDER OUTLET

The urethra and its sphincters are the best outlet and control mechanism. In the diverted patient cycling should reliably predict whether normal voiding will be possible, but only if a reasonable bladder capacity is achieved. The sphincteric function is not easy to test when bladder capacity is very small. Neurologically normal sphincters should allow complete emptying after enterocystoplasty. In patients with neuropathic bladders a combination of fluoroscopy of the internal sphincter and electromyography of the external sphincter can predict their behaviour accurately (Gonzalez & Sidi 1985).

In my experience young adults with normal sphincters have been continent after bladder substitution. However, in older patients some authors have found day or night incontinence after cystectomy. The main cause has been persistence of mass peristalsis even in detubularised bowel. Urodynamic studies have shown that the lowest pressures are achieved with an ileal patch augmentation of the colonic bladder (Lytton & Green 1989). In the reported patients most were elderly and all had had cystectomy, both of which may have had an adverse effect on sphincter function.

If the sphincters are continent but do not allow complete emptying, ICSC is generally the best management. There is sometimes pressure on the surgeon to arrange for 'normal' voiding. In this context it would be necessary to destroy the natural sphincters and to implant an AUS. In most cases this seems unwise. Even with an AUS complete voiding cannot be guaranteed after enterocystoplasty and ICSC may still be necessary. The long-term results of AUS are unknown.

Should the AUS become infected and require removal, the patient would be continually incontinent and worse off than he was originally: the options for further reconstruction would be more limited. Finally, in units performing large numbers of these operations, many of the patients come from remote parts of the world where 'servicing' of a faulty AUS might not be possible.

If the sphincters are incontinent, the options are to reconstruct the bladder outlet to create continence (and empty by ICSC) or to use an AUS. A good case can be made for either of these. However, it would seem that units have tended to use either one or the other and so it is difficult to establish indications for each. For example, Gonzalez has reported the use of the Young–Dees bladder neck reconstruction in eight patients with incompetent sphincters, seven of whom were continent on ICSC. The AUS had been used in other patients with success, but the need for 'servicing' and doubts about the mechanism's longevity favoured the Young–Dees (Gonzalez & Sidi 1985). Mitchell comments that the AUS is reserved for patients who can demonstrate complete bladder emptying (Mitchell & Piser 1987).

The long-term results of ICSC are good (see Chapter 9) but the urethra can be damaged so badly that the technique has to be abandoned. The risk is greater if the urethra has no sensation. Development of a false passage is a particular problem and can be difficult to treat: two of nine patients in one series had to have a continent diversion because of this complication (Koleilat *et al.* 1989).

Both Mundy and Stephenson have reported good results with undiversion using an AUS (Brantley Scott 792 or 800). There are 36 patients in their two series. It seems that virtually all were able to void to completion. Up to seven were at least partly incontinent. There were eight sphincter complications that required re-operation (Mundy *et al.* 1986, Galloway *et al.* 1987).

No real comparison can be made between these two alternatives. The patients were different; the relatively small numbers were spread over at least 7 years; the long-term results of ICSC are unrecorded. Although the spontaneous voiding that is usual with an AUS is very attractive, the surgical results are not sufficiently good to make it the automatic first choice.

Attempts to make a continent bladder neck and urethra which also allows complete spontaneous voiding have met with mixed results. It is difficult to balance the outflow resistance against the intravesical pressure. Furthermore, there must be enough good bladder tissue to allow the reconstruction to be done: not a common circumstance in patients presenting for undiversion.

In a series with 10 to 22 year follow-up on patients who had bladder neck reconstruction (but who had not been diverted) 19 of 27 children were completely dry. One child emptied by ICSC and one had stress incontinence, but the rest voided normally (Leadbetter 1985). This is probably the best result and longest follow-up available for such reconstructions. Those who claim success for more complex methods must compare themselves with it.

### Absence of urethra

If there is no urethra the choice lies between constructing one or using a technique of continent internal diversion with a suprapubic catheterisable stoma. It is possible completely to reconstruct the urethra from labia or from penile skin. The tube is then tunnelled into the bladder to make a continent outflow. The bladder is emptied by ICSC. Good results have been reported in six women and two men who had had radiation and/or surgery for pelvic cancer (Mundy 1988b).

This procedure is similar in principle to the Mitrofanoff, the difference being the point at which the meatus of the catheterisable tube is sited: the normal site of the external urinary meatus or a site on the abdominal wall. Apart from the philosophical problem of whether a boy should be invited to catheterise his penis discussed above, the site of a catheterisable stoma should be chosen chiefly for the patient's convenience. Those who are chair-bound, walk with crutches or lack manual dexterity find it difficult to catheterise the normally placed urethra.

### Reconstructed urethra and an artificial sphincter

The cuff of an artificial sphincter is designed to encircle a normal urethra or bladder neck. The risk of erosion is greater if these tissues have been damaged by surgery or radiation or if the 'urethra' is in fact skin. ICSC through an AUS also increases the risk of erosion though in one series 16 patients are reported with up to 6 years' follow-up and no complications (Strawbridge *et al.* 1989).

Experimental evidence suggests that AUS cuffs can be placed safely around intestine providing the pressure is low (Engelmann *et al.* 1985). An AUS with a cuff pressure 71 to 80 cm has been used successfully around large bowel in three of four children with follow-up to 11 years. Cuff erosion occurred twice, once when the cuff pressure was increased to 81 to 90 cm and in the other when a low pressure cuff became infected (Light 1989).

In the reconstructed urethra the most experience is in patients with exstrophy. In Scott's own series 10 of 16 patients retained their device, nine of whom were continent. Ten revision procedures were necessary to achieve even this result. Although these results are poor, the patients were a difficult group having failed numerous other attempts to achieve continence (Decter *et al.* 1988).

## CONTINENT INTERNAL DIVERSION

In the young adult it is a small step from 'undiversion' to continent internal diversion. With many of the undiversion techniques discussed above, the patient will have to empty the urine reservoir by ICSC. With continent internal diversion ICSC will always have to be used. The distinction between the two may only be in the site of the opening that is to be catheterised.

Several different systems of continent internal diversion have been described. It is preferable to be the master of them all so that the most appropriate system can be used for each patient. As with undiversion, selection of the three components can made from Table 11.2.

The urinary reservoir can be made from one or more of the items in the first column, including as much of the bladder as possible. The principles that have already been described apply.

The conduit can be any item in column two except, by definition, the urethra. The choice will partly depend on the type of continence mechanism that is to be used: narrow tubes are needed for the Mitrofanoff method, wide tubes for the Kock and terminal ileum for the Indiana.

The main discussion is in the choice of continence mechanism. The AUS has not yet reached a sufficient stage of development to be used routinely around bowel. The two most widely used systems are the Kock and the Mitrofanoff. In the Kock a segment of ileum is intussuscepted and used as a valve. In the Mitrofanoff a narrow tube is tunnelled into the urinary reservoir (as in the re-implantation of the ureter) to provide a valve.

As with undiversion, imagination must be used to produce the best system for each patient. It is a mistake to become addicted to a single complete system and to use it exclusively: the problems encountered in adolescents are very varied and the correct combination of reservoir, outlet and valve must be chosen for each.

### The choice of conduit

Our own studies have shown that the resting pressure generated within a Mitrofanoff conduit is two to three times the highest pressure generated by the reservoir. Furthermore, the conduit responds to pouch pressure rises with a considerable pressure rise of its own. The difference between the conduit pressure and the pouch pressure is large so that continence is reliably maintained. In Kock nipples the resting conduit pressure is only slightly higher than the pouch pressure and the response to pouch pressure rises is limited. The difference between conduit and pouch pressures is small and continence is tenuous (Malone *et al.* 1989). These experimental observations in patients have mirrored my clinical experience: it is much easier to make a continent Mitrofanoff than a continent Kock (Cumming *et al.* 1987).

### *The Mitrofanoff technique*

In 1980 Mitrofanoff described the use of the appendix as a continent vesicostomy for self-catheterisation in a child with a neuropathic bladder (Mitrofanoff 1980). Independently Innes Williams had made an appendiceal vesicostomy at about the same time though it was not reported until later (Frank *et al.* 1982). Mitrofanoff's name has now been given to operations in which a narrow lumen tube such as the appendix or ureter is implanted in a sub-mucosal tunnel into any urinary reservoir to form a continent catheterisable stoma.

The name does not imply any system of complete internal urinary diversion in the way that, for example, 'Kock pouch' does. I believe that the Mitrofanoff principle is the best choice for outlet and control mechanism if the urethra is not available, regardless of the type of reservoir.

The appendix is the best choice of conduit for the Mitrofanoff conduit. It commonly admits a 12 FG catheter. It has a good vascular pedicle. The wall is compliant and thin enough to allow easy submucosal implantation. If it is short, it can be lengthened with tubularised caecum.

The ureter has similar properties to the appendix and is the second choice. A ureter that is completely normal may only admit an 8 FG catheter but it can usually be dilated at least to 10 FG. A ureter that has been anastomosed to a conduit or has been obstructed will admit a 12 or 14 FG catheter without difficulty. The ureter may get its blood supply by several routes (Fig. 11.2).

Possibly the most common indication for the Mitrofanoff technique in the world at large involves the use of the bladder alone as the reservoir. Familiar to all urologists is the 'terminally

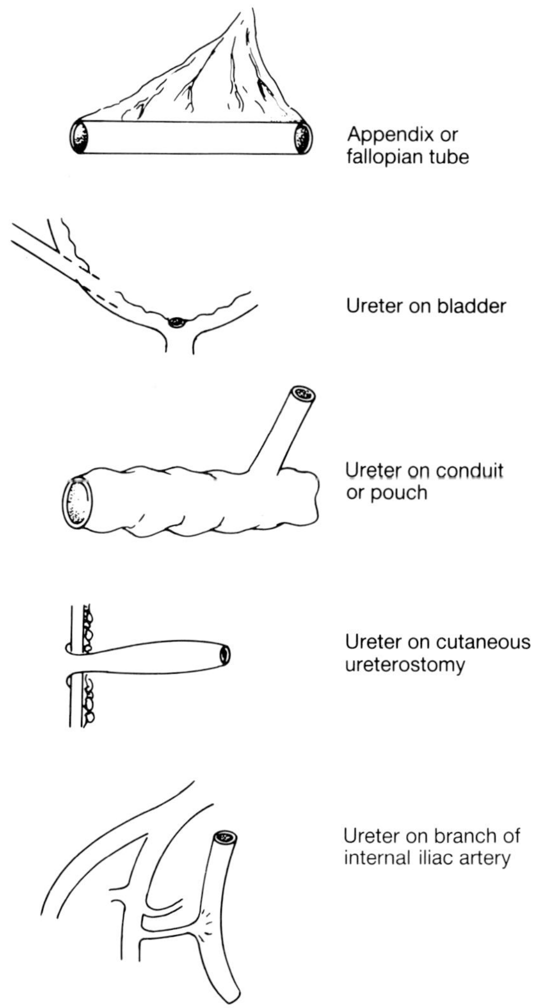


**Fig. 11.2** Sources of blood supply for structures used for Mitrofanoff continence systems.

incontinent girl'. She will have presented originally with sphincter incontinence and a stable detrusor. She will have had a number of procedures to achieve continence, usually including bladder neck reconstruction, Stamey-type sling and colposuspension. She is left with a rather rigid and scarred urethra which is incontinent. An AUS may be implanted if the tissues are thought adequate to support the cuff. If an AUS cannot be used (or afforded in some countries), the urologist may consider cutaneous diversion. For this patient a very simple Mitrofanoff is appropriate. The bladder neck is closed and the appendix implanted as a continent vesicostomy. If there is no appendix the ureters are joined by a trans-uretero-ureterostomy (TUU); the stump of the ureter thus liberated is used as a catheterisable stoma (Fig. 11.3).

The fallopian tube is a more delicate structure and is only of adequate calibre in its lateral two-thirds. It is a reasonable third choice.

A narrow tube can be made of skin. Its use as a substitute urethra has been mentioned. Although the procedure was described as 'total substitution of the lower urinary tract', it was identical to the Mitrofanoff principle (Mundy 1988b). I can see no theoretical reason why a pedicled skin tube should not be made at other sites, indeed I have used a skin tube as a part of the conduit when the appendix has been too short.

*Results of the Mitrofanoff.* The reported experience of the Mitrofanoff principle is limited and certainly much less than that of the Kock pouch. It must be remembered that the Mitrofanoff principle is a system of maintaining continence regardless of the type of pouch, and its results should be judged on that basis. Duckett and Snyder reported the first series of any size. The diagnoses and the reservoir types were varied. Nine of 10 patients were continent and one required a revision of the conduit implant to become so (Duckett & Snyder 1986).

In young patients with cancer undergoing radical cystectomy, a series of 11 having synchronous reconstructions has been reported. The pouches were made from the ileocaecal segment and the appendix used as the continent stoma. All were continent. Two required dilatation of the appendix at the outset before self-catheterisation could be established (Barker 1988).

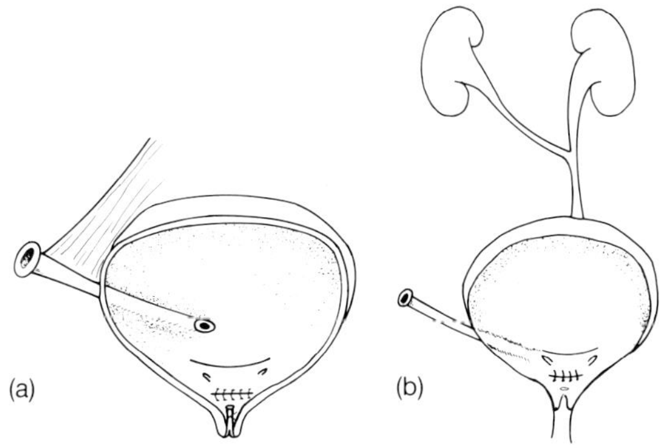


**Fig. 11.3** The simplest application of the Mitrofanoff principle. The bladder neck has been closed. (a) The appendix has been tunnelled into the bladder to form a continent stoma. (b) A right-to-left transuretero-ureterostomy has been made. The lower end of the right ureter is thus freed to form a continent conduit (from Woodhouse *et al.* 1989 with permission).

My own experience and technique have been reported in part (Cumming *et al* 1987, Woodhouse *et al.* 1989), and now extend to 46 patients. In 42 the Mitrofanoff principle was used primarily, four patients were converted to a Mitrofanoff when their Kock nipple became incontinent. The diagnoses and pouches were varied. The structures used as conduits are shown in Table 11.3.

Thirty-six patients were completely continent at the first attempt, three have had a revision to achieve continence (one unsuccessfully) and one

**Table 11.3** Conduits used in 46 personal cases of the Mitrofanoff procedure.

| | |
|---|---|
| Appendix | 29 |
| Ureter | 16 |
| Fallopian tube | 1 |

awaits revision. Follow-up is short at 6 to 58 months. Two patients have developed incontinence because the tunnel failed and have been revised. The conduit has become stenosed and difficult to catheterise in four, two of which responded to a dilatation; one required open revision and one eventually had a Kock nipple formed. One patient perforated his appendiceal conduit while drunk and had an appendicoplasty.

*The Kock nipple*

Kock originally described a pouch for the storage of small bowel contents after panproctocolectomy. Continence was maintained by an intussusception of the small bowel to form a nipple (Kock 1971). The system was subsequently modified to make a urinary reservoir (Kock *et al.* 1978, Skinner *et al.* 1984).

Although the term 'Kock pouch' implies a complete system of continent diversion, the essential ingredient is the nipple (Fig. 11.4). A nipple can be formed from an existing ileal conduit or from an isolated segment of ileum and used as a continence mechanism for any reservoir (Fig. 11.5).

The system has been developed and used extensively by Skinner with good results but a high complication rate. In my experience, the nipple can provide continence if it is constructed precisely according to Skinner's description (Skinner *et al.* 1989). I find it more difficult and less reliable than the Mitrofanoff and only use it as a last resort.

*Results of the Kock pouch.* Skinner's latest report includes 531 patients. It is not possible to discover how many would fit into the category of 'adolescents'. In 41 the operation was done for the symptoms and complications of neuropathic bladder and in 112 as a change of diversion (Skinner *et al.* 1989). In an earlier report from his unit 60 of 250 patients were young adults (Boyd *et al.* 1985). In all 531 patients, follow-up

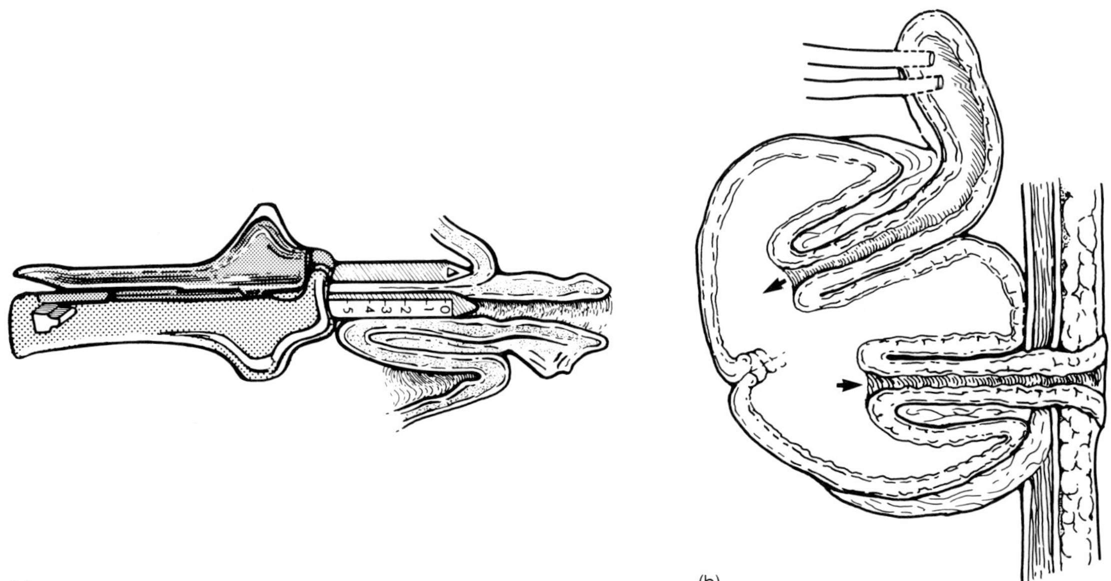

(a) (b)

**Fig. 11.4** Diagrams of the Kock nipple. (a) The ileum has been intussuscepted and the stapler is in position. (b) The completed pouch showing the afferent nipple with the ureters anastomosed and the efferent nipple as a continent cutaneous stoma (from Cumming & Woodhouse 1989 with permission).

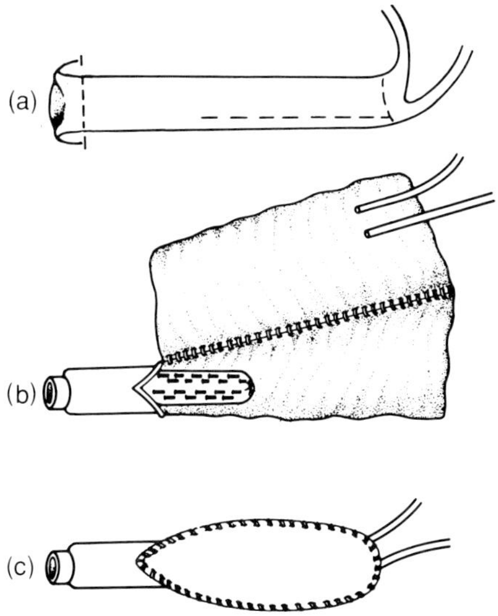


**Fig. 11.5** Formation of a Kock nipple from an existing ileal conduit. (a) The broken lines on the ileal conduit show the mobilisation and incisions. (b) The opened out conduit with the nipple may then be anastomosed face to face to any reservoir; in this example a length of detubularised bowel is used. The ureters are anastomosed to the reservoir. (c) The completed pouch.

was two to 69 months. The early complication rate was 15.2% in those who might be considered adolescents. The main late problem was incontinence affecting 10 to 15% of patients.

### *The ileocaecal valve*

The ileocaecal valve alone or with augmentation can be used as a continence mechanism. In the Indiana system the terminal ileum is tailored over a 12 FG catheter and the natural ileocaecal valve is said to provide continence (Rowland *et al.* 1987). It is a moot point whether the valve alone is responsible for continence or whether the narrowed ileum is also contributing. In the Mainz system the terminal ileum is intussuscepted through the ileocaecal valve to provide a Kock nipple as augmentation for the valve (Thuroff *et al.* 1988).

*Results with the ileocaecal valve.* The Indiana pouch has been reported in 29 young patients. Continence was achieved in 27 (Rowland *et al.* 1987). The results of the Mainz pouch were reported in 1988 and updated a year later. In 109 patients (42 of whom were children) a variety of techniques were used including, in some, the appendix as the stoma. Continence was achieved in 96% of patients with a complication rate of 15% (Thuroff *et al.* 1988, personal communication 1989).

### *Formation of the cutaneous stoma*

The long-term success of the procedure depends on this part of the operation more than any other. If the conduit cannot be catheterised, the whole system is useless.

The site for the cutaneous stoma should be selected before surgery. In the normally mobile patient it should be as low as possible. A site within the pubic hair area is good as the opening is invisible. In any case it should be below the normal bikini or underpant line. In patients who are chair-bound, any site below the umbilicus is likely to be inaccessible. I try to get the opening as high as possible, if necessary to a point just below the xiphisternum.

The conduit is tunnelled through the abdominal wall obliquely to make the track as straight as possible. The cutaneous end is spatulated and a long triangular skin flap (2–3 cm) sutured into the spatulation (Fig. 11.6). This allows the minimum of mucosa to be visible, forms a neat funnel for catheterisation and may contribute to prevention of stenosis (Fig. 11.7).

## GENERAL CONSEQUENCES OF AN INTESTINAL RESERVOIR

### Introduction

The large bulk of literature on bowel reservoirs for urine either as part of undiversion or as primary treatment for an abnormal bladder has

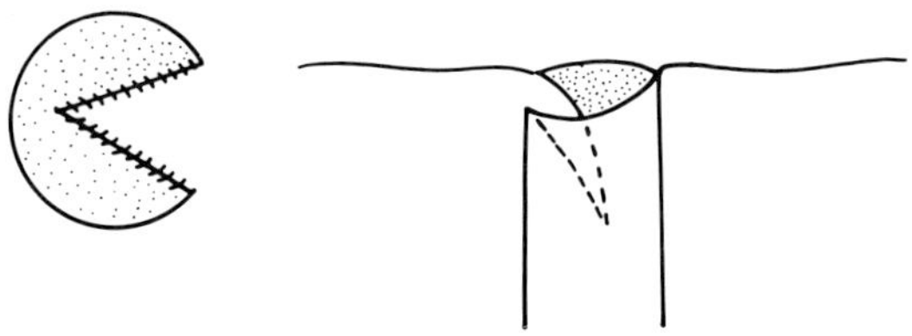

**Fig. 11.6** Formation of the stoma. A triangular flap of skin 2–3 cm long is mobilised and sutured into the spatulated end of the conduit. (From Woodhouse *et al.* 1989, reproduced with permission.)

shown that several systems work in the short-term. There is a high acceptance rate by the patients. In my group only one of 80 patients, having once got rid of their bag by any means, has volunteered to have it back again, no matter what complication has ensued.

There has been no long-term follow-up. It is not unreasonable to think that a closed system of urinary drainage will be better than an open one. Also, that as the results of cutaneous diversion are so poor, the new systems could hardly be worse.

Nevertheless, it took many years to realise the adverse long-term effects of the older diversions. It is essential that units that undertake this type of surgery also insist on the closest long-term follow-up. Imagination is essential to this as to the surgery: who can guess what the complications are likely to be?

## Psychological consequences

The psychological consequences have been generally good. However, most surgeons with wide experience of undiversion have the occasional patient who, while not wishing to have the bag back, is dissatisfied with the new arrangement. My own series includes two such patients. Their body image had, for as long as they could remember, included a stoma. The loss of the stoma altered their body image. They feel insecure, worried that the new system may leak (though it never has), unable to go to work and afraid of their peers. Both are responding slowly to psychotherapy.

Conversely, a problem arises with the 'disaffected teenager'. His or her many social and psychological problems are blamed by the family and doctors on 'growing up' and by the patient on his or her stoma. The greatest care must be taken in the assessment of these patients but occasionally I have found that the patient's view was correct: all was solved by getting rid of the stoma.

In a formal psychological assessment of his patients, Skinner found some surprising facts. He compared those who had had ileal conduits with those who had had a Kock pouch. A small sub-group had been converted from conduit to Kock. The majority of patients had cancer and were past middle age. There was little difference in the levels of satisfaction and of physical activity between the two main groups. Significantly for the adolescent, however, was the finding that the Kock patients had a better self-image, had more physical contact with others and more sexual activity. The sub-group who had had a conversion from conduit to Kock were almost uniformly extremely satisfied by the result (Boyd *et al.* 1987).

## Reservoir rupture

In a session of the Society of Pediatric Urology (Dallas, 1989), it was interesting to find that some units found late rupture of the bladder to be an important problem while others claimed never to have seen it. The explanation for this difference must lie in some matter of technique rather than in the closeness of follow-up.

It is clear, however, that when rupture of the reservoir occurs, the consequences are devastating. The patients are often well away from their usual hospital and there may be delay in diagnosis. They rapidly become very ill with generalised peritonitis.

'Cystogram' is commonly normal. Diagnosis is

(a)

(b)

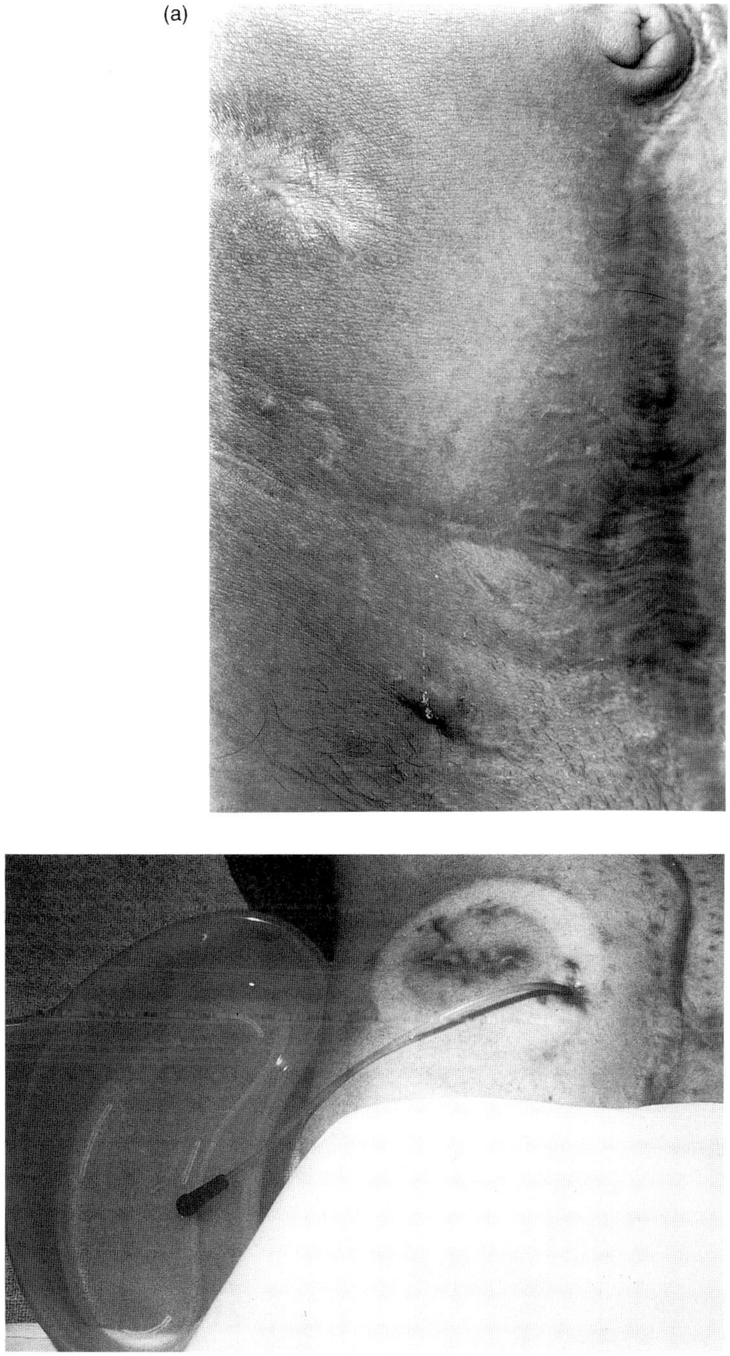

**Fig. 11.7** (a) Mitrofanoff stoma seen in the bottom left of the picture compared to the umbilicus in the top right. (b) Mitrofanoff stoma being catheterised. The shadow left by the urine bag for the previous ileal conduit is clearly seen.

best made by ultrasonography and peritoneocentesis of fluid collections. IVU may show a leak.

If diagnosed early, catheterisation and broad-spectrum antibiotics may lead to recovery. If the patient fails to respond rapidly on this regime or if there has been delay in diagnosis, laparotomy should be performed at once. In one series one of four patients died (Rushton *et al.* 1988).

Patients and their families should be warned of this possible complication and advised to return to hospital at once for any symptoms of acute abdomen, especially if the reservoir stops draining its usual volume of urine.

## Pregnancy

Pregnancies after any type of undiversion or lower tract reconstruction with bowel are rare so far. In doing the reconstruction in females it is essential to have a future pregnancy in mind. The 'bladder' should be made to lie anteriorly in the abdomen. The bowel pedicle should be fixed on one side to allow enlargement of the uterus on the other.

There must, by now, have been several pregnancies in women who have had simple undiversions. They are occasionally mentioned as a small footnote in some series. The lack of special comment suggests that there were no serious problems. At least two women in my own series have had pregnancies and vaginal deliveries without complications though one was 8 weeks premature.

Patients with augmented and substituted bladders have produced children. I agree with the published experience that they may be complicated and require the joint care of obstetrician and urologist (Bruce *et al.* 1979, Hill & Kramer 1989). Particular problems include upper tract obstruction and changes in bladder control as the uterus enlarges and damage to the bladder outlet during vaginal delivery. It is tempting to recommend caesarean section but only with a urologist present who can protect the bowel pedicle from damage.

Pregnancies after continent diversion have not been reported in writing yet. I know of a successful one following a Mitrofanoff (J.W. Duckett, personal communication 1989).

## Metabolic changes

In spite of an intensive search, most surgeons have not detected any serious abnormalities in the conventional haematological or biochemical parameters that are measured. In 183 children and young adults followed in our own unit we have found hyperchloraemic acidosis in 14% and anaemia in 8%. The type of bowel used in the reservoir was irrelevant (K.H. Wagstaff, *et al* 1990).

However, a warning note has been sounded by Nurse. She has made an experimental study of the handling of electrolytes instilled into the bladder and arterial blood gas analysis. Thirty-seven of 40 patients with reservoirs had ileum included while only three were made only of sigmoid colon. Eight further patients had ileal conduits and there were nine controls. One-third of all patients had hyperchloraemia, and 50% of those with an ileocaecal reservoir. All patients had abnormal blood gases, the majority having metabolic acidosis with respiratory compensation. All patients absorbed sodium and potassium from the reservoirs but the extent was variable. The findings were unrelated to renal function or the time since the reservoir was constructed (Nurse & Mundy 1989a). Conversely, in a study of 17 Kock pouch patients no changes in arterial base excess or pH were detected (Akerlund *et al.* 1989).

The significance of these findings is uncertain. It must be recognised that measurement of venous electrolytes gives only a crude view of the electrolyte status. The subtle changes in blood gases may be much more relevant in the long-term. In particular, in the growing child and adolescent and in the pregnant woman, chronic acidosis may have an adverse effect on bone mineralisation. Height and weight measurements have not been a routine part of our follow-up, but in those children in whom they have been measured, 20% have shown delayed linear growth in spite of normal growth in weight (Wagstaff *et al.* 1990).

A further area that might give concern is the consequence of using the ileocaecal valve and terminal ileum in the bladder reconstruction. Although the remainder of the ileum is known to have considerable ability to adapt, there have been fears that patients would develop macrocytic anaemia or chronic diarrhoea. In practice these fears seem to have been unfounded.

There have been no clinical problems in my own patients. In an experimental study in patients with reservoirs between 4 months and 8 years old, no disturbance of $B_{12}$ or carotene metabolism was found (Canning *et al.* 1989). In Kock pouch patients followed for 5 to 11 years six of 17 patients were found to have borderline or sub-normal $B_{12}$ levels requiring supplements (Akerlund *et al.* 1989).

Although these findings are encouraging, they give no cause for complacency. Nurse has shown that some important parameters are abnormal in these patients. The fact that they are difficult to detect in practice should not allow us to forget them.

It is particularly important to note that the reservoirs retain their ability to alter body metabolism for years. Where Nurse detected changes they were unaffected by the age of the reservoir. Furthermore, biopsy studies of caecal reservoirs have shown only minimal evidence of epithelial atrophy up to 9 years (Mansson & Willen 1988).

## Renal function

In the follow-up so far available, undiversion or continent diversion seems not to have affected renal function. In reports that function was improved after such surgery it is likely that pre-existing obstruction or high bladder storage pressure had been eliminated.

In the longer term, renal deterioration that has been found has been related to obstruction, reflux and stone formation. However, in one long-term study of Kock pouch patients, these complications occurred at the same rate as that found in patients with ileal conduits: 29% at 5 to 11 years (Akerlund *et al.* 1989).

## Cancer

It is the constant fear of surgeons who perform these operations on the young that history will repeat itself: the bowel segments will develop neoplasia in the same way that the ureterosigmoidostomy did. Animal evidence suggests that faecal and urinary streams must be mixed for neoplasia to occur. However, if it is chronic mixed bacterial infection, rather than the faeces *per se*, that is required, the bowel urinary reservoir may be at risk (see Chapter 10).

In patients with colonic and ileal cystoplasties high levels of nitrosamines have been found in the urine of all of 23 patients in one study. Biopsies of the ileal and colonic segments showed changes similar to those that have been found in ileal and colonic conduits and in ureterosigmoidostomies (see Chapter 10). More severe histological changes and higher levels of nitrosamines correlated with heavy mixed bacterial growth on urine culture (Nurse & Mundy 1989b). The inflammatory changes seen in these pouches and in conduits are probably innocent. The increased crypt staining with high iron diamine alcian blue seen in colonic pouches is seen in all ureterosigmoidostomies: it is not known whether it indicates that all are undergoing malignant change or whether it is a normal finding when urine is in contact with large bowel mucosa. Nitrosamines in urine are worrying under any circumstances.

Single cases of pouch neoplasms have been reported. In two cases the neoplasm occurred so soon after the reservoir construction (3 and 4 months respectively) and in elderly patients that a pre-existing lesion seems probable (Grainger *et al.* 1988, Stillwell & Myers 1988). A more worrying case was reported in a patient who had had an ileocystoplasty at 13 years old and developed an adenocarcinoma at the age of 43 (Hasegawa *et al.* 1988). A further worrying case was reported by Kirby and Lloyd-Davies (1985).

Cancer must remain a cause for great vigilance in the follow-up of patients. It is interesting to note that no cases have been reported from units routinely performing large numbers of these operations.

## REFERENCES


Adams M.C., Mitchell M.E. & Rink R.C. (1988) Gastrocystoplasty: an alternative solution to the problem of urological reconstruction in the severely compromised patient. *J. Urol.* **140**, 1152–6.

Akerlund S., Delin K., Kock N.G. *et al.* (1989) Renal function and upper urinary tract configuration following urinary diversion to a continent ileal reservoir (Kock pouch). *J. Urol.* **142**, 964–8.

Barker S.B. (1988) *Continent Diversion After Cystectomy.* Read at the Annual Meeting of the British Association of Urological Surgeons, Buxton, June 1988 (Abstract 140).

Boyd S.D., Feinberg S.M., Skinner D.G. *et al.* (1987) Quality of life survey of urinary diversion patients. *J. Urol.* **138**, 1386–9.

Boyd S.D., Skinner D.G. & Lieskovsky G. (1985) Ongoing experience with the Kock continent ileal reservoir for urinary diversion. *World J. Urol.* **3**, 155–8.

Bramble F.J. (1982) The treatment of adult enuresis and urge incontinence by enterocystoplasty. *Br. J. Urol.* **54**, 693–6.

Bruce P.T., Wheelahan J.B. & Buckham G.J. (1979) 'Undiversion' with colocystoplasty for neurogenic bladder. A report of 2 cases. *Br. J. Urol.* **51**, 269–74.

Canning D.A., Perman J.A., Jeffs R.D. & Gearhart J.P. (1989) Nutritional consequences of bowel segments in the lower urinary tract. *J. Urol.* **142**, 509–11.

Cumming J., Cox R. & Woodhouse C.R.J. (1988) Urinary undiversion in young adults. *Br. J. Urol.* **61**, 40–4.

Cumming J. & Woodhouse C.R.J. (1989) The role of the Kock pouch in adolescent urology. In: Spitz L. (ed) *Progress in Pediatric Surgery,* Vol 23. Springer Verlag, Berlin, pp. 126–34.

Cumming J., Worth P.H.L. & Woodhouse C.R.J. (1987) The choice of suprapubic continent catheterisable stoma. *Br. J. Urol.* **60**, 227–30.

Decter R.M., Roth D.R., Fishman I.J. *et al.* (1988) Use of the AS800 device in exstrophy and epispadias. *J. Urol.* **140**, 1202–3.

Dounis A. & Gow J.G. (1979) Bladder augmentation — a long term review. *Br. J. Urol.* **51**, 264–8.

Duckett J.W. & Snyder H.Mc. (1986) Continent urinary diversion: variations on the Mitrofanoff principle. *J. Urol.* **136**, 58–62.

Engelmann U.H., Felderman T.P. & Scott F.B. (1985) The use of the AMS-AS800 artificial sphincter for continent urinary diversion. 1. Investigations including pressure flow studies using rabbit intestinal loops. *J. Urol.* **134**, 183–90.

Frank J.D., Karthaus H.F.M., Johnston S.R. & Ransley P.G. (1982) An approach to undiversion in children. *Br. J. Urol.* **54**, 700–2.

Galloway N.T.M., Heathcote P.S., Gately C. Saloman J.R. & Stephenson T.P. (1987) Longer term results of undiversion. *Br. J. Urol.* **60**, 51–3.

Goldwasser B., Barrett D.M. & Kramer S.A. (1987) An alternative technique for undiverting the sigmoid conduit. *J. Urol.* **138**, 137–9.

Gonzalez R. & Sidi A.A. (1985) Preoperative prediction of continence after enterocystoplasty or undiversion in children with neurogenic bladder. *J. Urol.* **134**, 705–7.

Gonzalez R., Sidi A.A. & Zhang G. (1986) Urinary undiversion: indications, technique and results in 50 cases. *J. Urol.* **136**, 13–16.

Grainger R., Kenny A. & Walsh A. (1988) Adenocarcinoma of the caecum occurring in a caecocystoplasty. *Br. J. Urol.* **61**, 164–5.

Hasegawa S., Oshima S., Kinukawa T. *et al.* (1988) Adenocarcinoma of the bladder 29 years after ileocystoplasty. *Br. J. Urol.* **61**, 162.

Hill D.E. & Kramer S.A. (1989) Pregnancy after augmentation cystoplasty. *J. Urol.* **141**, 195A.

Kirby R.S. & Lloyd-Davies R.W. (1985) Adenocarcinoma occurring within a caecocystoplasty. *Br. J. Urol.* **57**, 357–8.

Kock N.G. (1971) Ileostomy without external appliances: a survey of 25 patients provided with intra-abdominal reservoir. *Ann. Surg.* **173**, 545–50.

Kock N.G., Nilson A.F., Norlen L. *et al.* (1978) Urinary diversion via a continent ileum reservoir: clinical experience. *Scand. J. Urol. Nephrol.* **49** (Supplement), 23–31.

Koleilat N., Sidi A.A. & Gonzalez R. (1989) Urethral false passage as a complication of intermittent catheterisation. *J. Urol.* **142**, 1216–17.

Leadbetter G.W. (1985) Surgical reconstruction for complete urinary incontinence: a 10 to 22 year follow-up.

*J. Urol.* **133**, 205–6.

Light K.K. (1989) Long term clinical results using the artificial sphincter around bowel. *Br. J. Urol.* **64**, 56–60.

Lytton B. & Green D.F. (1989) Urodynamic studies in patients undergoing bladder replacement surgery. *J. Urol.* **141**, 1394–7.

Malone P.R., Woodhouse C.R.J., Worth P.H.L. *et al.* (1989) Why are continent diversions continent? *J. Urol.* **141**, 303**A**.

Mansson W. & Willen R. (1988) Mucosal morphology and histochemistry of the continent cecal reservoir for urine. *J. Urol.* **139**, 1199–201.

Mitchell M.E. & Piser J.A. (1987) Intestinocystoplasty and total bladder replacement in children and young adults: follow-up of 129 patients. *J. Urol.* **138**, 579–84.

Mitrofanoff P. (1980) Cystostomie continente trans-appendiculaire dans le traitement des vessies neuro-logiques. *Chir. Pediatr.* **21**, 297–305.

Mundy A.R. (1988a) Detrusor instability. *Br. J. Urol.* **62**, 393–7.

Mundy A.R. (1988b) A technique for total substitution of the lower urinary tract without the use of a prosthesis. *Br. J. Urol.* **62**, 334–8.

Mundy A.R., Nurse D.E., Dick J.A. & Murray K.H.A. (1986) Complex urinary undiversion. *Br. J. Urol.* **58**, 640–3.

Nurse D.E. & Mundy A.R. (1989a) Metabolic complications of cystoplasty. *Br. J. Urol.* **63**, 165–70.

Nurse D.E. & Mundy A.R. (1989b) Assessment of the malignant potential of cystoplasty. *Br. J. Urol.* **64**, 489–92.

Pawar H.N. & Davenport T.J. (1986) Rehabilitation of the bladder after 32 years of suprapubic cystostomy. *Br. J. Urol.* **58**, 563.

Rowland R.G., Mitchell M.E., Bihrle R., Kahnoski R.J. & Piser J.E. (1987) Indiana continent urinary reservoir. *J. Urol.* **137**, 1136–9.

Rushton H.G., Woodard J.R., Parrott T.S., Jeffs R.D. & Gearhart J.P. (1988) Delayed bladder rupture after augmentation enteroplasty. *J. Urol.* **140**, 344–6.

Sheehan S.J., Duff F., Guiney E.J., Kelly D.G. & Smith J. (1984) Urinary tract undiversion. *Br. J. Urol.* **56**, 280–4.

Skinner D.G., Boyd S.D. & Lieskovsky G. (1984) Clinical experience with the Kock continent ileal reservoir for urinary diversion. *J. Urol.* **132**, 1101–7.

Skinner D.G., Lieskovsky G. & Boyd S. (1989) Continent urinary diversion. *J. Urol.* **141**, 1323–7.

Stillwell T.J. & Myers R.P. (1988) Adenomatous polyp in defunctionalised colonic segment used as a urinary bladder. *Urology* **32**, 538–40.

Stone A.R., Bary P.R., Holmes D.M., Salaman J.R. & Stephenson T.P. (1982) Assessment for and results of urinary undiversion. *Br. J. Urol.* **54**, 703–7.

Strawbridge L.R., Kramer S.A., Castillo O.A. & Barrett D.M. (1989) Augmentation cystoplasty and the artificial genitourinary sphincter. *J. Urol.* **142**, 297–301.

Thuroff J.W., Alken P., Riedmiller H., Jacobi G.H. & Hohenfellner R. (1988) 100 cases of Mainz pouch: continuing experience and evolution. *J. Urol.* **140**, 283–8.

Wagstaff K.E., Woodhouse C.R.J., Rose G.A. & Ransley P.G. (1990) *Biochemical and haematological profiles of patients with intestinal bladders.* Read at the Annual Meeting of the British Association of Urological Surgeons, Scarborough, July 1990 (Abstract 116).

Woodhouse C.R.J., Reilly J.M., Strachan J. & Malone P.R. (1989) The Mitrofanoff principle for continent urinary diversion. *Br. J. Urol.* **63**, 53–7.

# 12 *The prune belly syndrome*

## INTRODUCTION

The prune belly syndrome (PBS), sometimes called the triad syndrome, consists of bilateral undescended testes, absence of the muscle of the anterior abdominal wall and bizarre malformations of the urinary tract. By this definition it can only occur in males. Very rarely a similar condition may be seen in either sex consisting of megacystis and megaureter. In a review of the literature seven girls with 'prune belly syndrome' and 158 boys were identified (Burke *et al.* 1969). Some of the features of PBS are seen in several unrelated circumstances without producing the full blown syndrome.

An incomplete form of PBS occurs in which the muscle of the anterior abdominal wall is present to some degree — the pseudo-prune. Although the testes are lower and the renal parenchyma better preserved in pseudo-prunes, the urinary transport system is just as deficient. Surgical improvement is often necessary. In adulthood only one of seven pseudo-prunes in my group is in renal failure compared to nine of 22 complete examples (Malone *et al.* 1990).

In spite of references in the literature going as far back as 1839 (quoted by Burke *et al.* 1969), the cause of the syndrome is uncertain. If it is a chromosomal abnormality, a two-step autosomal dominant mutation with sex-linked expressions partially mimicking X-linkage is a likely explanation (Riccardi & Grum 1977). However, there are several other mechanical and embryological theories (Greskovich & Nyberg 1988). Innes Williams's series included a twin, the other of whom was not affected. Two patients also had posterior urethral valves (Woodhouse *et al.* 1982). Bladder outflow obstruction remains a possible cause, but although it may occasionally produce some similar results, I do not accept that it can be the cause of the classical syndrome. A case was reported of massive abdominal distension from urethral obstruction *in utero* leading to the birth of an infant who appeared to have prune belly syndrome (Pagon *et al.* 1979). In another similar case, the infant who appeared to have prune belly syndrome due to abdominal distension *in utero* was found to be normal clinically and on IVU examination at the age of 1 year (Smythe 1981). In spite of these two case reports, most infants with urethral obstruction, such as from posterior valves, do not have prune bellies.

The three features of the syndrome produce important effects in adult life and they are mutually independent. The overall prognosis is dependent on the renal anomalies. The minor associated anomalies seldom affect the child's life. Respiratory insufficiency has been reported as a post-operative complication and early physiotherapy recommended, but in adult life it seems not to be a problem and has not stopped patients being active in sport (Woodhouse *et al.* 1979).

In considering each of the three features of the syndrome, it must be remembered that it is rare. There are several unresolved controversies, especially in the management of the urinary tract, which will remain so as controlled trials would not be easy. Nonetheless, the prognosis in those who survive the neonatal period is good (except for fertility) and so it is reasonable to tread a fairly conservative path.

## THE URINARY TRACT

Innes Williams proposed a clinical classification of the syndrome based on the condition of the kidneys in the neonatal period (Table 12.1). Although it may be difficult to allocate an infant to the correct group immediately after birth, especially groups I and II, the classification has proved valuable in predicting prognosis both in the short- and long-term (Williams & Parker 1974, Woodhouse *et al.* 1982).

Patients in group I are born with insufficient nephrons to support life. The number of patients in this group is probably underestimated as some are lost in the general diagnosis of severe oligohydramnios and Potter's facies. Many others are so ill that they are never referred to specialist paediatric units and are not included in published reports. In the UK, the Great Ormond Street patients born between 1948 and 1977 included 8.5% in group I but Burke's estimate of 20% still-born or dying in the first month of life is probably a more accurate figure (Burke *et al.* 1969). Although renal transplantation in this syndrome has been reported in infants less than 1 year old (Reinberg *et al.* 1989), babies in group I have so many other problems that they are unlikely ever to be suitable candidates.

Group II patients present early in life with renal failure and septic complications unless they are identified at birth and treated in specialist units. Group III patients are well in infancy in spite of their obvious abnormalities. It is in these two groups that there is controversy on surgical management. Group II patients have impaired renal function anyway and a urinary tract that promotes inadequate drainage and predisposes to infection. They certainly require some reconstruction, often after temporary diversion by vesicostomy. The argument between the aggressive reconstructors and the conservatives will not be answered except by a controlled trial. Some useful guidance can be gleaned from the long-term results of each group.

**Table 12.1** Classification of prune belly syndrome and relative incidence of groups (Williams & Parker 1974).

Group I
Complete urethral obstruction leading to stillbirth or neonatal death: *c.* 20%

Group II
Infant emergency presentation requiring diversion and some reconstruction of the urinary tract: *c.* 20%

Group III
Well in the neonatal period with good renal function in spite of frightening radiology: *c.* 60%

### Conservative approach

In group III patients Innes Williams followed a policy of minimal surgical interference. It was assumed that the most important level of resistance to urine flow was from the external sphincter distally. It is still unclear whether there is real obstruction or only a relative one. In other words, the urethra and sphincter may be adequate for the normal bladder but too tight for the feeble power of the prune bladder. 'Functional obstruction' seems an appropriate term (Perlmutter & Retik 1970). There may be differences between patients: some have a visible urethral abnormality such as concentric rings or even valves while others are normal. Urodynamics have given conflicting results, most patients having a low pressure system while a few, especially those presenting late, have detrusor instability. The urethral pressure is also low and is lowered further by urethrotomy (Snyder *et al.* 1976). The reflux into hugely dilated upper tracts in the untreated state makes interpretation of intravesical pressures difficult.

After radiological assessment, the policy was to work upwards from the urethra. After each operation further evaluation was made and the next level of potential obstruction was not operated on until it had become clear that the previous surgery had failed to establish adequate emptying of the whole system (Williams & Burkholder 1967).

When I reviewed 27 group III patients from two to 30 years old, the results were good. There were differences between those who presented in the first year of life and those who presented later, sometimes after treatment elsewhere.

Six of 11 who presented early were found to have partial urethral obstruction and incomplete bladder emptying. Urethrotomy was done in five and urethroplasty in one. Five were then able to empty the bladder completely and the sixth required a bladder plication to do so. In four of the six proper emptying allowed the upper tracts to improve while in two apparent vesico-ureteric obstruction was treated by remodelling and reimplantation of the ureters. Five of 11 had no early surgery; three remained well and two had later renal deterioration corrected by urethrotomy.

In the 16 who presented to the unit later in life renal function was less good though none had a plasma urea above normal. Eleven required urethrotomies and one had a partial cystectomy as well. Upper tract surgery was avoided if possible but various operations for reconstruction were done in six.

Successful relief of bladder outflow obstruction produced improved emptying although the bladders remained large (Fig. 12.1). The upper tracts were improved in six of 12 patients for whom complete sets of X-rays were available for retrospective review (Fig. 12.2). Renal growth occurred in unobstructed kidneys providing they had reasonable function to begin with. Upper tract reconstruction seldom improved the X-ray appearances, at best it prevented deterioration. Tailoring of a wide aperistaltic ureter merely resulted in a narrower aperistaltic ureter. In both early and late presenters infected and non-functioning kidneys were removed (two patients in each group).

This policy of minimal surgical interference produced a good result — normal micturition, normal creatinine and little or no infection — in nine of 11 early presenters and 11 of 16 late presenters. Of the other two early presenters, one was lost to follow-up at 15 years old at which time he had a good result; and one was lost from 2 to 7 years old when he re-presented in renal failure and was diverted. In both groups 77% had a good result.

The bad results were one patient in end-stage and one in early renal failure, two hypertensive and one with stones. One patient had a respiratory arrest postoperatively from which he never recovered. No feature could single out boys who would do badly, but there were two pointers. Two boys with parenchymal scars did badly, one becoming hypertensive and the other developing renal failure; four of seven boys with calyceal dilatation have had renal deterioration (Woodhouse *et al.* 1979).

The same group of patients has been reviewed again 10 years later. The good results have been largely maintained. Three men have had recurrent cystitis for which no cause was found. Seventeen of 21 adults (mean age 24.2 years) have normal renal function with a mean GFR of 84.8 ml/min corrected for surface area.

Four adults are in renal failure, three of whom have been transplanted. Four patients are now hypertensive, unrelated to renal failure, so that the rate is 19% (Malone *et al.* 1989).

Although other authors have advocated a conservative approach, there is no large group of patients who have been treated by similar protocols. Palmer and Tesluk emphasised the common finding of urethral stenosis. However, their conservative surgery in four patients consisted of diversion in two (one after failed total reconstruction), limited ureteral reconstruction in one and none in one (1974).

Burke's approach was similar to our own. In a spectrum of 19 patients two were diverted, five had transurethral resections (presumably of some obstructing urethral lesion) and five had no surgery. Only one patient had upper tract reconstruction. With this very conservative approach, seven of 14 patients who were followed up were alive and well at more than 14 years old and five beyond 20 years old. The survivors

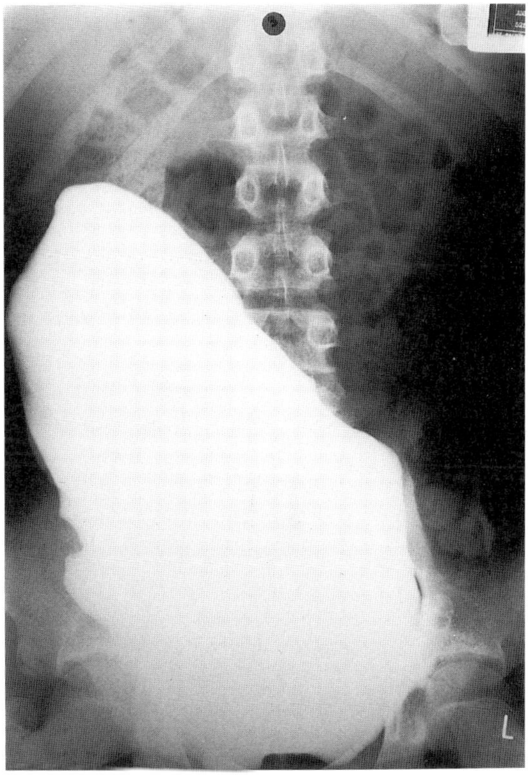


(a)

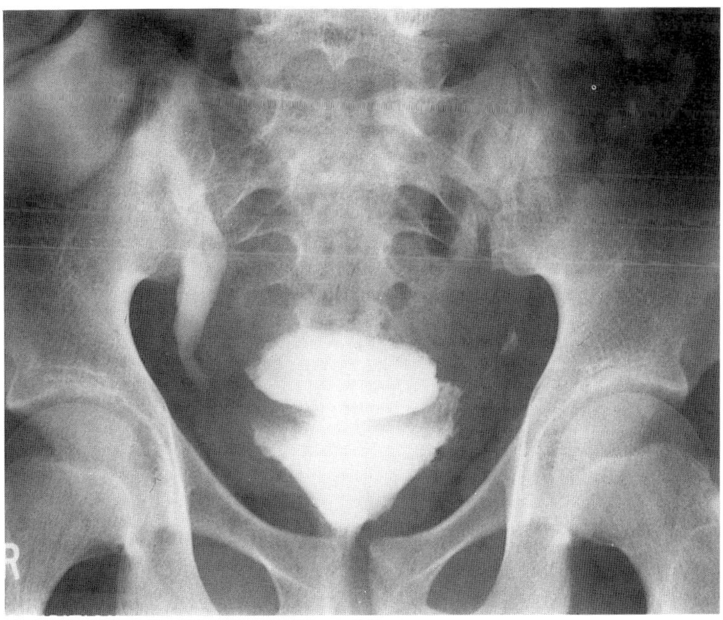


(b)

**Fig. 12.1** Cystograms of a patient with PBS after urethrotomy: (a) before micturition and (b) after micturition.

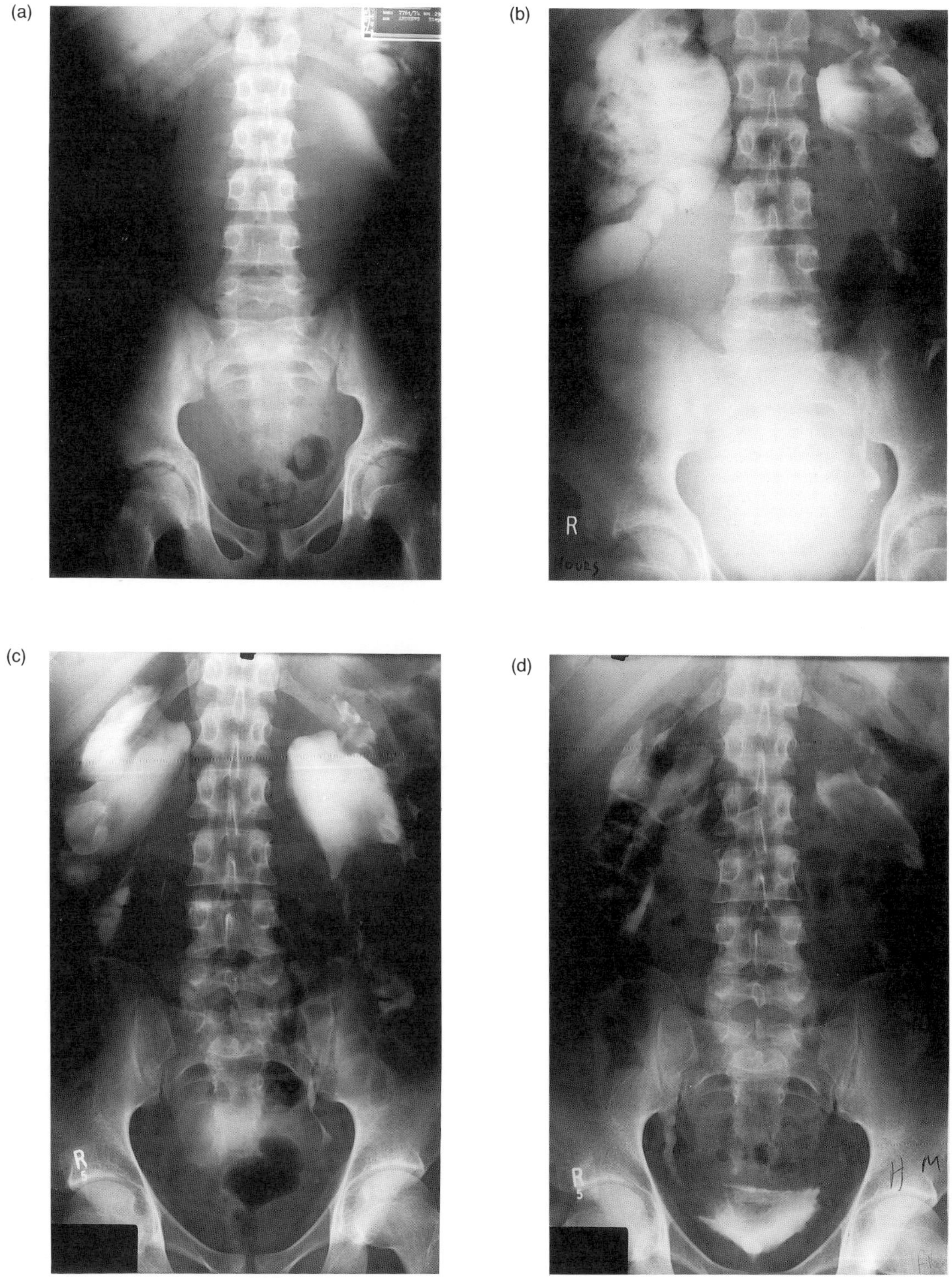
(a)
(b)
(c)
(d)

included three who had TURs and five who had no operation (Burke *et al.* 1969).

The weakness of all of these studies, including our own, is that complete knowledge of the state of the urinary tract, especially of renal function, was not known at the outset or at follow-up. It is possible that the uncorrected urinary tracts are slowly destroying the kidneys and that the normal plasma creatinines do not reflect a stable glomerular filtration rate. It can only be said that late deterioration has not been detected by creatinine measurement or the onset of hypertension and proteinuria. Patients who have done badly started to do so in early childhood.

### Aggressive approach

In group II patients at Great Ormond Street who presented as neonatal emergencies, the management was more aggressive. High diversion was carried out in 12 of 13 cases (though now a vesicostomy would be more likely). In 10 renal function was stabilised. Reconstruction was attempted in six though normal voiding and stable renal function were only achieved in three. In one child stable renal function was never achieved and management was complicated by tuberculosis in mother and child. The boy died of uraemia at 14 years old (Woodhouse *et al.* 1982). Eight are now adults. Three have remained normal with a mean GFR of 58 ml/min (corrected). Five are in renal failure, three of whom have been dialysed or transplanted (Malone *et al.* 1989).

The policy is still to follow a conservative policy. Thirty-one new patients were seen from 1978 to 1988. Eight required diversion and reconstruction and 17 were treated conservatively, usually with a urethrotomy. Six were identified *in utero*, two of whom had vesico-amniotic shunts. Four of these six (including the two shunted patients) developed renal failure soon after birth (H.F. Parkhouse, personal communication 1988).

Lattimer followed an intermediate path. The mortality of 32% occurred within the perinatal period. Twenty-one of his 34 survivors had upper tract reconstruction but in 10 only after preliminary diversion. Eleven patients had no surgery other than orchiopexy. Eight had urethral surgery either alone or as part of overall treatment: it is commented that no urethral surgery had been done since 1977 and it had not been missed. Throughout the 35 years of the series upper tract surgery had only been done for specific indications, mainly reflux and infection. In the later years there was emphasis on full urodynamic assessment. All but two patients were well at follow-up with stable renal function; the two in renal failure had had transplants (Burbige *et al.* 1987).

Other authors have advocated a more aggressive surgical approach in virtually all cases. It is easy to see why: the results of treatment up until the 1950s were very poor. Waldbaum and Marshall pointed out that 86% of patients in their literature review were dead or dying (1970). Welch and Kearney treated their early cases by high or low catheter drainage and 14 patients died of sepsis (1974).

Early and complete reconstruction of the urinary tract has been promoted by these and other authors (Woodard and Parrott 1978, Fallat *et al.* 1989). However, even they include the occasional patient having little or no surgery and others having permanent diversion. Fallat selected obstructed or refluxing ureters for reconstruction. In these series combined, radical

**Fig. 12.2** IVU of the same patient as Fig. 12.1a. Before urethrotomy (July 1974), showing poor excretion on the left and none on the right. (b) After urethrotomy (January 1975), film with bladder full but showing better drainage on the left and good excretion on the right, even allowing for minor right-sided reflux. The GFR at this time was 100 ml/min. (c) IVU in 1985 having had no further treatment, bladder full. (d) Same IVU, film taken after micturition.

reconstruction was done on about 71 patients, 42 of whom did well. Apart from patients who would obviously have fitted into grade I of Williams's classification, all patients appear to have been operated. The earlier two series included several patients from the 1950s when the surgical techniques were being learnt and antibiotics were not so good. The two later series reported good results in 24 of 25 patients between them. Follow-up, particularly in Woodard and Parrott's series, was often short.

The same criticisms can be made of these reports as of those advocating conservative surgery. It has been shown that the surgery can be carried out safely and that renal function, measured by plasma creatinine, is preserved. Late deterioration, in spite of normal creatinine, may occur. It has not been shown whether such surgery is necessary. It is interesting that Fallat comments on her more conservative approach in later cases wtih the advent of more sophisticated methods of investigation.

## Conclusion

Unfortunately, a definite conclusion cannot be drawn. Both approaches are feasible. The fact that a conservative approach appears to have as good results as an aggressive one in correctly selected patients suggests that this is the path to follow first. There is even a difficulty over the role of urethrotomy: one unit finds it to be the mainstay of treatment, while another never uses it! The only approach that can be recommended with confidence is surgery based on sound investigation of urinary tract function rather than anatomy.

Complete reconstruction may be used early for those who are in group II and later for those who fail on conservative management. Whichever path is chosen patients must be closely followed as infection and renal deterioration can occur swiftly in childhood. After puberty the urinary tract seems much safer, infections and renal deterioration are rare.

## Renal failure and transplantation

Up to 30% of prune belly patients who survive infancy develop renal failure. In the infants who die, renal histology shows dysplasia and overall there is insufficient renal parenchyma to support life. The picture in renal failure acquired later is different. In some patients, as our own 'late presentation' group shows, inadequate correction of the urinary drainage system causes slow but continuous damage to the kidneys. In some there is, presumably, hyperfiltration of surviving nephrons leading to nephrosclerosis. In most patients, however, Reinberg has shown gross and histological features of reflux nephropathy and obstruction in renal biopsies of patients in failure (Reinberg *et al.* 1990). The implication of this finding is that attention to the prevention of reflux, obstruction and infection in childhood may prevent later renal failure.

Transplantation with an abnormal lower urinary tract is considered in more detail in Chapter 5. The question that arises in the PBS is whether the renal failure is the end result of inadequately developed kidneys or damage by the bladder and ureters. Before putting a transplant into a prune patient, the bladder must be reassessed, including urodynamically, and consideration given to removing the native kidneys and ureters.

Our own experience has been similar to that of Gonzalez, except that we retained the native upper tracts and he always removed them. In Gonzalez's series of 32 PBS cases from 1970 to 1987, 21 patients survived infancy of whom 10 developed renal failure and eight were transplanted. There was no difference in patient or graft survival between these patients and two age matched controls selected for each patient. Patients were aged 18 or younger except one who was 50 years old. Mean follow-up was 46 months (range three to 126). Patient survival was 87% and graft survival 75% (Reinberg *et al.* 1989).

We have done six transplants in five patients.

There was one acute rejection. One was lost by chronic rejection at 7 years and one when the patient developed a lymphoma at 5 years. All patients are alive and three kidneys survive (at 5, 5 and 6 years respectively).

## THE TESTES

Males with PBS have normal erections, intercourse and orgasms. Most have limited ejaculation and all who have been investigated have had azoospermia. None has fathered a child. The patients who are now adults had orchiopexies relatively late in life, seldom before 8 years old. The results of early orchiopexy, especially using the Fowler–Stephens method of preliminary ligation of the testicular artery, are awaited.

We have investigated 18 patients aged 16 to 28 years old. All but the youngest patient had developed to complete and normal puberty, though three were anorchic and had testosterone supplements. Serum testosterones were normal in 14 and low in four. Serum LHs were normal or high but FSHs were all high, in four cases more than four times normal. A high pituitary drive appears necessary for the rather poor testicles.

The sexual activities of nine were investigated in more detail. Libido was normal. All patients claimed to have normal erections and orgasms (though one did not admit to masturbation or to having intercourse). Seven had retrograde ejaculation. Five were having regular intercourse (Woodhouse & Snyder 1985).

Ejaculated semen was provided by five, all having azoospermia. Six produced urine after masturbation, one of which showed some sperm, 30% with sluggish movement. One of six testicular biopsies showed some early spermatogenesis. The rest showed sertoli cells only with Johnson counts of one or two and no carcinoma *in situ* (Woodhouse & Snyder 1985, Malone *et al.* 1989).

It is not known whether the prune testis is doomed from its formation or has potential for fertility if it were brought down early. Histology of fetal testes in prune belly syndrome shows some spermatogonia in all cases but in smaller numbers than normal (Orvis *et al.* 1988). The fact that the fetuses were available for postmortem study suggests that they were from the worst group and others might have better spermatogenesis. The presence of any spermatogonia in the fetal testes and a few sperm in one of my patients are encouraging signs.

One of our patients has developed a classical

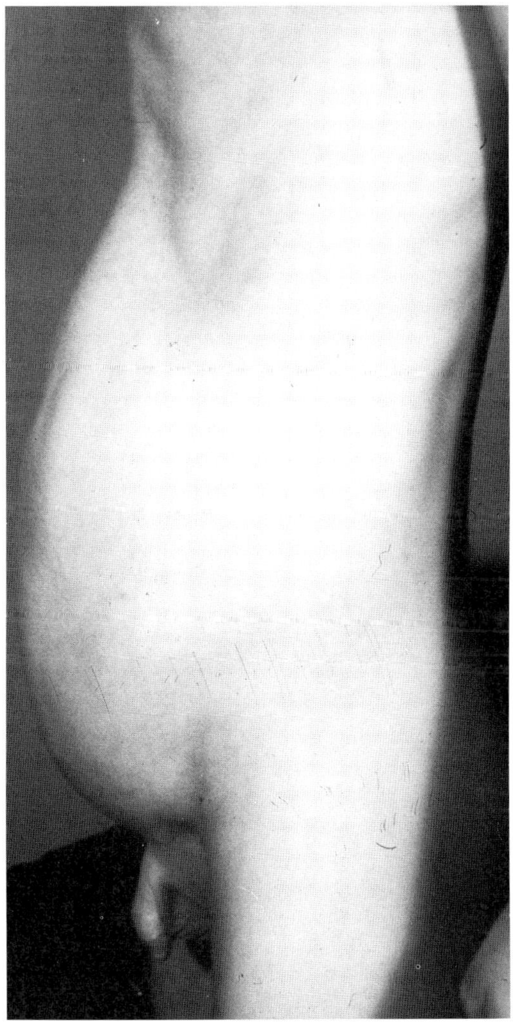

**Fig. 12.3** Abdominal wall of a PBS patient at 12 years old.

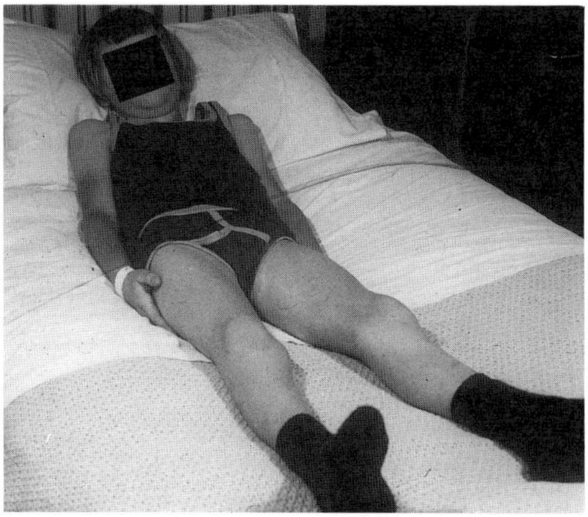

(a)

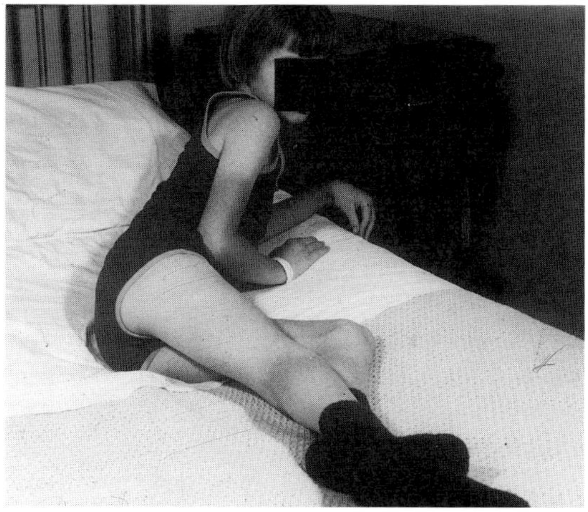

(b)

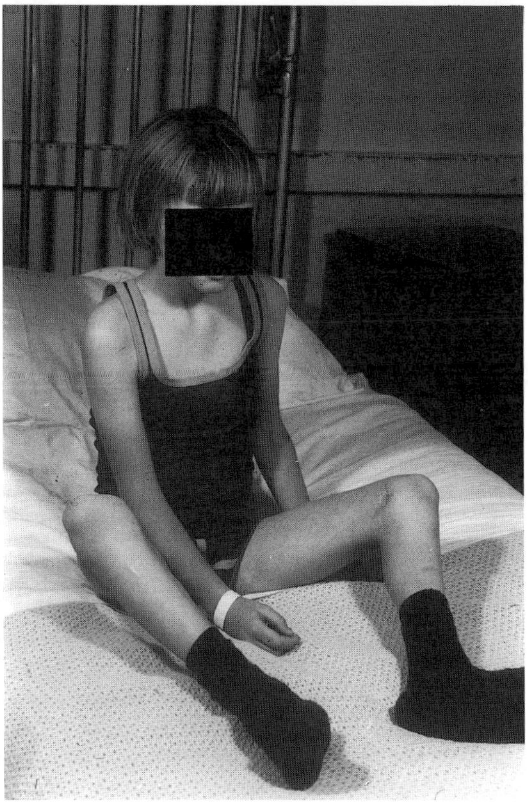

(c)

**Fig. 12.4** Sequence to show how a PBS patient sits up from the lying position. (a) Supine. (b) Rolls to one side. (c) Sitting up.

non-seminomatous germ cell tumour of the testis. He was treated by orchiectomy and chemotherapy and remains well at 10 years' follow-up (Woodhouse & Ransley 1983). A retroperitoneal germ cell tumour has also been reported (Sayre *et al.* 1986).

## THE ABDOMINAL WALL

Early experience suggested that the absence of muscle in the anterior abdominal wall was not of functional importance. In our series three boys had abdominal wall plications but it seemed to make little difference to function or appearance. By the end of childhood the wrinkled skin is smoothed out and replaced by a premature 'beer belly' (Fig. 12.3). Adults are often strikingly tall and athletic. The only action that they cannot make is to sit up directly from the supine position: they have to roll to one side first (Fig. 12.4). They can flex their hips while supine as this is a function of the iliacus and psoas muscles (Fig. 12.5).

In a more recent review of this subject, Ehrlich has suggested that abdominal wall reconstruction is an important part of management. The wrinkled appearance was thought to be offensive to children. Correction by an overlapping repair (similar to the Mayo repair of umbilical hernias) led to better social adjustment and, probably, fewer respiratory infections in eight boys. This style of repair was said to be more effective than simple plication or than excision of the lower abdominal wall. Recurrence of the laxity of the abdomen did not occur at least in the 2 years of follow-up available (Ehrlich *et al.* 1986).

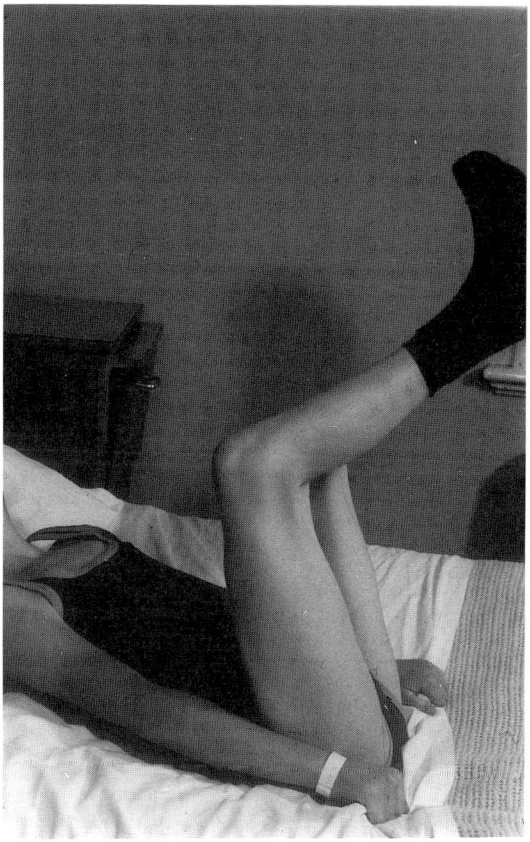

**Fig. 12.5** PBS patient showing hip flexion while lying supine.

**Table 12.2** Social development in 27 prune belly patients surviving to adulthood.

| Outcome | Patients | Occupation/state | Number |
|---|---|---|---|
| Good | 23* | Higher professional | 3 |
| | | Nurse | 1 |
| | | Skilled technician | 2 |
| | | Semi-skilled | 3 |
| Poor | 4 | Mentally retarded | 1 |
| | | Pethidine addict | 1 |
| | | Alcoholic | 1 |
| | | Behavioural problems | 1† |

* Excluding students and those with inadequate information.

† Patient thought to be normal at 18 years old.

## SOCIAL DEVELOPMENT

In series where the information is given and certainly my own, the boys have grown up normally. They have gone to normal schools and played normal games. Amongst my patients are a rock climber and a long distance competition cyclist. Later development has been in keeping with education and social background in 23 of 27 surviving adults (details are shown in Table 12.2).

## REFERENCES


Burbige K.A., Amodio J., Berdon W.E. *et al.* (1987) Prune belly syndrome: 35 years of experience. *J. Urol.* **137**, 86–90.

Burke E.C., Shin M.I. & Kelalis P.P. (1969) Prune belly syndrome. *Am. J. Dis. Child.* **117**, 668–71.

Ehrlich R.M., Lesavoy M.A. & Fine R.N. (1986) Total abdominal wall reconstruction in the prune belly syndrome. *J. Urol.* **136**, 282–5.

Fallat M.E., Skoog S.J., Belman A.B., Eng G. & Randolph J.G. (1989) The prune belly syndrome: a comprehensive approach to management. *J. Urol.* **142**, 802–5.

Greskovich F.J. & Nyberg L.M. (1988) The prune belly syndrome: a review of its etiology, defects, treatment and prognosis. *J. Urol.* **140**, 707–12.

Malone P.R., Parkhouse H.F., Duffy P.G., Ransley P.G. & Woodhouse C.R.J. (1989) Prune belly syndrome: a long term follow-up. *Paper read at the Annual Meeting of the British Association of Urological Surgeons*, Jersey, June 1989, (Abstract 128).

Orvis B.R., Bottles K. & Kogan B.A. (1988) Testicular histology in fetuses with the prune belly syndrome and posterior urethral valves. *J. Urol.* **139**, 335–7.

Pagon R.A., Smith D.W. & Shepard T.H. (1979) Urethral obstruction malformation complex: a cause of abdominal muscle deficiency and the prune belly syndrome. *J. Pediatr.* **94**, 900–6.

Palmer J.M. & Tesluk H. (1974) Ureteral pathology in the prune belly syndrome. *J. Urol.* **111**, 701–7.

Perlmutter A.D. & Retik A.B. (1970) Prune belly syndrome (letter). *Am. J. Dis. Child.* **119**, 191.

Reinberg Y., Manivel J.C., Fryd D., Najarian J.S. & Gonzalez R. (1989) The outcome of renal transplantation in children with the prune belly syndrome. *J. Urol.* **142**, 1541–2.

Reinberg Y., Manivel C., Pettinatto G. & Gonzalez R. (1990) Development of renal failure in children with prune belly syndrome. *J. Urol.* (in press). (personal communication).

Riccardi V.M. & Grum C.M. (1977) The prune belly anomaly. *J. Genet. Med.* **14**, 266–70.

Sayre R., Stephens R. & Chonko A.M. (1986) Prune belly syndrome and retroperitoneal germ cell tumour. *Am. J. Med.* **81**, 895–6.

Smythe A.R. (1981) Ultrasonic detection of fetal ascites and bladder dilatation with resulting prune belly. *J. Pediatr.* **98**, 978–80.

Snyder H.M., Harrison N.W., Whitfield H.N. & Williams D.I. (1976) Urodynamics in the prune belly syndrome. *Br. J. Urol.* **48**, 663–70.

Waldbaum R.S. & Marshall V.F. (1970) The prune belly syndrome: a diagnostic therapeutic plan. *J. Urol.* **103**, 668–74.

Welch K.J. & Kearney G.P. (1974) Abdominal musculature deficiency syndrome: prune belly. *J. Urol.* **111**, 693–700.

Williams D.I. & Burkholder G.V. (1967) The prune belly syndrome. *J. Urol.* **98**, 244–51.

Williams D.I. & Parker R.M. (1974) The role of surgery in the prune belly syndrome. In: Johnston J.H. & Goodwin W.E. (eds). *Reviews in Paediatric Urology.* Excerpta Medica, Amsterdam, pp. 315–31.

Woodard J.R. & Parrott T.S. (1978) Reconstruction of the urinary tract in prune belly uropathy. *J. Urol.* **119**, 824–8.

Woodhouse C.R.J., Kellett M.J. & Williams D.I. (1979) Minimal surgical interference in the prune belly syndrome. *Br. J. Urol.* **51**, 475–80.

Woodhouse C.R.J., Ransley P.G. & Williams D.I. (1982) Prune belly syndrome — a report of 47 cases. *Arch. Dis. Child.* **57**, 856–9.

Woodhouse C.R.J. & Ransley P.G. (1983) Teratoma of the testis in prune belly syndrome. *Br. J. Urol.* **55**, 580–1.

Woodhouse C.R.J. & Snyder H.M. (1985) Testicular function in adults with prune belly syndrome. *J. Urol.* **133**, 607–9.

# 13 *Exstrophy and epispadias*

## INTRODUCTION

Exstrophy of the bladder is part of a spectrum of congenital anomalies of the lower urinary tract. The most minor form is an epispadiac position of the urethra on a normal penis with a normal prepuce. The most extreme examples have cloacal exstrophy with anomalies of the genitalina, bladder and hindgut. The most numerous group have classical exstrophy as a largely isolated anomaly. An intermediate group have major epispadias with a split symphysis pubis: they are likely to be incontinent from deficient urethral sphincters and to have the same genital deformities as the classical exstrophy patient. About two-thirds of the patients are male.

Classical exstrophy has been recognised for about 2000 years and has been the subject of voluminous surgical literature since the middle of the last century. It is not surprising to find that there is little new in the contemporary surgery for this condition. The posterior pelvic osteotomy and bladder reconstruction used by Trendelenburg in Leipzig at the turn of the century is similar to that used today. He also mentioned that Thiersch had implanted a 'special mechanical contrivance' to maintain continence after reconstruction, which sounds like a fixed pressure artificial sphincter (Trendelenburg 1906). The photographs in Trendelenburg's paper show a very acceptable cosmetic result and a young boy able to void with a most impressive stream. As so often, it is not the surgical ideas that have changed with time, but the materials and drugs necessary to support those ideas.

## MORTALITY

Exstrophy is not, in itself, a lethal abnormality but the complications and treatment often were. In 1926 it was recorded that, historically, 50% of patients were dead by 10 and 67% by 20 years old. The contemporary series of 66 patients reported a 28% mortality but nearly half the living patients were under 10 years old. There was long-term follow-up on 20 patients from 30 to 73 years old (Mayo & Hendricks 1926).

All the advances in paediatric medicine and surgery have contributed to a dramatic fall in mortality. In 140 cases in New York from 1945 to 1970, only five deaths are recorded, three of which were in patients with ureterosigmoidostomies. Obviously the follow-up was short in some cases and 39 were lost altogether so the overall mortality may have been higher (Megali & Lattimer 1973).

It is interesting to look at the causes of death and to note that it is difficult to relate some to the exstrophy. Our own adult series includes 101 cases with a minimum follow-up of 18 years with only 10 patients lost before puberty. There were nine deaths and as their follow-up has continued no more have died since the original report. The causes and times of death are shown in Table 13.1; only four can be attributed to the exstrophy and its treatment (Woodhouse *et al.* 1983).

Late deaths show a similar pattern. In a group of 87 patients presenting between 1912 and 1935 and reviewed in 1974, the 25 deaths could all be attributed to the urinary diversion by ureterosigmoidostomy or to non-urinary tract causes (Segura & Kelalis 1975).

**Table 13.1** Causes of death and ages at death in 101 cases of exstrophy (Woodhouse *et al.* 1983).

| Cause of death | Number | Age |
|---|---|---|
| *Urological* | | |
| Renal failure* | 2 | 8 months |
| | | 12 years |
| Ca. bladder* | 1 | 29 years |
| *Non-urological* | | |
| Intestinal obstruction | 2 | 7 years |
| | | 10 years |
| Inhalation of vomit | 1 | 5 years |
| Carcinoma of colon* | 1 | 30 years |
| Poliomyelitis | 1 | 3 months |
| Unknown (?accident) | 1 | 17 years |

* Deaths related to exstrophy and its treatment

## THE BLADDER

Although good functional results have been reported for bladder closure by several authors over the last 100 years, the percentage of fully continent exstrophy patients was small. Reviewing the literature over the previous 60 years Marshall and Muecke found that only 5% had a 'good' result and 14% a 'fair' result from bladder reconstruction. Their own series had a 20% 'good' result rate but follow-up was short (1970). In 1973, with experience of 140 patients, Megali and Lattimer recommended ileal conduit diversion to give the best social and psychological results with the least morbidity (1973).

The policy at Great Ormond Street, UK at that time was to close only those bladders that appeared to have a reasonable size and to have good tissue. The decision was usually taken at 6 to 18 months of age. With this policy an attempt was made to close 62 of 101 bladders. Many techniques were tried but the outcome appeared to depend more on the original bladder size than anything else; performance of a pelvic osteotomy and age at surgery were irrelevant. Indeed, most of the patients who had an osteotomy had re-established a widely open symphysis by adult life without adverse effect on their continence. Completely reliable continence was achieved in five of 21 girls and five of 41 boys. One other girl had partial continence requiring the use of one pad per day. One other boy, who later died, was enuretic though dry by day (Woodhouse *et al.* 1983). The greater success rate in girls has been noted by others and remains unexplained.

The continent exstrophy bladder in adult life has maintained its function but is beginning to give me some concern. Four patients have now formed stones. When they are cystoscoped, the bladder looks like the inside of an egg shell even though it does not appear calcified on plain X-ray. I presume that fragments break off the wall from time to time and form the nucleus for a proper stone. There have been no renal stones so far.

Stone formation has usually, but not always, been associated with persistent infection with urea splitting bacteria. In one patient treatment with the urease inhibitor acetohydroxamic acid abolished the symptoms of severe frequency and intermittent dysuria but has not prevented stone formation.

Bladder sensation and voiding frequency appear to be normal. However, one 24 year old female developed a dilated kidney due to progressive deterioration in compliance. She is now on intermittent clean self-catheterisation (ICSC). Another girl is showing early signs of the same problem. None of the patients treated at that time had bowel augmentations.

In the long-term, once continence is established, it is maintained. In the few patients with borderline continence, there does not seem to be improvement with time. Although prostatic growth at puberty is said to produce continence in the 'semi-continent' boy (Duckett & Caldemone 1984), I have not had this happy experience and two boys have passed through puberty without any improvement.

Although the long-term outcome for exstrophy patients is excellent, constant vigilance, even in those who appear to have been stable for years, is essential.

Now, reconstruction in the first day or so of life has produced continence and good bladder function in 60–86% of patients. In patients who do not become continent or whose bladders are unsuitable for closure, bladder augmentation with or without an artificial urinary sphincter are useful additional techniques (Arap *et al.* 1980, Duckett & Caldemone 1984, Light & Scott 1984, Diamond & Ransley 1986). There is no long-term follow-up on these patients, but there is no reason to doubt that the results will be a further improvement in the quality of life for the exstrophy patient.

There is little independent evidence of the results in patients with epispadias and sphincter deficiency, mainly because the number of patients is so small. It is certainly easier to make them continent than the classical exstrophy patients. In my experience about half the patients have a working bladder and I have not encountered the same long-term problems as occur in exstrophy. In more recently treated patients a continence rate of 87% has been reported (Peters *et al.* 1988).

## Failed bladder reconstruction

Many centres will be unable to achieve the spectacular results of reconstruction reported by the great hospitals. Even amongst the greats there may be some failures. Mucosal cystectomy and urinary diversion will be necessary. Many of the techniques discussed in Chapter 11 are appropriate. My own preference is to form a bowel reservoir and implant the appendix using the Mitrofanoff technique. The patients practise ICSC. Paediatric urologists should resist the temptation to remove the appendix in case it should become useful later. Patients with cloacal exstrophy may have two appendices, one of which has been used for a Mitrofanoff and the other retained as a spare, in a recent difficult case (P.G. Ransley, personal communication 1989).

There is still a place for the ureterosigmoidostomy. The short-comings and complications are discussed in Chapter 10. This form of diversion is occasionally used in Europe and remains popular in developing countries where the support necessary for any form of major reconstruction is lacking. Even in America it still enjoys some support (King 1984, Zabbo & Kay 1986).

## Bladder cancer

The histology of the bladder mucosa in untreated exstrophy has been described. Below the ureteric orifices it is transitional cell, in the middle it shows glandular metaplasia and at the top there is squamous metaplasia merging into normal skin (Williams 1977). With time all bladders develop acute and chronic inflammation. About 45% show generalised squamous metaplasia (Engel & Wilkinson 1970).

Up to 1955, 40 carcinomas had been reported in untreated exstrophy bladders, 33 adenocarcinomas, two squamous and five of unknown origin (McIntosh & Worley 1955). In 1944 the incidence of carcinoma in the exstrophy bladder was calculated to be 4% (Wattenburg *et al.* 1956).

There have been few reports since that time. The only case that I have encountered was in a 40 year old with untreated exstrophy. A case was reported in 1979 in a 71 year old patient who had remained untreated until 59 years old when he had had a diversion leaving the bladder *in situ* (Yannopoulos & Kyriakidis 1979).

If the glandular area is in the middle of the bladder, it would be expected that patients treated by early cystectomy and diversion would not be at special risk of adenocarcinoma. If the patient has been diverted but the bladder left behind after closure, there may be a theoretical risk remaining but in practice cases do not seem to occur.

Strachan has reviewed the cancers occurring

in our patients. He divided the adult patients into those who had ever had urine and faeces mixed (high-risk group — 42 patients) and those who had early ileal or colonic loop diversions (low-risk group — 61 patients). No cancers occurred in the low-risk group. In the 'high-risk' group eight patients developed colonic neoplasms (see Chapter 10). Interestingly two other patients in the 'high-risk' group are said to have died of adenocarcinoma of the bladder at 28 and 34 years old though both had had cystectomies in early childhood. In one the information came only from the family doctor's record and there was no postmortem. The other had a postmortem and it is said that the ureterocolonic anastomoses were normal, the cancer arising from the bladder remnant (Strachan & Woodhouse 1990). Although the evidence, at least in the second case, strongly supports a bladder origin, the niggling doubt remains that the ureterosigmoidostomy had something to do with the cancers.

I have been worried that recurrent pyocystis might initiate cancer in such bladders and have encouraged patients to have mucosal cystectomies. In one bladder removed after nearly 30 years of recurrent infection there were changes in the mucosa that the histopathologist thought might be a premalignant change; the patient remains well at 5-year follow-up. Chronic infection usually induces squamous metaplasia and only occasionally an adenomatous change (Polsky *et al.* 1976) and so the cancer, if it occurred, would be squamous cell in origin, as in other bladders left behind.

A bladder that has never been exposed to urine is unlikely to develop transitional cell carcinoma (TCC). The absence of the carcinogens in urine would be protective. Indeed, even in bladders that have already developed TCC, diversion of the urine alone may cause regression (Everson & Cole 1966).

Whether or not the epithelium returns to normal after successful bladder closure is not known. In the functioning exstrophy bladder the risk of TCC is, presumably, the same as for any normal individual. It might be increased if the bladder was chronically infected or had repeated stones. The augmented bladder might have a risk of carcinoma for the reasons discussed in Chapter 10, but there is no evidence so far.

## THE KIDNEYS

Most exstrophy patients have normal kidneys at birth. In our adult series one child had a solitary normal kidney and two had bilateral hydronephrosis (Woodhouse *et al.* 1983). Most series do not record the condition of the kidneys at birth and it may be that the short-comings of neonatal investigation 20 or more years ago mean that even the kidneys reported in our series were not as normal as we thought. Lattimer reports that 33% of his patients had dilated ureters at the time of presentation (not at birth), but does not comment on the kidneys. However, the pyelograms of many of these patients were normal after diversion, suggesting that the preoperative hydro-ureter was not significant (Lattimer *et al.* 1960).

It is clear, however, that subsequent renal deterioration is the result of surgery and its complications. In the short-term diversion or reconstructive surgery may damage about 20% of normal kidneys. Turner calculated a figure of 15% for patients at Great Ormond Street, UK having primary reconstructions of the bladder (Turner *et al.* 1980). Lattimer's view that dilated upper tracts improve with diversion must be accepted, but is probably not relevant to current patients having reconstructions on the first day or so of life. The early renal complication rate is probably the same whether the surgery is for reconstruction or diversion (Demaria *et al.* 1980).

The late results are dependent on the ultimate fate of the bladder. The incidence of upper tract damage is high, though renal failure is rare at least in the first 30 years of life. Looking at our own patients retrospectively, I have found it difficult always to find at exactly which point renal damage occurred. The long-term results shown in Table 13.2 indicate that an ileal conduit carries a worse prognosis for the kidneys than a ureterosigmoidostomy. This may be a false assumption because many patients had a ureterosigmoidostomy first, then a switch to an ileal loop for 'failure' which may have included unrecognised structural damage to the kidneys. Thus the ileal loop may have got the blame for the short-comings of the ureterosigmoidostomy.

In the long-term (up to 25 years), the kidneys do much better with a working bladder: the Toronto group found renal damage in 13% of 51 patients successfully reconstructed against 82% with ileal conduits, 22% for non-refluxing colonic conduits and 33% for ureterosigmoidostomies (Husman *et al.* 1988). All diversions have a high rate of renal damage (Table 13.2).

## THE PENIS

Reconstructive surgery of the basic bladder condition has progressed so much that patients can now live a normal life and, in the last 15 years, can expect to have a normally working bladder. Although it has always been recognised that the penis required reconstruction as well, a good functional result for sexual intercourse was not always achieved. It will be seen that the exstrophy patient now grows up in ordinary society and has the same sexual and reproductive aspirations as his more normal peers.

It is clear both from my own patients and from the experience of other groups that exstrophy patients grow up very well. They are highly motivated and hard-working people who make light of their problems. Their libido is high. It is a matter of priority to reconstruct the genitalia to allow normal intercourse to take place.

Patients with epispadias with a split symphysis have the same genital anomalies as are found in exstrophy. In this section the terms 'exstrophy penis', 'exstropy pelvis', etc. include the same anomalies in epispadiac patients.

**Table 13.2** The renal consequences of exstrophy management for 151 *kidneys* in 76 patients. All *kidneys* were believed to be normal at birth, one infant had congenital absence of a kidney. (Woodhouse *et al.* 1983).

| Lower tract | Normal kidneys | Damaged kidneys | | Change of diversion | % with any renal damage |
|---|---|---|---|---|---|
| | | Mild/moderate | Severe | | |
| Continent | 18 | 6 | | | 25 |
| Incontinent | 2 | 2 | | | 50 |
| Ureterosigmoidostomy | | | | | |
| Failed bladder reconstruction | 14 | 6 | | 8 | 50 |
| Primary | 10 | 3 | 1 | 8 | 55 |
| Ileal loop | | | | | |
| Failed bladder reconstruction | 5 | 14 | 9 | 2 | 83 |
| Primary | 9 | 11 | 4 | | 63 |
| Rectal bladder* | | | | | |
| Failed bladder reconstruction | | 2 | 2 | 2 | 100 |
| Primary | 3 | 1 | | | 25 |
| Colon loop | | | | | |
| Failed bladder reconstruction | 1 | 3 | | | 75 |
| Primary | 6 | | | | 0 |
| Cutaneous ureterostomy | 2 | 3 | | | 60 |

## Penile anatomy

The typical exstrophy penis is short and broad. When seen in the flaccid state it certainly does not 'dangle'. Its shortness is emphasised by the normal size of the scrotum and the recession of the lower abdominal wall (Fig. 13.1). Except in the rare cases where the penis has become buried in the scrotum due to previous surgery, no operation will make the exstrophy penis significantly longer.

The orientation of the inferior pubic rami and the attachments of the deep parts of the corpora are unlike those of normal males. The findings by cavernosogram, by computerised tomography (CT) and at anterior exenteration of an exstrophy patient with bladder carcinoma are consistent (Woodhouse & Kellett 1984). The symphysis is not only open but the pelvis is rotated caudally so that the inferior pubic ramus is parallel to the floor when the patient is standing (Fig. 13.2).

The oblique view of the pelvis gives a true lateral view of the inferior pubic ramus. The orientation of the inferior pubic rami is seen in Fig. 13.3. Cavernosogram in this projection shows that the deep parts of the corpora are similarly lying horizontally.

Comparison of the cavernosogram in exstrophy with that of anatomically normal men shows the reason for the shortness of the penis (Fig. 13.4). It is not, as might be thought, that the symphysis is open causing most of the penis to be buried in the perineum. The corpora are actually deficient in length although of normal calibre.

Further evidence for this view has been provided by the results of surgical apposition of the pubic bones in infancy. In cases reported by Johnston and in my own cases, those who had successful apposition of the pubis as part of their original bladder closure do not have a longer penis than others (Johnston 1974).

It would be wrong to draw firm conclusions from the single patient who has had CT of the pelvis, but the pictures do, at least, confirm the cavernosographic findings. The patient illustrated in Fig. 13.5 had had no treatment of any kind for his exstrophy until he presented with carcinoma of the bladder. Comparison with the CT of a normal pelvis at about the same level shows the shortness of the deep part of the corpora between the attachment to the inferior pubic ramus and the anterior border of the perineum. When this patient came to anterior

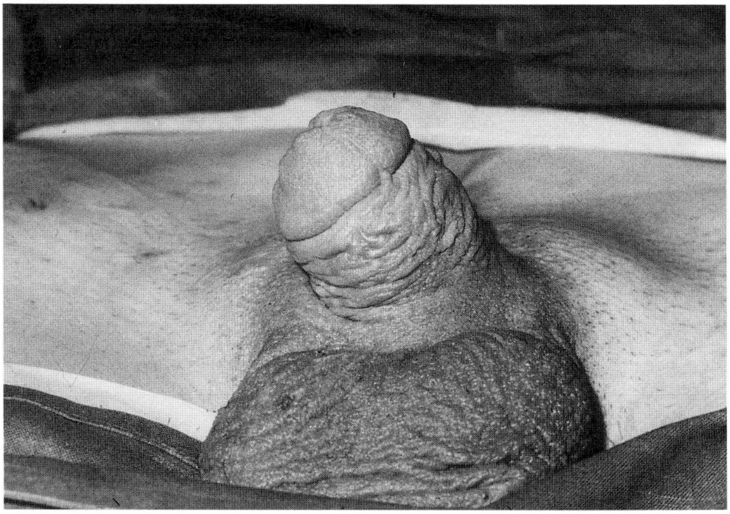

**Fig. 13.1** Typical exstrophy penis, flaccid.

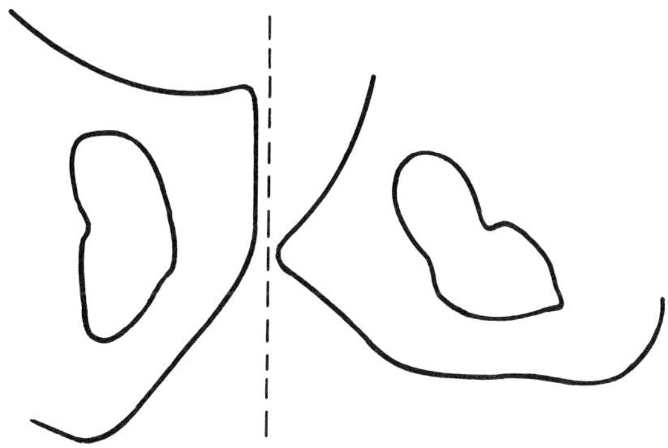

**Fig. 13.2** Diagram of the pelvic orientation: left, normal and right, exstrophy (from Woodhouse & Kellett 1984, with permission).

pelvic exenteration the pelvic anatomy confirmed the radiographic appearances and in particular the orientation of the inferior pubic ramus.

I have not had an opportunity to do pelvic arteriography. The flow of contrast into the veins that occurs with cavernosography and the operative findings suggest that the blood supply of the exstrophy penis is normal. The main supply (and certainly the main venous drainage) appears to come from the pudendal vessels passing through Alcock's canal.

These anatomical findings have important implications for any proposed penile lengthening procedure. Firstly, no dissection posterior to the junction with the pubic body will give any penile lengthening. Secondly, the suggestion that the corpora could be completely detached from the inferior pubic rami and pulled forward (Kelley & Eraklis 1971) seems a theoretically dangerous procedure because of the risk of devascularising the corpora.

The position of the superficial neurovascular bundles reflects the lateral rotation or 'kippering' of the corpora. They lie in the true lateral position in the distal and middle portions of the corpora, moving dorsolaterally as they pass proximally (Fig. 13.6). These positions were found to be constant in five primary cases and 13 revision cases dissected at surgery in our unit (Hurwitz *et al.* 1986).

## Investigation

An artificial erection, either by intracorporeal injection of papaverine or by infusion, will demon-

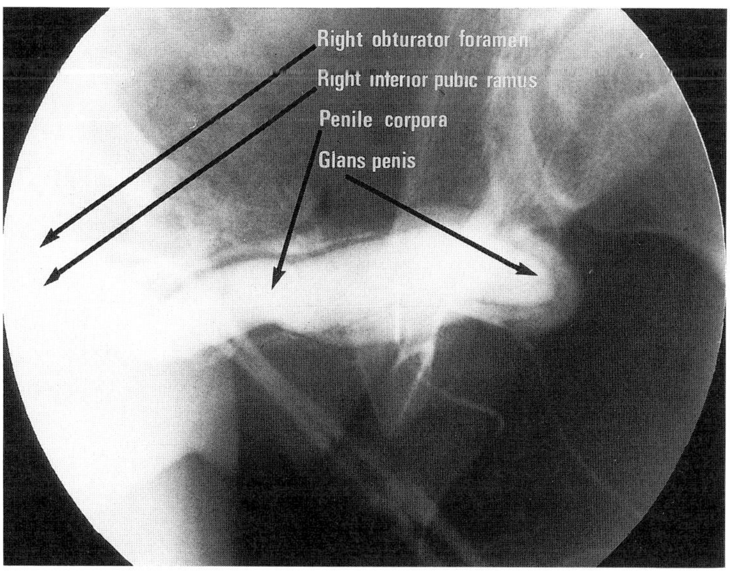


**Fig. 13.3** Oblique view of a cavernosogram in an exstrophy patient showing the relationship of the corpora to the pubis. Note that the penis is parallel to the floor (from Woodhouse & Kellett 1984, with permission).

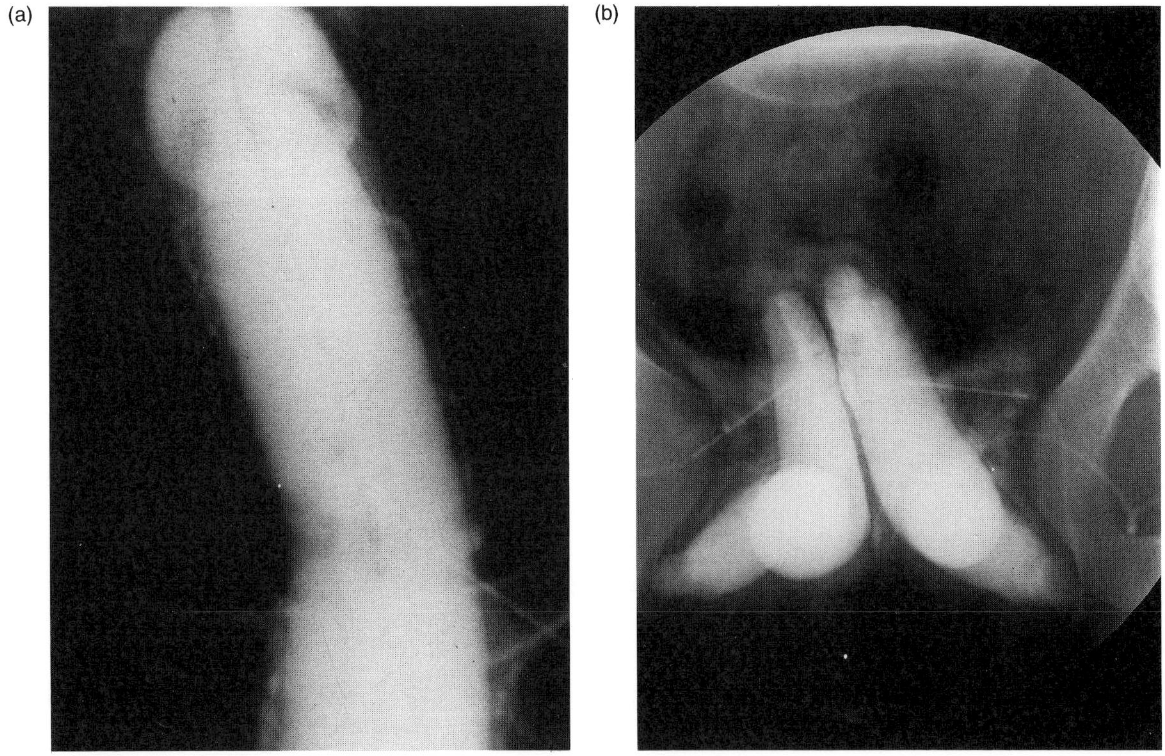


**Fig. 13.4** Cavernosograms of (a) a normal penis, and (b) an exstrophy penis (from Woodhouse & Kellett 1984, with permission).

strate the erectile deformity. It will not define the anatomy of the deep portion of the corpora. Unless the patient describes an uncomplicated dorsal chordee and the deep parts of the corpora are palpably normal, a cavernosogram is essential.

The cavernosogram technique is modified from that described by Herzberg (Herzberg *et al.* 1981). The corpora must be infused separately because there is no cross-circulation. 120 ml of 65% urograffin in 250 ml of physiological saline is used. A pressure of 300 mm of mercury is generated by Fenwall bags (Fig. 13.7). The corpora are punctured with 19 gauge butterfly needles. No tourniquet should be used as it would obscure the true chordee which occurs in the deep part of the corpora.

### Erectile deformities

All exstrophy males complain of dorsal chordee on erection (Fig. 13.8). The degree of chordee is variable. In some the angle is such that sexual intercourse is possible either in the conventional position or in one that brings the female introitus in more direct apposition to the penis (Fig. 13.9).

Chordee is such a constant finding that I regard it as a part of the exstrophy/epispadias complex. It is found in epispadiacs who have had little or no surgical dissection at the base of the penis. It was seen in two classical exstrophy patients who had no surgical procedure of any kind until they were past 35 years old. On erection the penis is tightly curved and almost digs into the anterior abdominal wall. It might be thought that this deformity was due to the scar tissue around the

(a)

(b)

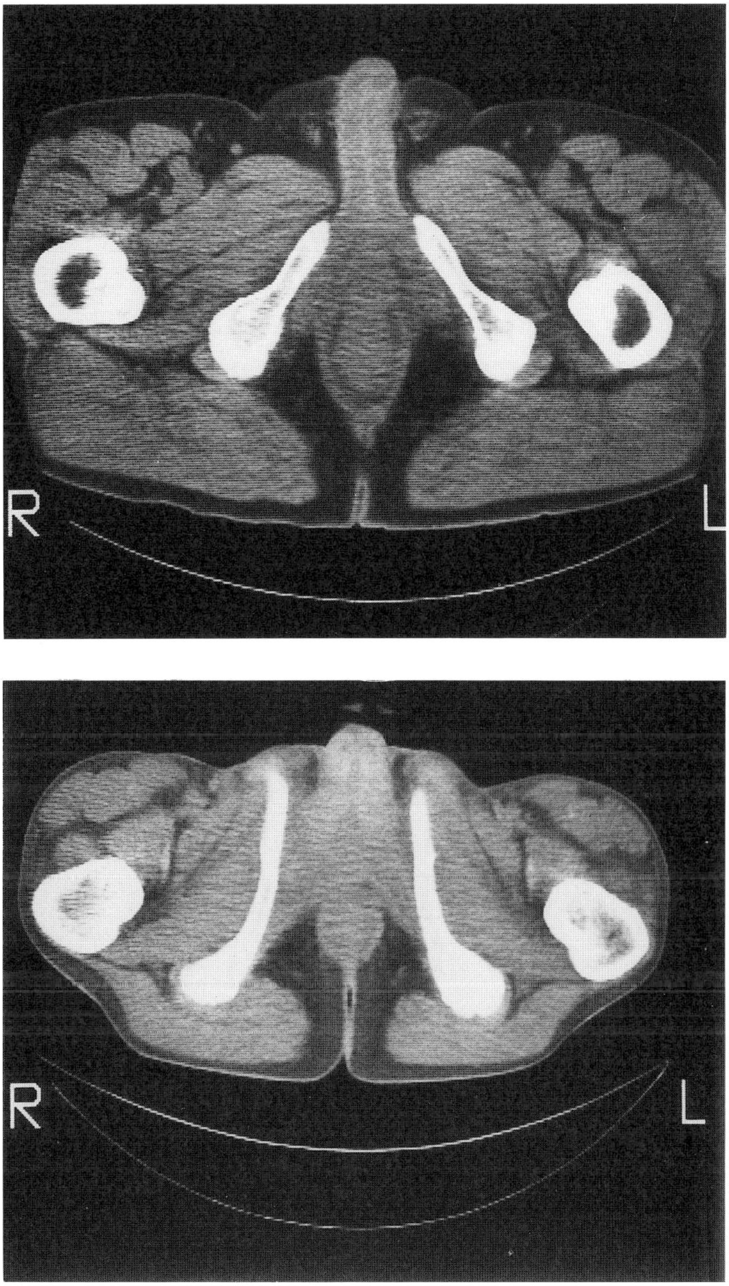


**Fig. 13.5** CT at approximately the same level, showing sections through the lower pelvis of (a) a normal man, and (b) an exstrophy patient. Note how short the deep parts of the corpora are, especially from the anterior end of the inferior pubic ramus to the surface, in the exstrophy patient (from Woodhouse & Kellett 1984, with permission).

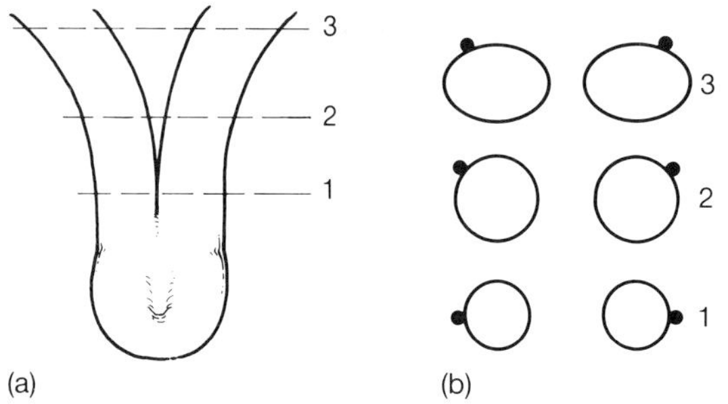


**Fig. 13.6** Diagrams of the anatomy of the superficial neurovascular bundles in exstrophy. Dorsal view of the penis (a). Transverse sections at the levels indicated showing the bundles (b) (from Hurwitz *et al.* 1986, with permission).

dorsally placed urethra. It has been said that clearance of the scar and detachment of the urethra correct the chordee. I have only found this to be so in one of 32 operated cases. Although the original problem may have been a congenitally short urethral plate, by adulthood the basic problem is intrinsic curvature of the corpora. Cavernosogram in these cases shows that the site of the maximum curvature is at the point where the corpora emerge from the perineum (Fig. 13.10).

A more complex deformity occurs when one or both of the corpora are abnormal. If one corpus fails to fill on erection it acts as a 'bow-string' on the other and causes lateral deviation in addition to the dorsal chordee (Fig. 13.11).

If both corpora are rudimentary, the visible or exophytic part of the penis is normal except that it is a little higher than usual on the abdomen. On cavernosography the corpora appear to have no attachment to the pubic rami. Erection is very limited and the penis unstable (Figs 13.12 and 13.13). In one patient the whole of one corpus and the exophytic part of the other is missing so that there is no visible penis at all.

Only one of the patients with this abnormality has intercourse and he managed to fracture his corpus during vigorous penetration (Fig. 13.13). It failed to heal spontaneously after 4 weeks. After localised surgical repair he was impotent for several months but then returned to normal. This patient is the only example I have found with cross-circulation between the corpora and I think it must have been a result of the trauma.

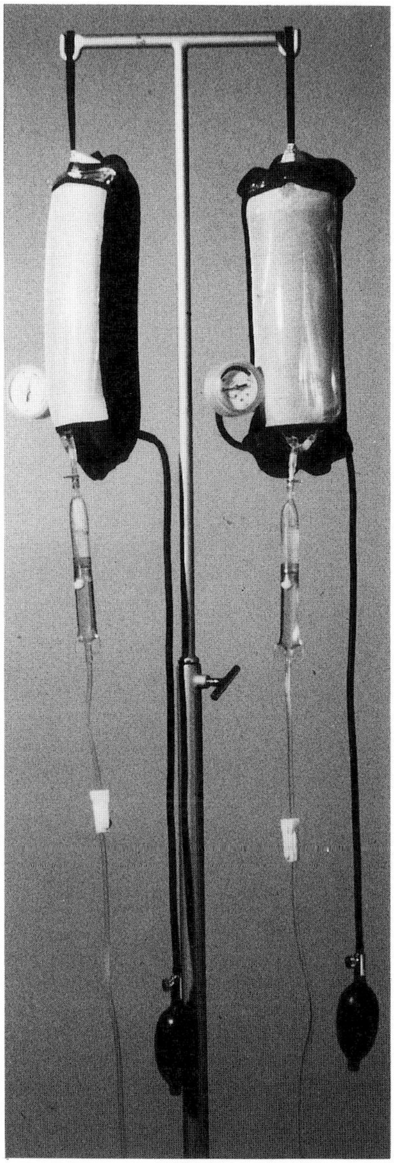

**Fig. 13.7** Apparatus for artificial erection: infusion of saline under pressure from Fenwall bags.

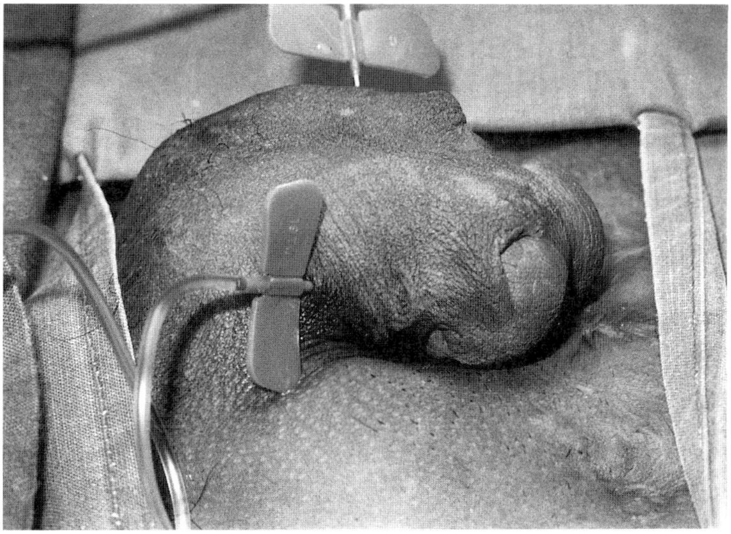

**Fig. 13.8** Artificial erection showing the tight dorsal chordee that is the most common erectile deformity in exstrophy. (From Woodhouse 1988, reproduced with permission.)

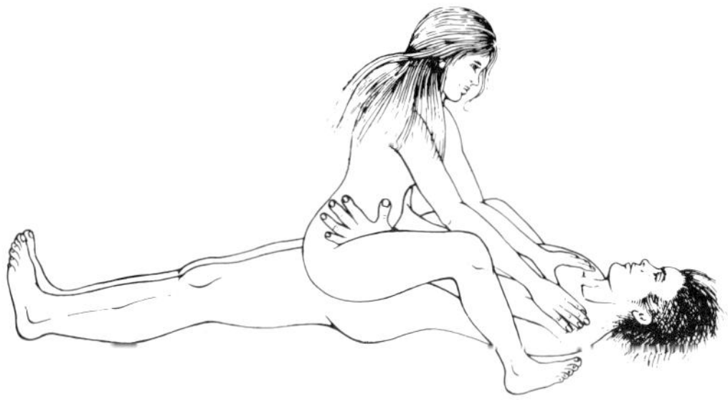

**Fig. 13.9** Sketch of a position adopted for intercourse when the dorsal chordee is uncorrected (from Woodhouse 1988, with permission).

I believe that these rudimentary corpora were normal (for exstrophy) at birth and were damaged at the reconstructive surgery (Woodhouse & Kellett 1984, Brzezinski *et al.* 1986).

If a young man with exstrophy has a short penis that is otherwise all right and has no chordee, there is nothing that can be done. A review from the Mayo Clinic, USA suggests that modern techniques of reconstruction do lead to just this situation: a short but normal penis (Mesrobian *et al.* 1986). Thus the management in adolescence in the future may only be concerned with helping

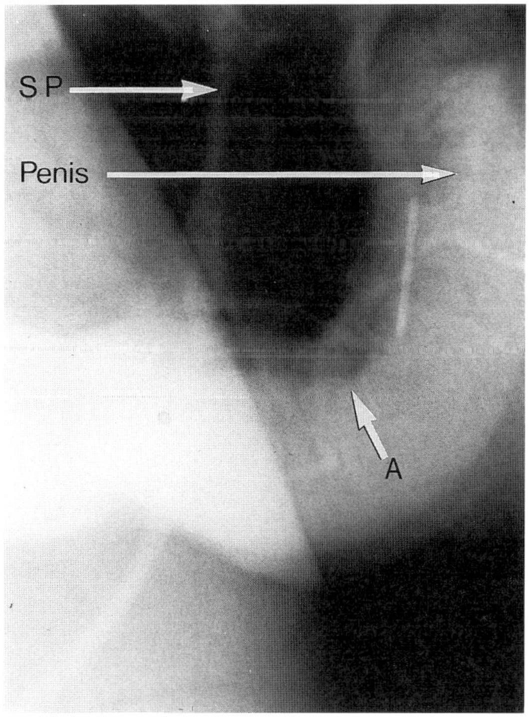



**Fig. 13.10** Lateral view of a cavernosogram showing dorsal chordee. SP = fibrous symphysis pubis. A = point of maximum curvature (adapted from Woodhouse 1986, with permission).

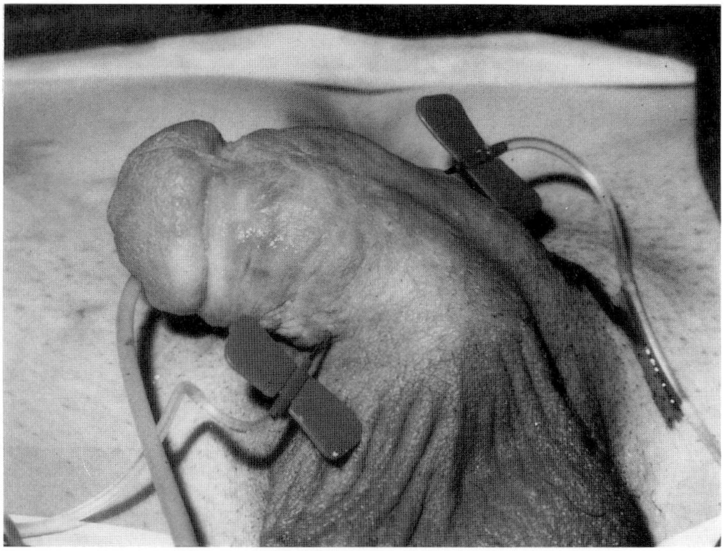

(a)

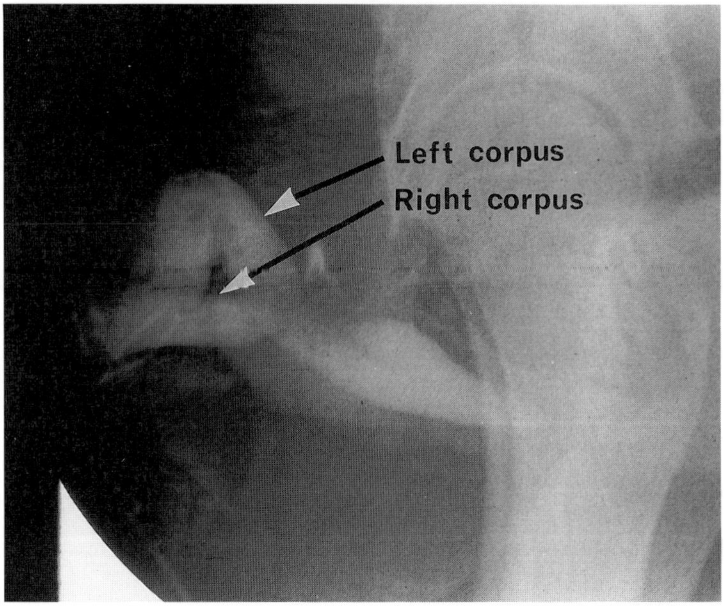


(b)

**Fig. 13.11** (a) Artificial erection showing 90° of deviation to the right. (b) Lateral view of the cavernosogram shows the 'bowstring' effect of the rudimentary right corpus (from Woodhouse 1988, with permission).

the boys to adjust to their abnormality. However, my experience with patients who are now young adults is that nearly all have an erectile deformity.

The three main types of erectile deformity that I have identified are shown in Table 13.3. The first description was based on cavernosograms in 16 patients but subsequent cases have confirmed the findings and have given me no cause to modify the classification (Woodhouse & Kellett 1984).

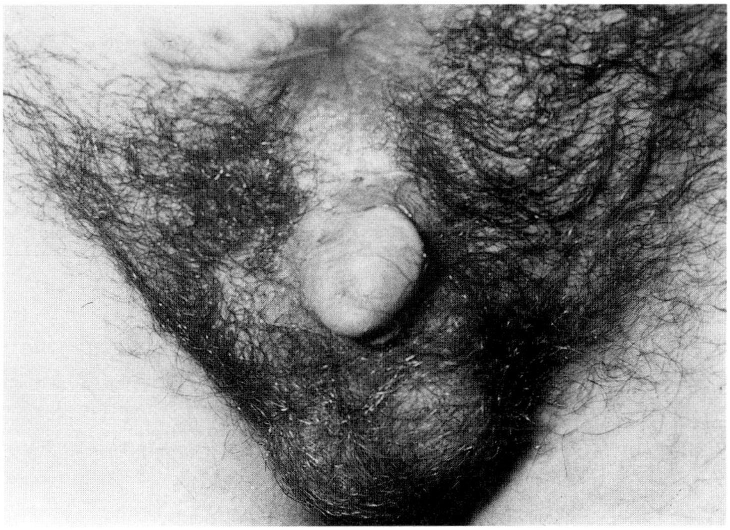

**Fig. 13.12** Exstrophy penis with bilateral rudimentary corpora.

*Lengthening procedures*

The anatomical evidence, outlined above, shows that the corpora are deficient in length. Increase in the length of the visible penis can only be achieved by making the best use of the corpora distal to their attachment to the inferior pubic ramus. Additional length is not achieved by osteotomy to close the pubic symphysis (Johnston 1974). However, it has been pointed out that the penis is longer if the divarication of the pubic bones is 3 cm or less and it is shorter if the divarication is 4 cm or more (Schillinger & Wiley 1984). Whatever the situation in infants, pelvic osteotomy does not seem to be a very attractive option for adults. Those who had an osteotomy in infancy as a part of their primary repair have not retained the apposition into adolescence and do not have a longer penis than others.

In some patients the corpora may have been 'concertina-ed' by contraction and scarring of the urethral plate and pericorporeal tissue. Considerable lengthening can be achieved in children by clearing it all away and cleaning the corpora (Hendren 1979). This dissection is the first step in chordee correction but in my experience in adults it has not allowed any penile lengthening; it may be that by this stage in life, secondary and irreversible changes have occurred in the corpora.

The horizontal plane in which the inferior pubic rami lie prevents the lengthening of the penis by partial detachment of the corpora. Some length is gained by dissection from the body of the pubis but it is useless to continue it posterior to the junction with the inferior ramus. Complete detachment of the corpora from the inferior pubic rami is said to have given good lengthening in nine of 11 children (Kelly & Eraklis 1971, King 1984). However, there has been no follow-up.

Thus it seems that in adolescents and adults there is no worthwhile procedure to lengthen the penis. Good chordee correction will give a little increase in length and will allow the best use to be made of the length that is available.

## Correction of erectile deformities

*Selection and investigation*

Ideally the penile anomaly should be corrected at the time of the initial reconstruction in infancy. It would seem that modern techniques can

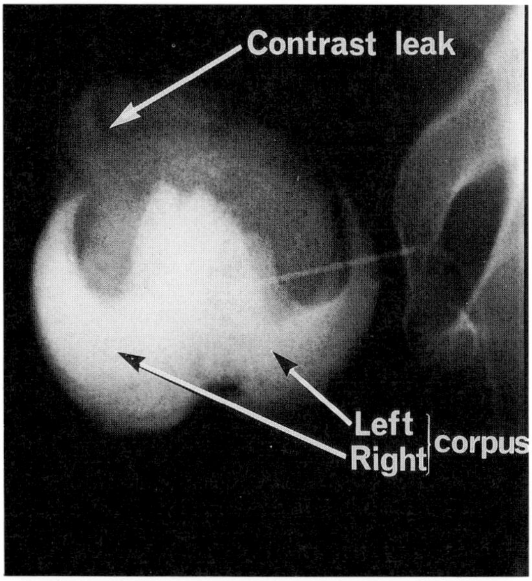


(a)

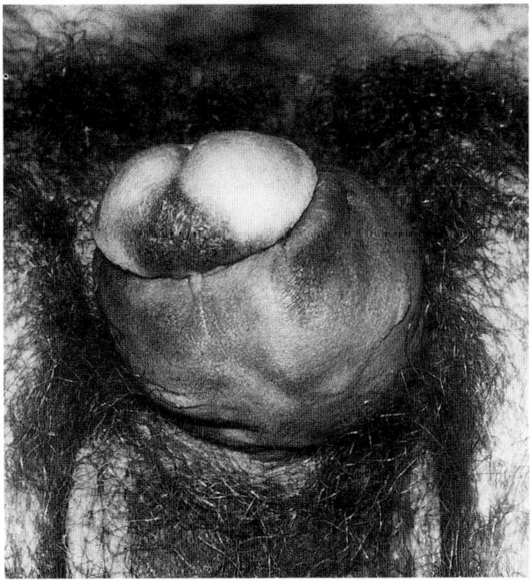

(b)

**Fig. 13.13** (a) Cavernosogram of a penis with bilateral rudimentary corpora which was fractured during intercourse 4 weeks earlier. (b) Photograph of the same penis.

achieve this goal so that phalloplasty in adulthood may become unnecessary. Mesrobian has reported 24 of 44 patients reconstructed in in-

**Table 13.3** Distribution of types of erectile deformity in exstrophy and epispadias.

| Deformity | Figure | Number |
|---|---|---|
| Dorsal chordee | 13.8 and 10 | 27 |
| Unilateral rudimentary corpus | 13.11a and b | 3 |
| Bilateral rudimentary corpora | 13.12 and 13 | 5 |

fancy who had a straight penis when reviewed as adults. Release of the urethral plate and chordee and partial detachment of the corpora from the pubis were considered essential steps. It was rare for correction to be completed in a single stage, the mean being 1.62 operations (range one to four) (Mesrobian *et al.* 1986). Ransley has anticipated the need for later chordee correction by inserting ellipses of dura in the dorsum at the primary reconstruction (P.G. Ransley, personal communication 1986), though it remains to be seen whether the correction achieved will be maintained as the penis grows.

It is clearly best to achieve complete reconstruction in infancy and to allow the child to grow up looking as much like his peers as possible. The appearance and function of the penis are of paramount importance to the adolescent with exstrophy (Feinberg *et al.* 1974). There must be a word of caution, however. The complex erectile deformities that I have seen in some patients are due to rudimentary corpora; it is most likely that they were normal at birth and were damaged by surgery in infancy. Although there are now many techniques to reconstruct a near normal bladder from scratch, so far we have no operation to restore the corpora, let alone construct a penis with sexual sensation and function.

The patients who are now adults have some degree of erectile deformity and many require phalloplasty. Careful selection is important. It is preferable to wait until penile growth is complete at the end of puberty and also until the boy has developed emotionally so that he understands the purpose of the operation. It is not satisfactory to embark on a programme of cosmetic operations if the patient cannot see anything wrong with the existing situation. If he has an understanding partner and has tried to have intercourse, it is a help, but I certainly would not wait until repeated failures have damaged the ego.

In the early cases a cavernosogram was always done, to assess the nature of the problem before surgery. If two good corpora are palpable in the perineum and there is no lateral deviation on erection, it seems unnecessary. Cavernosogram is reserved for cases in which there is doubt about the nature of the deformity or the condition of the deep part of the corpora.

### *Theory*

Several methods of correcting the deformities of the exstrophy penis have been described. If the deformity is considered as a curve in a parallel-sided cylinder, two basic methods are available for its correction: lengthening of the concave side or shortening of the convex side. The techniques developed for Peyronie's disease are applicable.

Shortening of the convexity is relatively simple by Nesbit's procedure. No dissection on the dorsum is required. The urethra normally lies on the dorsum and so will not be affected by the surgery. I have used this method successfully in an exstrophy patient who did not wish to have an implantation of dura. The disadvantage is that there is slight shortening of an already short penis.

Lengthening of the concavity by implantation of some material in the corpora produces slight lengthening (Fig. 13.14). In Peyronie's disease many autologous and heterologous materials have been used. In exstrophy only skin and lyophilised dura mater have been reported. These operations are tedious and bloody. The position and shortness of the urethra on the dorsum are a considerable problem. Ultimately, I believe that they provide the best results.

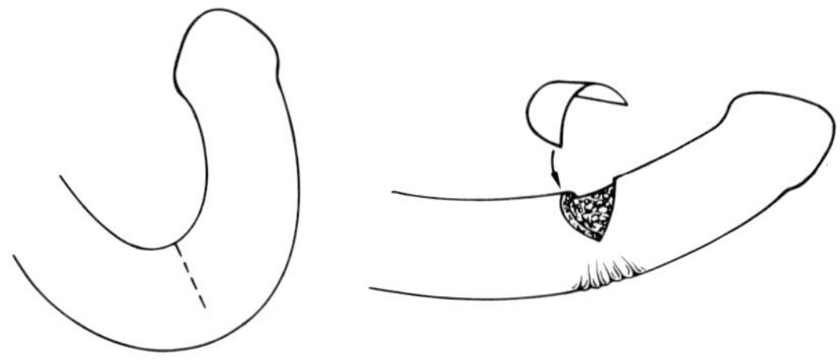

**Fig. 13.14** Diagram of penile straightening by transverse incision of the concavity of the corpus and insertion of an elliptical graft (from Woodhouse 1986, with permission).

The Koff procedure is an ingenious method of rotating the corpora so that their curvatures cancel out and the resulting angle of erection is satisfactory (Koff & Eakins 1984). This method and an important modification suggested by Ransley will assume greater importance in the future if the dangers of lyophilised dura are confirmed.

My approach includes some elements of most of these methods but relied until recently on the implantation of a patch of lyophilised human dura into the corpora. The results of using dura have been good and so it is disappointing to find that the sterilisation procedures may not kill all the viruses in the material. A case has been reported of Jacob–Creutzfeld disease developing in a 28 year old woman who had received a dural graft 22 months earlier (Editorial 1987). Although different processes are followed by manufacturers, the American Food and Drug Administration considers that all preparations carry a risk of transmitting this viral disease. If one virus can be carried, presumably others can also.

When an implant is needed, skin, rectus sheath or tunica vaginalis may be used instead of dura (Bruschini & Mitre 1979, Das 1980, Brzezinski *et al.* 1986).

### *Surgical technique*

The techniques of chordee correction are described in detail elsewhere (Woodhouse 1986, 1988).

The base of the penis and the junction of the corpora with the pubis are exposed. The urethra in these older patients still lies on the dorsum; it is mobilised, divided as far distally as possible and retracted cranially. All the scar tissue is then cleared from the dorsum of the corpora (Fig. 13.15). The superficial neurovascular bundles which are not in the usual position must be identified and protected.

In only one case have I found that this dissection was sufficient to eliminate the chordee, though others have found that the chordee is relieved at this stage (Spehr & Melchior 1985).

Until recently I have lengthened the concavity on the dorsum of the penis by inserting a gusset of lyophilised human dura but now I use rectus sheath. Each corpus is incised transversely, the penis straightened and the implant sutured in place (Fig. 13.14).

An alternative to insertion of any material is a

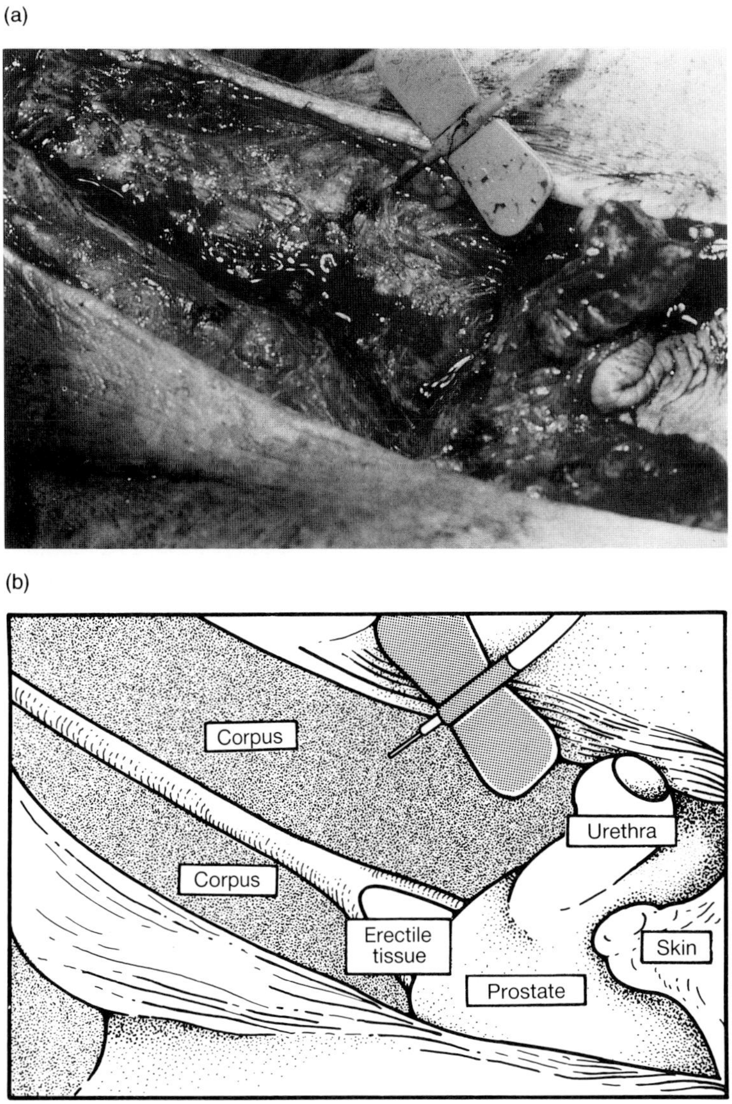


**Fig. 13.15** (a) Operative photograph after clearance of all tissue from the dorsum of the penis. (b) Diagram of the operative field.

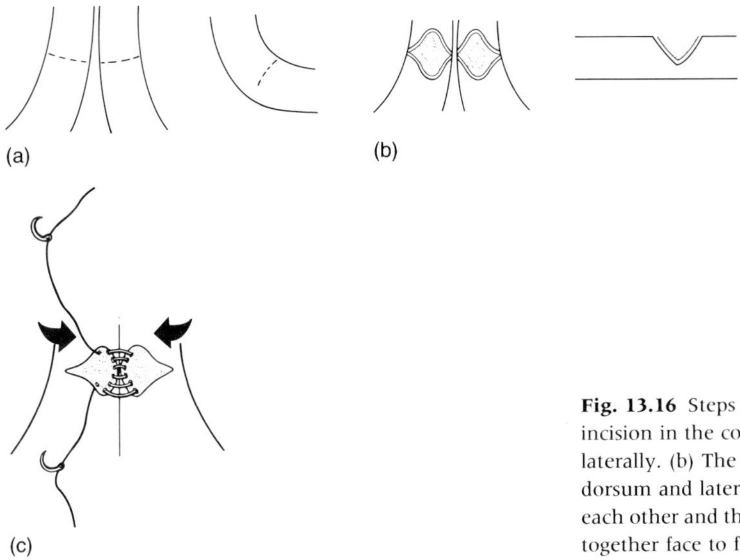


**Fig. 13.16** Steps in a rotational phalloplasty. (a) The incision in the corpora seen from the dorsum and laterally. (b) The corpora straightened out seen from the dorsum and laterally. (c) The corpora rotated towards each other and the openings in the corpora partly sutured together face to face, seen from the dorsum.

caverno–cavernostomy which might be considered a variation of the Koff procedure (P.G Ransley, personal communication 1987). After the corpora have been incised the corpora are rotated towards each other and the cavernotomies sutured to each other face to face (Fig. 13.16). The curvatures of each corpus will then cancel out. In effect each corpus is incised transversely and sutured longitudinally.

The urethra is brought through to the ventrum of the penis. If there is sufficient good skin a urethroplasty is done straight away but usually I leave it until healing of the phalloplasty is complete.

### *The urethra*

The urethral plate in exstrophy is on the dorsum of the penis and is too short. Current techniques of reconstruction allow for division of the plate and urethroplasty. I share the view of Turner-Warwick, that the urethra should be transposed to the ventrum (personal communication 1987). When doing a phalloplasty in an adult the urethra is nearly always too short; I use the length available to form a urethrostomy at the penoscrotal junction.

At a second stage, if the patient wishes, I do a urethroplasty by rolling a tube out of ventral skin to bring the meatus to the tip of the glans. I have found the complication rate to be high. Even when the short-term result is good, it is difficult to keep a 'dry' urethra patent; patients frequently develop strictures resulting in dry and sometimes painful ejaculation.

There is seldom enough skin to allow urethroplasty at the same time as penile straightening. On two occasions in diverted patients there has been enough remaining bladder to mobilise a strip of urothelium and detrusor on a pedicle from the bladder neck area. The strip is rolled into a tube and brought to the tip of the glans as a urethra (Woodhouse 1988).

Of 13 urethroplasties only six have achieved a complete urethra without any fistula or stricture. The remainder have been left with at least one small fistula (or worse) and have declined further reconstruction. Such poor results do not encourage patients to undergo secondary urethroplasty.

*Results*

The series now has 30 phalloplasties of which 20 are assessable. Thirteen have had an excellent result on the first occasion and three only after a revision (Fig. 13.17).

Three patients have had a moderate result in that there is less curvature and more flexibility even though the angle of erection is not the 40° to 45° that I would like to achieve. Two have not been improved.

Follow-up is from 1 to 5 years. In all but one case the chordee correction, once achieved, has been maintained. The exception developed a new chordee distal to the site of the original implant 18 months postoperatively. It was corrected by a further dural phalloplasty. I cannot say why this should have happened and certainly the chordee of exstrophy has not been progressive in any other case.

Afterwards, all those who were improved and who have had an appropriate opportunity have been able to achieve limited vaginal penetration. The limitation is the overall penile length.

A similar procedure using skin instead of dura has been reported to have a satisfactory result in all of three children. It is important to use non-hairy skin (Brzezinski *et al.* 1986). There must always be a slight reservation on the results of implants in childhood which might not grow at puberty and thus cause recurrence of the chordee.

Caverno–cavernostomy has been done on five adolescents or children over 10 by myself and Ransley. It has proved technically satisfactory and chordee has been corrected in all cases in the immediate postoperative period. There is no long-term follow-up and no conclusions can be drawn.

## Complex erectile deformities

When the penis is deviated to one side (Fig. 13.11), the fault lies in the rudimentary corpus which does fill and acts as a 'bow-string' on the normal side. In the first case that I saw I divided the rudimentary corpus. This resulted in a straight erection but it was very unstable: a proper erection requires the two corpora to support each other like the gables of a house. For the second case the rudimentary corpus was straightened with dura in the way described for the common deformities and this worked well. The third case has not come to surgery yet.

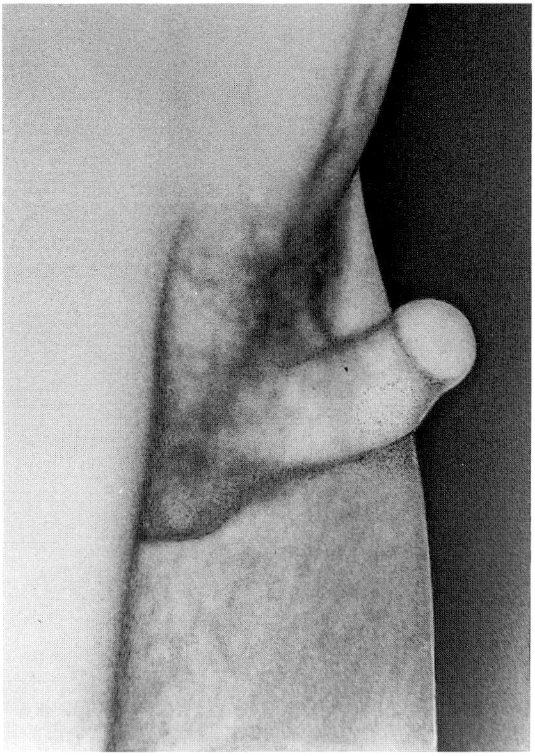

**Fig. 13.17** Natural erection of a patient showing a good result from chordee correction by dural inlay (from Woodhouse 1986, with permission).

When both corpora are rudimentary they have no attachment to the pubic rami. The venous drainage is into the superficial veins and not into the pudendal veins through Alcock's canal; the arterial supply presumably follows the same route. Penile surgery is likely to damage that little blood supply which remains and thus abolish any erection. Complete reconstruction, as is done for female to male gender reassignment, would be a possibility but has not been attempted on any of my patients.

## SEXUAL FUNCTION

With or without surgical correction the men appear to have a normal libido. They have fewer casual sexual partners than would be expected. They appear to form very stable partnerships with normal girls and have a normal family life. Thirty-three of 43 for whom full information is available have been married or lived with a partner.

Only one patient is known to be homosexual and he is one of three who have gone into the priesthood. One boy has doubts about his sexual identity and he is an epispadiac rather than a true exstrophy: he may come to gender reassignment eventually. The remaining patients of all ages do not admit to any sexual contact and for many of them the combination of abnormal genitalia and an external urinary diversion seems to be too overwhelming. Internal continent diversions may help such patients. For the next generation a working bladder and counselling of children and parents may further improve sexual function.

A case has been made for early gender reassignment for male infants with grossly deficient penis and exstrophy, especially cloacal exstrophy. In the view of King this might cover 20% of cases (1982). Cases have been cited where refusal of such advice by the parents has resulted in poorly adjusted adolescents who commit sexual offences (McLorie *et al.* 1989). One of my own patients whose penis is reasonably sized for exstrophy has served a prison sentence for attempted rape. Male exstrophy patients can certainly be made into girls (King 1984). However, there has been no long-term follow-up of exstrophy patients re-assigned to the female gender and it is possible that they will make equally unhappy female adolescents.

My experience has been that, with proper help, males with a very small penis from whatever cause can have a satisfactory life as a male. Sexual intercourse and other relations with female partners have been normal. The exstrophy patient with no remaining penis mentioned above was well-adjusted and, aged 23, started a stable sexual relationship with a woman. They appear to have a mutually satisfactory sex life. I do not think that male infants should be turned into girls just because the penis is small.

Sexual counselling is a very important aspect of patient care at all ages. Some patients have been told peculiar stories about their condition that make them think that either intercourse or fertility is impossible. These myths have to be gently laid to rest. I give an optimistic view of the possibility of paternity.

The presence of an external urinary diversion is a considerable barrier to intercourse for obvious reasons. The only advice that can be given is to let the partner know in advance what to expect. Thus longer relationships are the norm and casual partnerships uncommon.

### Paternity

Ejaculation has been assessed continuously during follow-up. In the first review of adult patients all but two of 31 patients ejaculated (Hanna & Williams 1972). Absence of ejaculation is still rare in spite of the more extensive reconstructions that are done, but the emission that does occur is slow and may continue over several hours after orgasm. Some patients describe a more or less continuous urethral discharge of semen-like fluid. In another series 16 of 25 patients had ejaculation but its quality is not recorded (Mesrobian *et al.* 1986).

Although the genital tract up to the verumontanum is normal, there is a high incidence of poor or absent sperm. It is not known whether this is due to obstruction or repeated infection. The figures in Table 13.4 show that patients who had an early diversion have better sperm than those in whom reconstruction was attempted.

**Table 13.4** Seminal analysis of patients with exstrophy or epispadias (data from Hanna & Williams 1972, Lattimer *et al.* 1979b and current series). Men who claim to have fathered children have not had semen analyses.

| | Exstrophy | | Epispadias | |
|---|---|---|---|---|
| Semen | Reconst. | Diversion | Reconst. | Diversion |
| No ejaculation | 1 | — | — | — |
| Azoospermia | 9 | 16 | — | — |
| Poor | 5 | 6 | — 4* | — |
| Good | 2 | 11 | 3 | 6 |
| Paternity | 1 | 5 | — | — |

Reconst. = reconstructed bladder
* Diversion or reconstruction not stated

Seven of my patients have initiated one or two pregnancies from which there have been five children. A further 13 are known to be infertile. These figures are broadly in line with those reported elsewhere: Mesrobian reports 12 of 53 patients married, five of whom had fathered children.

The main cause of infertility appears to be repeated prostatic and bladder infections. Thus, ironically, the boys who underwent early urinary diversion have the best record for fertility.

## FEMALES

### The vagina

Because the bladder and anterior abdominal wall are effectively missing, the vagina and anus are displaced forwards (Fig. 13.18). Indeed in some patients even after successful bladder reconstruction, the introitus appears to be on the lower abdomen rather than in the perineum (Fig. 13.19). The introitus is usually narrow. In most cases the narrowed part is short and is easily opened by an episiotomy. Only six patients have required a formal vaginoplasty (Table 13.5). Similar figures are reported from Lattimer's series (Krisiloff *et al.* 1978). When vaginoplasty is necessary, the posterior wall is incised deeply and the resulting defect covered by rotating a flap of labia minora from each side.

The vagina runs directly posteriorly so that when the patient is standing the vagina is almost parallel with the floor. It is also rather shorter than usual. These arrangements do not interfere with intercourse: 14 of 23 women have normal intercourse and none report any difficulties (six are virgins and there is no information for the remaining three). Orgasm is said to be normal in all patients (Krisiloff *et al.* 1978).

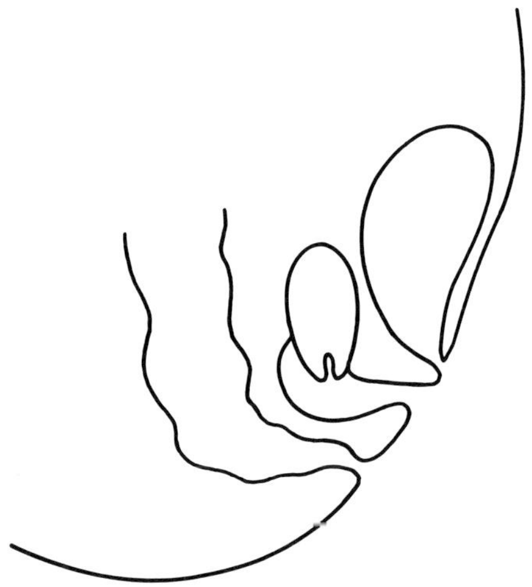

**Fig. 13.18** Diagram of a sagittal section of a female with exstrophy to show the relationship of the pelvic organs. From left to right: rectum and anus, vagina and uterus, bladder. (From Woodhouse 1989, reproduced with permission.)

### The uterus

The cervix enters the superior wall of the vagina

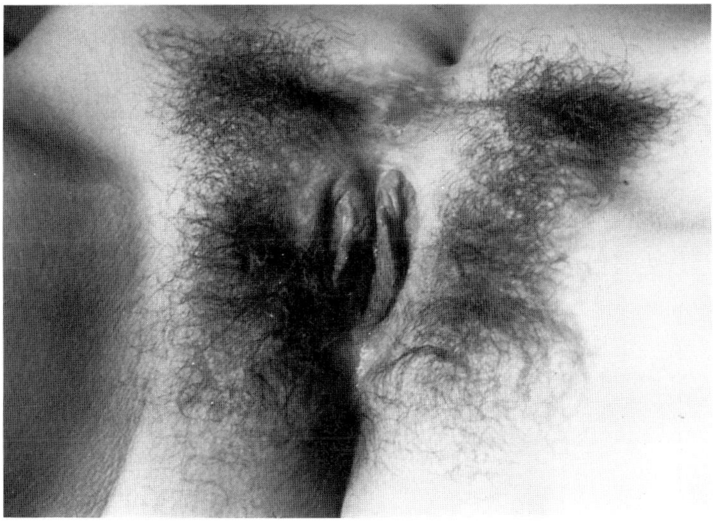

**Fig. 13.19** The vulva in exstrophy: note how anterior the structures are compared to normal. The pubic hair is on either side of the vulva and deficient in the mid-line over the mons due to the distribution of skin at the time of original bladder closure. The reconstructed umbilicus is seen at the top. (From Woodhouse 1989, reproduced with permission.)

**Table 13.5** Vaginal surgery required in 23 patients.

| Procedure | Patients |
|---|---|
| Episiotomy | 6 |
| Vaginoplasty | 6 |
| None (normal sexual intercourse) | 6 |
| None (no sexual intercourse or no information) | 5 |

and is very close to the introitus (Fig. 13.18): this must contribute to the ease with which the women get pregnant. It is essential to explain to the patients at an early stage that fertility is normal. Some women have thought that they were so abnormal that conception was impossible. Two of the 20 pregnancies in our patients have occurred because of this view, one of the women having an intact hymen at the time of conception.

The defective pelvic floor and poor uterine supports make prolapse common. It is a considerable problem to correct. Three of our patients have had a total procedentia, one of whom has never had intercourse or a pregnancy. The uterus should not be removed as it is the only solid organ in the pelvis that has any hope of holding up the pelvic floor. The simplest procedure for prolapse is to suture the lower segment of the uterus to the anterior abdominal wall with silk. If this fails or in cases of procedentia, some form of sling should be put around the uterus: abdominal wall fascia or gracilis has been used. It must be said, however, that the management of uterine prolapse has presented great difficulty for the gynaecologists (Dewhurst *et al.* 1980, Blakeley & Mills 1981). Our present practice is to make a sling from Goretex. It is sutured to the promontory of the sacrum after mobilisation of the rectum and wrapped around the uterus at the level of the cervix. It has been curative at least in the short-term (up to 5 years), in the four cases in which it has been used (J.H. Shepherd, personal communication 1990).

## Pregnancy

Fertility is unimpaired. One of the women with procedentia conceived (before correction) and had a difficult pregnancy: in-patient bedrest was necessary for almost the whole of the pregnancy. Patients with diversion may have more infections, stoma prolapse or, in one of our cases, uretero-ileal obstruction (Krisiloff *et al.* 1978). Some degree of uterine prolapse is almost invariable. Malpresentation seems to be common, for example three of five patients having a breech delivery in Krisiloff's series, but for the most part pregnancies have been uncomplicated.

Nine women in my series have had 17 children, one termination, one spontaneous abortion and one intra-uterine death of twins. These last two complications and the uretero-ileal obstruction all occurred in the same patient. Krisiloff reports seven pregnancies in 28 patients producing six children and one termination.

Three of my patients and four of Krisiloff's who have urinary diversions were delivered vaginally without difficulty. Five with a functioning bladder and the one with uretero-ileal obstruction have had caesareans which is safer than risking damage to the bladder outlet.

All the 22 offspring from my patients (male or female) have been normal. It has been reported from a postal survey of clinics all over the world that one in 70 offspring have exstrophy or epispadias (Shapiro *et al.* 1984). This figure must represent the worst that can be expected.

Cloacal exstrophy can be identified *in utero* while screening for neural tube defects because the maternal serum alpha-fetoprotein is elevated (Gosden & Brock 1981). Classical exstrophy should be identified on maternal ultrasound.

## SOCIAL DEVELOPMENT

As an unsupported and unscientific observation I would say that exstrophy patients are good looking, well-motivated and well-adjusted people. There is no doubt that the occurrence of exstrophy or epispadias in a child puts a heavy burden on the whole family. Their many anxieties can be helped by careful and informed counselling. It is certainly helpful to have a specially trained team, as suggested by Lattimer, for this work. But even less well endowed units can guide the patients safely into adult life (Lattimer *et al.* 1979a).

Special schooling is not required. It is important that the exstrophy child grows up with his or her peers. Their educational achievements have been satisfactory and not different from those of other children (Table 13.6).

Exstrophy patients seem to be hard working and proud of their jobs. I reviewed their work in 1983 at a time when the unemployment rate in young adults was particularly high in the UK; I found that the unemployment rate was considerably lower than the national average. Simi-

**Table 13.6** Educational achievements of exstrophy patients.

| Type of education | Number of children |
|---|---|
| Normal | 69 |
| University | 8 |
| Professional or apprenticeship | 8 |
| Special school | 9 |
| Tutor at home | 2 |
| Inadequate information (probably normal) | 21 |

**Table 13.7** Jobs held by exstrophy patients comparing my patients and Cleveland Clinic patients (Zabbo & Kay 1986).

| Occupation | UK | USA |
|---|---|---|
| *Males* | | |
| Professional | 8 | 7 |
| Business | | 9 |
| Skilled labour | 21 | 14 |
| Unskilled labour | 22 | 3 |
| Clown | | 1 |
| Disabled | | 1 |
| Student | 11 | |
| Unemployed | 5 | |
| Criminal | 1 | |
| *Females* | | |
| Professional | | 5 |
| Office work | | 3 |
| Housewife | 5 | 9 |
| Croupier | 1 | |
| Unknown (male & female) | 29 | |

lar findings have been reported from the USA though the group selected had ureterosigmoid diversions and excluded patients with ileal conduits which may have influenced the figures (Zabbo & Kay 1986). The occupations are shown in Table 13.7.

## REFERENCES


Arap S., Giron A.M. & Menzes de Goes G. (1980) Initial results of the complete reconstruction of bladder exstrophy. *Urol. Clin. North Am.* **7**, 477–91.

Blakeley C.R. & Mills W.G. (1981) The obstetric and gynaecological complications of bladder exstrophy and epispadias. *Br. J. Obstet. Gynaecol.* **88**, 167–73.

Bruschini H. & Mitre A.I. (1979) Peyronie's disease: surgical treatment with muscular aponeurosis. *Urology* **13**, 505–6.

Brzezinski A.E., Homsy Y.L. & Laberge I. (1986) Orthoplasty in epispadias. *J. Urol.* **136**, 259–61.

Das S. (1980) Peyronie's disease: excision and autografting with tunica vaginalis. *J. Urol.* **124**, 818–19.

Demaria J.E., Alton D.J., Krueger R.P. *et al.* (1980) Renal function in continent patients after surgical closure of bladder exstrophy. *J. Urol.* **124**, 85–8.

Dewhurst J., Topliss P.H. & Shepherd J.H. (1980) Ivalon sponge hysteropexy for genital prolapse in patients with bladder exstrophy. *Br. J. Obstet. Gynaecol.* **87**, 67–9.

Diamond D.A. & Ransley P.G. (1986) Bladder neck reconstruction with omentum, silicone and augmentation cystoplasty — a preliminary report. *J. Urol.* **136**, 252–5.

Duckett J.W. & Caldemone A.A. (1984) *Bladder Exstrophy.* AUA Update Series, Lesson 13, Vol. III. American Urological Association Inc., Office of Education, Houston.

Editorial (1987) Update: Creutzfeld–Jacob disease in a patient receiving a cadaveric dura mater graft. *J.A.M.A.* **258**, 309–10.

Engel R.M. & Wilkinson H.A. (1970) Bladder exstrophy. *J. Urol.* **104**, 699–704.

Everson T.C. & Cole W.H. (1966) *Spontaneous Regression of Cancer.* W.B Saunders Co., Philadelphia, pp. 320–37.

Feinberg T., Lattimer J.K., Jeter K., Langford W. & Beck L. (1974) Questions that worry children with exstrophy. *Pediatrics* **53**, 242–6.

Gosden C. & Brock D.J.H. (1981) Prenatal diagnosis of exstrophy of the cloaca. *Am. J. Med. Genet.* **8**, 95–109.

Hanna M.K. & Williams D.I (1972) Genital function in males with vesical exstrophy and epispadias. *Br. J. Urol.* **44**, 169–74.

Hendren W.H. (1979) Penile lengthening after previous repair of epispadias. *J. Urol.* **121**, 527–34.

Herzberg Z., Kellett M.J., Morgan R.J., & Pryor J.P. (1981) Method, indications and results of corpus cavernosography. *Br. J. Urol.* **53**, 641–4.

Hurwitz R.S., Woodhouse C.R.J. & Ransley P.G. (1986) The anatomical course of the neurovascular bundles in epispadias. *J. Urol.* **136**, 68–70.

Husmann D.A., McLorie G.A. & Churchill B.M. (1988) A comparison of renal function in the exstrophy patient treated with staged reconstruction versus urinary diversion. *J. Urol.* **140**, 1204–6.

Johnston J.H. (1974) Lengthening of the congenital or acquired short penis. *Br. J. Urol.* **46**, 685–7.

Kelley J.H. & Eraklis A.J. (1971) A procedure for lengthening the phallus in boys with exstrophy of the bladder. *J. Pediatr. Surg.* **6**, 645–9.

King L.R. (1982) The inadequate penis in some males with exstrophy — a plea for early sex conversion. Paper presented at the American Urological Association Annual Meeting (Abstract 153) p. 116.

King L.R. (1984) Editorial — exstrophy and epispadias. *J. Urol.* **132**, 1159–60.

Koff S.A. & Eakins M. (1984) The treatment of penile chordee using corporeal rotation. *J. Urol.* **131**, 931–2.

Krisiloff M., Puchner P.J., Tretter W., Macfarlane M.T. & Lattimer J.K. (1978) Pregnancy in women with exstrophy. *J. Urol.* **119**, 478–9.

Lattimer J.K., Dean A.L., Dougherty L.J. *et al.* (1960) Functional closure of the bladder in children with exstrophy: a report of 28 cases. *J. Urol.* **83**, 647–55.

Lattimer J.K., Hensle T.W., Macfarlane M.T. *et al.* (1979a) The exstrophy support team: a new concept in the care of the exstrophy patient. *J. Urol.* **121**, 472–3.

Lattimer J.K., Macfarlane M.T. & Puchor P.J. (1979b) Male exstrophy patients: a preliminary report on the reproductive capability. *Trans. Amer. Assoc. Genito-Urinary Surg.* **70**, 42–6.

Light J.K. & Scott F.B. (1984) The artificial urinary sphincter in children. *Br. J. Urol.* **56**, 54–7.

McIntosh J.F. & Worley G. (1955) Adenocarcinoma arising in exstrophy of the bladder: report of 2 cases and review of the literature. *J. Urol.* **73**, 820–9.

McLorie G.A., Khoury A.E. & Husmann D.A. (1989) Surgery for the small penis. *Dial. Ped. Urol.* **12**(7), 6–7.

Marshall V.F. & Muecke E.C. (1970) Functional closure of typical exstrophy of the bladder. *J. Urol.* **104**, 205–12.

Mayo C.H. & Hendricks W.A. (1926) Exstrophy of the bladder. *Surg. Gynecol. Obstet.* **43**, 129–34.

Megali M. & Lattimer J.K. (1973) Review of the management of 140 cases of exstrophy of the bladder. *J. Urol.* **109**, 246–8.

Mesrobian H-G.J., Kelalis P.P. & Kramer S.A. (1986) Long

term follow-up of cosmetic appearance and genital function in boys with exstrophy: review of 53 patients. *J. Urol.* **136**, 256–8.

Peters C.A., Gearhart J.P. & Jeffs R.D. (1988) Epispadias and incontinence: the challenge of the small bladder. *J. Urol.* **140**, 1199–201.

Polsky M.S., Weber C.H., Williams J.E. *et al.* (1976) Chronically infected and postdiversionary bladders: cytological and histopathological study. *Urology* **7**, 531–5.

Schillinger J.F. & Wiley M.J. (1984) Bladder exstrophy penile lengthening procedure. *Urology* **24**, 434–7.

Segura J.W. & Kelalis P.P. (1975) Long term results of ureterosigmoidostomy in children with bladder exstrophy. *J. Urol.* **114**, 138–40.

Shapiro E., Lepor H. & Jeffs R.D. (1984) The inheritance of the exstrophy-epispadias complex. *J. Urol.* **132**, 308–10.

Spehr Ch. & Melchior C. (1985) *Operative Correction of the Penis Deformity in Bladder Exstrophy.* XXth Congress of the International Society of Urology, Vienna (Abstract 1008) p. 320.

Strachan J.R. & Woodhouse C.R.J. (1990) Malignancy in exstrophy patients. *Paper read at the Annual Meeting of the British Association of Urological Surgeons.* Scarborough, July 1990, (abstract 61).

Trendelenburg F. (1906) The treatment of ectopia vesicae. *Ann. Surg.* **44**, 281–9.

Turner W.R., Ransley P.G. & Williams D.I. (1980) Patterns of renal damage in the management of vesical exstrophy. *J. Urol.* **124**, 412–6.

Wattenberg C.A., Beare J.B. & Tormey A.R. (1956) Exstrophy of the urinary bladder complicated by adenocarcinoma. *J. Urol.* **75**, 583–93.

Williams D.I. (1977) Epispadias and exstrophy. In: Eckstein H.B., Hohenfellner R. & Williams D.I. (eds) *Surgical Paediatric Urology.* Georg Thieme, Stuttgart, pp. 298–312.

Woodhouse C.R.J. (1986) The management of erectile deformity in adults with exstrophy and epispadias. *J. Urol.* **135,** 932–5.

Woodhouse C.R.J. (1988) Dural phalloplasty in exstrophy and epispadias. In: Mundy A.R. (ed) *Current Operative Surgery — Urology.* Bailliere Tindall, London, pp. 106–18.

Woodhouse C.R.J. (1989) Sexual rehabilitation in bladder exstrophy. In: Eicher W. (ed). *Plastic Surgery in the Sexually Handicapped.* Springer-Verlag, Berlin, pp. 34–46.

Woodhouse C.R.J., Ransley P.G. & Williams D.I. (1983) The patient with exstrophy in adult life. *Br. J. Urol.* **55**, 632–5.

Woodhouse C.R.J. & Kellett M.J. (1984) Anatomy of the penis and its deformities in exstrophy and epispadias. *J. Urol.* **132**, 1122–4.

Yannopoulos P. & Kyriakidis A. (1979) Bladder exstrophy complicated by carcinoma. *Acta Urol. Belgica* **47**, 28–30.

Zabbo A. & Kay R. (1986) Ureterosigmoidostomy and bladder exstrophy: a long term follow-up. *J. Urol.* **136**, 396–8.

# 14 *Posterior urethral valves*

## INTRODUCTION

Boys presenting with posterior urethral valves appear to have a simple abnormality that is simple to treat. The immediate improvement seen in the condition of the child and his urinary tract is gratifying to all. It may be little thought that, in many cases, the ground is laid for life-long trouble with the genito-urinary tract. It is one of the few conditions for which prenatal diagnosis (and possibly prenatal treatment) will be helpful.

No matter how good the initial result, follow-up must be vigilant and must continue well into adult life.

## DEATH

The results of treatment have improved considerably in the last 40 years. In his large series of 172 boys presenting between 1951 and 1970, Innes Williams recorded a mortality of 16% which was probably the best at the time. Early presentation carried a poor prognosis: 40% of 54 boys presenting before 3 months of age died and all but three of the deaths occurred in those who presented before 1 year old. However, the death rate fell steadily as more knowledge and experience were gained: from 36% from 1956 to 1960, 20% from 1961 to 1965 to 15% from 1966 to 1970 in patients presenting before 1 year of age (Williams *et al.* 1973). Ten years later the mortality had fallen to 7.4% and again the deaths were in infants presenting before 3 months (Atwell 1983). An early mortality of less than 5% is now found in most units (Warshaw *et al.* 1985).

## LONG-TERM PROBLEMS

It has long been recognised that the most common late problems were incontinence and renal failure. It is now becoming clear that these two are interrelated.

The other problems include urinary infection, urethral stricture and sexual dysfunction.

### Renal function

Poor renal function is recorded in all series. In Innes Williams's series 17 of 144 survivors had an elevated plasma urea at a mean age of 8.5 years. In more modern series similar results have been recorded but the mean follow-up times have been 6 or 7 years. It is only with follow-up to the end of childhood and beyond that the progressive nature of the renal damage can be appreciated.

Warshaw has found that the 'final' plasma creatinine is related to the best creatinine level achieved in the first year of life. In 22 infants presenting at under 1 year old and followed for a mean of 5.8 years, those who had a creatinine nadir of 0.8 mg/dl or better had a 'final' level of 1.1 mg/dl or better. Those whose nadir level was worse than 0.8 mg/dl had progressive deterioration to the time of follow-up. At final review one patient was in end-stage renal failure and five had a creatinine above 1.5 mg/dl (Warshaw *et al.* 1985).

These figures are typical of those quoted in the literature and are similar to our own. However, we have realised two important points; firstly there is nothing 'final' about renal function in valve patients at follow-up in mid-childhood;

secondly, normal creatinine at the end of childhood does not guarantee normal creatinine at the end of puberty.

It has also been pointed out that plasma creatinine is not an accurate measure of overall renal function. Scott found that glomerular filtration rate (GFR) as measured by creatinine clearance was better and more predictive. He identified two groups of patients who had renal failure. Group 1 had an initial GFR that was less than 50% of normal when corrected for age and surface area; they did not recover renal function and nine of 10 remained in chronic renal failure. Group 2 had a GFR between 50 and 80% of normal at presentation; they recovered initially but went back into renal failure in early childhood or at puberty (Scott 1985).

In a preliminary review of the long-term results of Innes Williams's patients it was found that two patients had died of renal failure and its complications between 5 and 10 years of follow-up. The patients in chronic renal failure were (J.D. Frank, unpublished data):

**1** At 5-year follow-up: 6.5%.
**2** At 10-year follow-up: 25%.
**3** At 15-year follow-up: 50%.

The only long-term review available is our own from Great Ormond Street and the Institute of Urology (Parkhouse *et al.* 1988). Although it lacks corroboration from the literature, it is believed to reflect the outcome for valve patients in adult life as the results follow the trend set in reviews of younger patients. Ninety-nine survivors of initial treatment for type 1 valves have been followed for 11 to 22 years with a mean of 15 years. Twenty-one patients are in chronic renal failure and all but one of them had a normal plasma creatinine after their initial surgery. Deterioration began between 6 and 14 years after diagnosis. Several factors were examined as predictors of poor prognosis and three were found to be significant, although they were not always mutually independent.

### *Vesico-ureteric reflux*

As with most reports, it was found that bilateral reflux carried a poor prognosis. It occurred significantly more often in those presenting before 1 year old. Unilateral reflux occurred in about 30% of patients presenting at all ages.

With bilateral reflux 58% of boys developed chronic renal failure while only 15% of non-refluxers did. Upper tract surgery for reflux did not appear to have any positive influence, though it is impossible to tell whether it prevented late deterioration.

Although reflux carries a poor prognosis, it must be remembered that 15% of patients without reflux still went into renal failure. This is the same percentage as those with unilateral reflux, and the figures do not confirm the view of Hoover and Duckett that unilateral reflux is protective. They have postulated that gross reflux into a kidney that ultimately ceases to function protects the other kidney from any damage (1982).

The kidneys may be dysplastic from a very early age because of maldevelopment. It has been suggested that this associated anomaly occurs when the ureteral bud arises from an unusually cranial position on the Woolfian duct. The renal parenchyma fails to develop in whole or in part and the ureter may reflux. In these cases it is thought that the reflux is not the cause of the dysplasia (Henneberry & Stephens 1980).

### *Age at presentation*

All of the patients who have died and 16 of 21 patients who have, so far, developed renal failure presented before their first birthdays. This observation has been made by all authors but it may not be possible to separate the effect of age from the presence of reflux.

### *Incontinence*

The most important prognostic indicator was

incontinence by day at 5 years old. Information was only available for 87 boys, the others being dead or diverted. Only 4% of boys who had daytime continence at 5 years old developed renal failure compared to 46% who were incontinent.

### Other parameters of renal function

Even the GFR does not tell the whole story of renal function. Other parameters may be abnormal without necessarily leading to end-stage renal failure. For example seven of 67 of our patients who are not in renal failure have hypertension and 14 have more than 0.3 g/l of protein in the urine. Although proteinuria usually precedes renal failure and hypertension often accompanies it, the associations are not invariable.

An abnormality that we believe is of greater importance is polyuria. The association of polyuria with posterior urethral valves has been known for many years (Baum *et al.* 1974). If, as appears likely, progressive renal damage is caused by high intravesical storage pressure, the more urine that is produced, the more bladder cycles there will be in a day and the longer time will be spent with a detrusor pressure above a critical safety level.

Data on 24 boys attending Great Ormond Street, UK who were not in renal failure have suggested that tubular dysfunction may still be present. Thirteen had corrected GFRs of more than 80 and 11 of less that 80 ml/min. The lower GFR group were characterised by 24-hour urine volumes above a litre with an osmolality below 802 mmol/kg and pH above 6. However, even the boys with GFR above 80 were not always normal. Six had urine osmolalities below 800 mmol/kg. Six, including two with normal urine osmolalities, were unable to acidify their urine to less than a pH of 6. The 24-hour urine volume ranged from 380–1400 ml (Parkhouse & Woodhouse 1990).

Thus there seem to be renal functional abnormalities which may not lead directly to the need for dialysis but may exacerbate the functional problems of the bladder.

## BLADDER FUNCTION

Incontinence has been recorded in a proportion of patients in most series. It has been attributed to sphincter weakness; either in the distal mechanism due to surgery or the bladder neck mechanism due to the known dilatation or surgical resection. Continence has usually come spontaneously with puberty.

Bauer pointed out that some of the incontinent boys had abnormal filling cystometrograms and suggested that sphincter weakness was not the only explanation for incontinence (Bauer *et al.* 1979). Others have confirmed these findings and associated them with poor renal function.

It has also been shown that treatment of some bladder dysfunction will improve renal function. In a series of four boys with high pressure bladders and incomplete emptying, three had improvement in renal function and one was stabilised when intermittent clean selfcatheterisation (ICSC) was started (Campaiola *et al.* 1985).

Instability is not the only abnormality that can be found. In 42 consecutive valve patients at Great Ormond Street from 1 month to 14 years old a wide range of urodynamic abnormalities has been found. All had had the valve destroyed and none had residual obstruction. Twenty were unstable, eight had reduced compliance, 10 were stable and four were acontractile (Parkhouse, 1990).

The links between detrusor dysfunction, incontinence and renal failure have been further strengthened by work in our own patients. Parkhouse compared the urodynamic findings in 15 boys who had been treated for valves and 15 incontinent children with gross reflux but no outflow obstruction. The valve patients were all in the highest risk group having presented in the first year of life with bilateral reflux and having continued incontinence. Thirteen of 15 valve patients had significantly higher detrusor pressures than the simple reflux patients; their functional capacities were lower but the difference did not reach significance. The relationship between the maximum detrusor pressure and GFR for the children is shown in Fig. 14.1: the correlation is statistically significant (Parkhouse, 1990).

## HYPOTHESIS FOR THE CAUSE OF LATE RENAL FAILURE

The explanation of late renal failure that best fits the present data begins with the idea that prolonged bladder outflow obstruction *in utero* causes irreversible damage to the detrusor. The bladder lacks compliance, has a high pressure and a small functional volume. The principal cause of incontinence in these severely affected boys is the detrusor instability, and not external sphincter weakness.

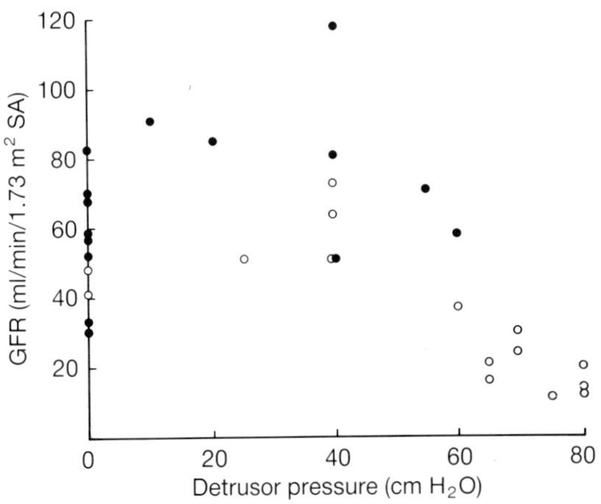


**Fig. 14.1** A plot to show the relationship between corrected GFR and maximum detrusor pressure in 30 children. ○ represent the 15 boys who had been treated for posterior urethral valves and who had no residual outflow obstruction. ● represent 15 age-matched patients with severe vesico-ureteric reflux without neuropathy or outflow obstruction (courtesy of H.F. Parkhouse, unpublished data).

The high storage pressures are transmitted back to the kidneys leading to renal failure. Although reflux will help this process, it is not essential at least in the patients with polyuria: it has been shown the during diuresis the renal pelvic pressure mirrors the bladder pressure even in the absence of reflux.

The speed of renal deterioration will be greatest in those with highest pressures, largest residual urine and greatest polyuria. Those incontinent boys whose renal function survives until puberty become exposed to a further danger as the prostate grows. The outflow resistance from the bladder increases so that continence develops but there is a further deterioration in conditions within the bladder.

Beware the boy with detrusor instability who becomes continent spontaneously: he loses one problem but puts his renal function at risk.

## MANAGEMENT

Boys with obvious bladder dysfunction leading to incontinence have been treated symptomatically with anticholinergic drugs and occasionally by surgery. If it is accepted that renal failure is a consequence of detrusor instability and hypocompliance, sometimes aggravated by polyuria, investigation and treatment must be more vigorous. A case could be made for urodynamic investigation of all valve patients at least once after valve ablation. Those in high-risk categories may need repeated investigations.

Instability and hypocompliance must be treated in their own right rather than because of their symptoms. Boys with substantial residuals can be managed by ICSC. However, the urethra is normally innervated and the regime can be difficult to enforce. It is a particularly difficult regime for adolescents who are continent because they can see no obvious advantage to themselves and the concept of late renal failure is not a sufficient driving force.

Anticholinergic drugs or augmentation cystoplasty may be more attractive.

## Undiversion in posterior urethral valve patients

In our own series of valve patients treated between 1966 and 1975, five of 98 had 'permanent' diversions. In addition we have been referred some diverted boys with 'bladder outflow obstruction' from other hospitals whose primary diagnosis is unknown though most probably had valves. In considering undiversion, four factors must be considered:

**1** Is there any residual obstruction?
**2** What is the function of the bladder?
**3** What is the function of the sphincters?
**4** What is the normal 24-hour urine output?

None of these can be ignored in valve patients. In particular, the bladder storage pressure must be considered in relation to the daily urine output: if the output is large, the proportion of the day spent at damagingly high bladder pressure is increased leading to accelerated renal damage.

We have found the assessment of the valve bladder particularly difficult both for undiversion and in anticipation of renal transplantation (see Chapter 11). If the criteria defined in Chapter 11 are not achieved by cycling, undiversion is not ruled out but the surgery must incorporate steps to achieve them. If such steps may result in the need for ICSC, it is essential to find out that the boy is willing and able to do it before operating.

The results of undiversion in valve patients are difficult to determine. The reported series of undiversions include valve patients within a larger group and follow-up periods have been short. Our awareness of the particular problems of poor compliance and polyuria in the valve bladder is recent. In future valve patients should be considered separately from other non-neuropathic undiversion patients.

Four recent publications have included 21 valve patients operated for undiversion. Follow-up was 6 months to 9 years with a mean that was impossible to determine but probably no more than 2 to 3 years. The outcome was described as satisfactory in 19. One patient was incontinent and one suffered deterioration of renal function (Frank *et al.* 1982, Stone *et al.* 1982, Sheehan *et al.* 1984, Gonzalez *et al.* 1986).

Although these figures look encouraging, they must be considered in the light of the very short follow-up: enough time has not yet passed to know if the bladders newly brought into use are going to damage the kidneys.

## Renal transplantation

If a bladder has been responsible for the destruction of two native kidneys, it is likely to make short work of a transplanted kidney unless the underlying defect has been corrected. In the valve bladder, correction of the outflow obstruction may not always be sufficient. This problem is discussed further in Chapter 5.

The results of transplantation into the valve bladder are less good than those using a normal bladder. It can be difficult precisely to attribute the cause of graft loss, but in many cases the poor bladder function seems to be the main problem. Better results may follow more aggressive correction of the bladder anomalies of which we are now aware. Transplantation has been managed successfully in patients with augmentation cystoplasties and in patients using ICSC (Barnett *et al.* 1985, 1987). There seems no reason why these techniques should not be applied to valve patients.

# SEXUAL FUNCTION AND FERTILITY

There are several reasons why valve patients might have impaired sexual and reproductive function. The high pressure developed in the bladder behind the valve produces an open bladder neck, posterior urethral dilatation and, sometimes, vasal reflux. As a result prostatic, seminal, vesicular or testicular components of semen may be affected. Retrograde ejaculation may occur. The libido and sexual function may further deteriorate with renal failure. Finally, surgical treatment might damage the nerves of erection around the prostate.

It is, therefore, pleasing to find that valve patients have good sexual function and some are fertile.

I have recently reviewed 21 adults previously treated for valves (Woodhouse *et al.* 1989). Eighteen had normal erections, one on dialysis had poor erections and one man had life-long impotence. All (except the impotent patient) had normal intercourse.

Ejaculation was normal in 11 and dry in one. Eight patients had slow ejaculation; that is an apparently normal orgasm but a slow trickle of ejaculate thereafter over a variable period.

Nine men provided semen for analysis (Fig. 14.2). The findings fell into two distinct groups. Four had essentially normal semen. Five patients had very viscous semen with high pH (range 8.4 to 9.2); three of these had low sperm counts with only moderate motility.

Seven men also provided a specimen of urine passed after masturbation (Fig. 14.3). In only one was the sperm count higher than our laboratory normal, suggesting that retrograde ejaculation is uncommon. It mattered not whether the patient had viscous or normal semen or whether he was a slow or normal ejaculator. On these results it is likely that valve patients do ejaculate whatever semen they produce, albeit rather slowly. This conclusion supports the findings of an earlier study of patients with loss of bladder neck function in whom ejaculation was normal (Ochsner *et al.* 1970).

Six of 21 men were married. Two of their wives had produced children and a third had had a miscarriage at 4 months after many years of trying. One of the putative fathers had viscous ejaculate with a poor count; he was on dialysis at the time of the review but not at the time of

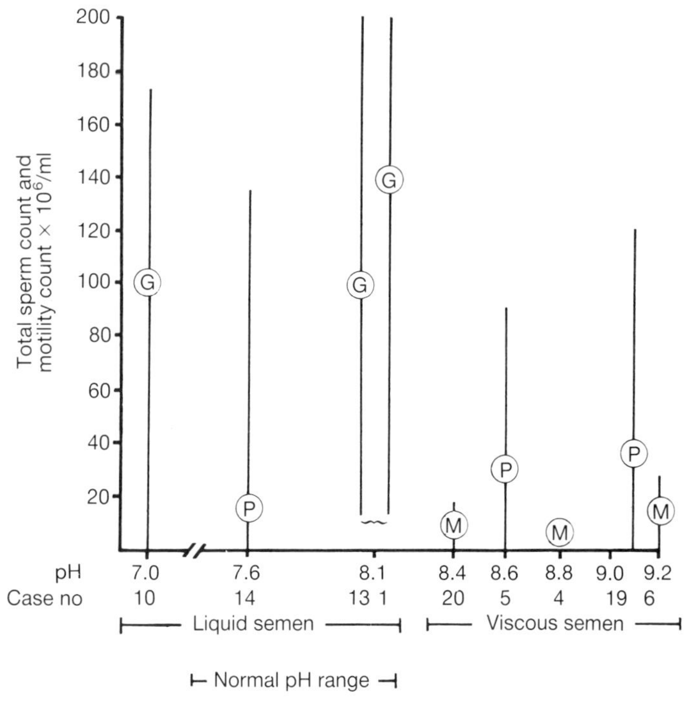


**Fig. 14.2** Results of semen analysis in nine adults previously treated for valves. The vertical lines represent the total count; the rings represent the number of motile sperm; G, M and P indicate that the motility was good, moderate or poor. The case numbers refer to the whole series (from Woodhouse *et al.* 1989, with permission).

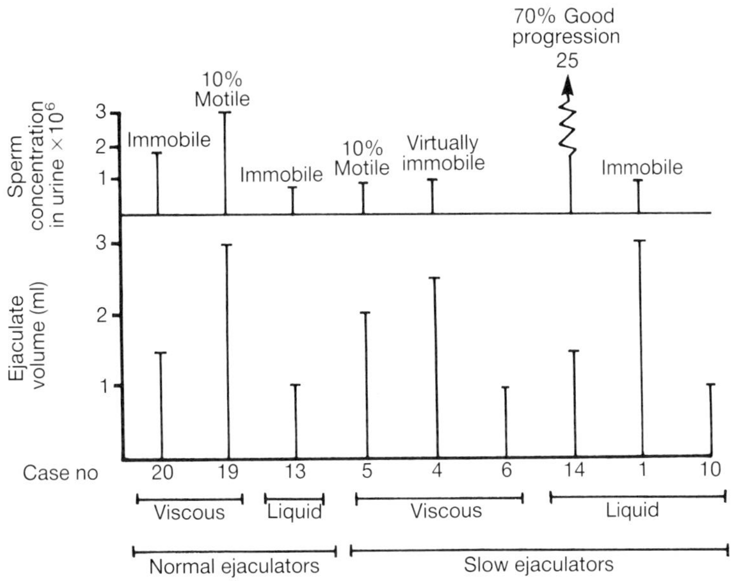


**Fig. 14.3** Comparison of the characteristics of ejaculated semen and urine voided after masturbation in seven of the adults illustrated in Fig. 14.2 (from Woodhouse *et al.* 1989, with permission).

conception. None of the other patients had complained of infertility. No very definite conclusions can be drawn except that it is possible for valve patients to father children.

## URETHRAL STRICTURE

The incidence of urethral stricture has declined steadily with better instruments and less manipulation of the urethra with catheters. Most series have reports of some cases. Churchill considers that the incidence is highest in patients treated before 1 year of age when it may reach 50%. With older instruments which required a perineal urethrostomy for use, the incidence was also high (19% with a perineal urethrostomy against 9% without, in Churchill's series). Overall, Churchill's incidence of stricture was 12% in 173 patients from 1957 to 1978 (Churchill *et al.* 1983). The use of the hook to disrupt valves may lead to fewer strictures.

Some strictures are fairly trivial affairs which only need a dilatation. Others are more troublesome. I agree with Crooks (1982) that a stricture in a defunctioned urethra is very difficult to manage. It is safest to undivert a valve patient with a stricture and use a perineal urethrostomy at a first stage. The urethra can be reconstructed at a second stage.

## RETARDED GROWTH

Boys with posterior urethral valves are small at presentation. Regardless of age they are nearly always below the 25th percentile for weight. After treatment they grow but rarely get above the 50th percentile. As usual, the younger the age at presentation and the worse the renal function, the less good is the prognosis. In younger patients the outcome for weight and height is significantly better if there is a period of upper tract diversion before surgery, rather than proceeding directly to valve ablation (Krueger *et al.* 1980).

## LATE PRESENTATION

The typical valve patient presents in infancy. Older patients are likely to have less severe obstruction and better renal function. It is likely that very minor valves will not produce sufficient symptoms to draw attention to themselves. Presentation in adult life is, therefore, rare.

Forty-eight cases presenting as adults have been reported (Mueller & Marshall 1983). The majority of cases had irritative bladder symptoms that had been attributed to chronic prostatitis and normal IVUs. Two patients were reported who presented in renal failure, both had been extensively investigated in childhood but the diagnosis had been missed.

The diagnosis must be difficult to make, especially considering the large number of men in urology clinics with urinary frequency and perineal pain. It seems unlikely that many have unrecognised valves. Suspicion would be aroused by a history of life-long non-competitive stream confirmed by measurement of a low flow rate. In difficult cases of bladder outflow obstruction it may be helpful to cystoscope the patient by passing the instrument through a suprapubic stab incision and looking at the outflow in an antegrade direction.

## REFERENCES

Atwell J.D. (1983) Posterior urethral valves in the British Isles: a multicentre B.A.P.S. review. *J. Ped. Surg.* **18**, 70–4.

Barnett M.G., Bruskewitz R.C., Belzer F.O., Sollinger H.W. & Uehling D.T. (1987) Ileocecocystoplasty bladder augmentation and renal transplantation. *J. Urol.* **138**, 855–8.

Barnett M.G., Bruskewitz R.C., Glass N. *et al.* (1985) Long-term clean intermittent self-catheterisation in renal transplant recipients. *J. Urol.* **134**, 654–7.

Bauer S.B., Dieppa R.A., Labib K.K. & Retik A.B. (1979) The bladder in boys with posterior urethral valves: a urodynamic assessment. *J. Urol.* **121**, 769–803.

Baum N.H., Burger R. & Carlton C.E. (1974) Nephrogenic diabetes insipidus associated with posterior urethral valves. *Urology* **4**, 581–3.

Campaiola J.M., Perlmutter A.D. & Steinhardt G.F. (1985) Noncompliant bladder resulting from posterior urethral valves. *J. Urol.* **134**, 708–10.

Churchill B.M., Krueger R.P., Fleisher M.H. & Hardy B.E. (1983) Complications of posterior urethral valve surgery and their prevention. *Urol. Clin. North Am.* **10**, 519–30.

Crooks K.K. (1982) Urethral strictures following transurethral resection of posterior urethral valves. *J. Urol.* **127**, 1153–6.

Frank J.D., Karthaus H.F.M., Johnston S.R. & Ransley P.G. (1982) An approach to undiversion in children. *Br. J. Urol.* **54**, 700–2.

Gonzalez R., Sidi A.A. & Zhang B. (1986) Urinary undiversion: indications, technique and results in 50 cases. *J. Urol.* **136**, 13–16.

Hennerby M.O. & Stephens F.D. (1980) Renal hypoplasia in infants with posterior urethral valves. *J. Urol.* **123**, 912–15.

Hoover D.L. & Duckett J.W. (1982) Posterior urethral valves, unilateral reflux and renal dysplasia: a syndrome. *J. Urol.* **128**, 994–7.

Krueger R.P., Hardy B.E. & Churchill B.M. (1980) Growth in boys with posterior urethral valves. *Urol. Clin. North Am.* **7**, 265–72.

Mueller S.C. & Marshall F.F. (1983) Spectrum of unrecognised posterior urethral valves in the adult. *Urology* **22**, 139–42.

Ochsner M.G., Burns E. & Henry H.H. (1970) Incidence of retrograde ejaculation following bladder neck revision as a child. *J. Urol.* **104**, 596–600.

Parkhouse H.F. (1990) The relatioship between renal function and bladder function after relief of congenital obstructive uropathy. *Ann. Roy. Coll. Surg. Engl.* (in press).

Parkhouse H.F., Barrett T.M., Dillon M.J. *et al.* (1988) Long-term outcome of boys with posterior urethral valves. *Br. J. Urol.* **62**, 59–62.

Parkhouse H.F. & Woodhouse C.R.J. (1990) Long-term of patients with posterior urethral valves. *Urol. Clin. North Am.* **17**, 373–78.

Scott J.E.S. (1985) Management of congenital posterior urethral valves. *Br. J. Urol.* **57**, 71–7.

Sheehan S.J., Duff F., Guiney E.J., Kelly D.G. & Smith J. (1984) Urinary tract undiversion. *Br. J. Urol.* **56**, 280–4.

Stone A.R., Bary P.R., Holmes D.M., Salaman J.R. & Stephenson T.P. (1982) Assessment for and results of urinary undiversion. *Br. J. Urol.* **54**, 703–7.

Warshaw B.L., Hymes L.C., Trulock T.S. & Woodard J.R. (1985) Prognostic features in infants with obstructive uropathy due to posterior urethral valves. *J. Urol.* **133**, 183–7.

Williams D.I., Whitaker R.H., Barrett T.M. & Keeton J.E. (1973) Urethral valves. *Br. J. Urol.* **45**, 200–10.

Woodhouse C.R.J., Reilly J.M. & Bahadur G. (1989) Sexual function and fertility in patients treated for posterior urethral valves. *J. Urol.* **142**, 586–8.

# 15 *Hypospadias*

## INTRODUCTION

Most hypospadias operations are entirely cosmetic. There are some patients whose chordee is so severe that sexual intercourse would be impossible. Some patients with penoscrotal hypospadias may have difficulty voiding. In general, however, the operations are done to make boys look like their peers, to enable them to void standing up and through their flies and to give them a straight penis for intercourse when the time comes. The results must, therefore, be examined very critically.

The techniques of repair have changed considerably over the last 40 years. The single most common operation was the buried strip of Denis-Browne. Many variations have been described marking the evolution to the single stage, pedicled tube urethroplasty that is popular in 1990.

Such is the success of the modern repair that even minor degrees of hypospadias are corrected. The Mental Advancement and Granuloplasty Incorporated (MAGPI) operation seems to be an almost foolproof technique for advancing the very distal meatus. Even 10 years ago minor hypospadias was commonly left alone or treated by a modified circumcision to disguise the coronal meatus.

Hypospadias appears to be an isolated abnormality. It is possible that the defect that causes it might cause psychological disturbances as well. It is more likely that any such problems are the consequence of the physical defect and its treatment.

Because the surgical techniques have changed so radically there is little justification for dwelling on the long-term results of the past. Some common problems in older patients are seen that require correction now. Some targets can be identified for the future.

## SURGICAL RESULTS

It seems that some surgeons have different criteria of success to others. The assessments may be subjective and depend on the original aims of the surgeon. It is best to rely on the reviews done by surgeons who were not involved in the original treatment.

Taken at their best, the results of the Denis-Browne operation are very good. Johanson has reviewed his own cases at a mean age of 18.4 years and at a mean of 7.1 years from the last operation. All of 220 cases had a straight erection, a formed stream with normal flow rate and a urethra that had grown appropriately with the rest of the penis. One hundred and forty-two patients had reached 'fertile age' and apparently had a normal ejaculate. Seven of 220 patients had a hypoplastic penis but four of them had other causes of developmental failure (Johanson & Avellan 1980).

Only 76 of 220 had a terminal meatus; in 133 it was in the coronal sulcus and in 11 it was 'directly proximal' to the sulcus. In other words, 144 patients had a proximally placed meatus that, were it a primary case, would have been an indication for hypospadias correction by today's standards.

In another series from Austria 24 of 36 adults operated as children were considered to have a perfect result with a penis indistinguishable from normal. The remainder were said to have minor cosmetic problems but these did include three with meatal stenosis and four with fistulae. The patients with meatal stenosis had abnormal ejaculation and reduced volume of ejaculate (Marberger & Pauer 1981).

These results are considered satisfactory by the surgeon. The views of the patients are unknown. Certainly if the surgeon, the patient and his parents regard them as satisfactory, then that is what they are.

When patients who have had such surgery are reviewed by an independent surgeon, the results are not so good. Summerlad attempted to trace 113 patients operated in one unit who would have been 17 or more years old. Sixty were actually found and seen. Thirty had had Denis-Brownes (27 having a meatus in the middle third of the penis or worse) and 24 had had Ombredannes for a distal meatus. Six had had a meatotomy alone. The patients having the Denis-Browne operation fared worse but, of course, were worse to start with.

Summerlad thought that 13 penises were not straight in the flaccid position, but only 10 patients complained of chordee on erection (two of whom had a straight penis when examined flaccid). The meatus was 'rarely' at the tip of the penis but was within 1 cm of the tip in 54. Very similar results were found in a series of patients operated at Great Ormond Street, UK (Kenawi 1976).

Almost none of the patients had normal voiding. At the least, the stream was deflected downwards. More than two-thirds had a stream that sprayed and 16 of 60 had difficulty in using a lavatory bowl when standing.

Sexual intercourse was difficult because of pain in four patients and because of hypoplasia of the penis in two (one of whom also had chordee). Twenty patients had weak or incomplete ejaculation (Summerlad 1975).

Since 1980 the majority of hypospadias repairs have used pedicled preputial skin or bladder mucosa. The operation is done in a single stage. The published results are excellent: a complete urethra with a normal appearance of the penis can be achieved in up to 95% of children (Duckett 1981, Hendren & Reda 1986, Elder *et al.* 1987). It is not only the technique that has led to the good cosmetic result. There has been recognition that the meatus must be brought to the tip of the glans; that the glans must be reconstructed; and that the operation is difficult and should not be done by the 'amateur'. Few of these children have become adults yet. However, the surgical results are so much better that it is reasonable to assume that they will be preserved into adult life. A single operation done in the first year or 2 of life should eliminate the psychological problems unless they have a basis beyond the physical appearance of the penis.

## PSYCHOLOGICAL RESULTS

Several authors have suggested that there might be psychological consequences from hypospadias or from its treatment. There have been few formal studies of adults.

Summerlad found that 20% of patients appeared to have suffered from their several admissions. However, most patients underestimated the number of admissions that they had had and that number was not particularly high by the standards of major urological anomalies: a mean of four for the Denis-Browne operation and 1.9 for the Ombredanne. Only eight remembered being altered by surgery and all felt that they were improved.

It was more striking to find that, of 60 patients, 21 avoided changing in public and 31 admitted to anxieties during adolescence, mainly about sexual function and fertility. Forty-three thought that their penis was abnormal. Two patients who could not be interviewed (and were not part of the series) were in prison, both for sexual offences (Summerlad 1975).

The difficulty of following up these patients is illustrated by the series from Great Ormond Street, UK where many of the cases had been personally operated on by Denis-Browne. Of 351 patients only 82 could be contacted as adults.

The main object of this review was to assess the patient's sexual function. Unlike the Berg and Berg survey (see below), sexual function was largely normal and in particular the age of sexual debut was normal (41% by the age of 18). Four of five patients who had sexual difficulties had residual chordee as the cause and only one had psychological problems (Kenawi 1976).

A very extensive psychoanalysis has been made of 33 men who were operated on for hypospadias as children. Thirty-six men who had had an appendicectomy in the same hospital, at the same time and at the same age were investigated as controls. There were no significant differences between the groups in general health, IQ or socioeconomic background. Obviously there was considerable difference in the type and number of operations that they had undergone although the details are not given. The analyses were made without knowledge of the patient's diagnosis.

The patients who had hypospadias fared badly. They had lower ego strength and poor utilisation of mental resources. They had reduced capacity for social and emotional relationships. Their levels of hostility, general anxiety and castration anxiety were higher and they had lower self-esteem. The severity of these abnormalities was not related to the original severity of the hypospadias.

In childhood the patients had been shy, timid, isolated and mobbed. As adults they were prone to neurotic (but not psychotic) disturbances and abnormal social relationships. They were less secure in their gender identity, had delayed sexual debut and a smaller number of sexual partners. Eventually they settled down in secure and lasting sexual partnerships. In the long run, they had less rewarding and less demanding jobs. The modern jargon for such men might be 'under-achievers' (Berg *et al.* 1982, Berg *et al.* 1983a,b, Berg & Berg 1983a,b).

These studies are open to several criticisms:

**1** The control subjects were, presumably, chosen because they had been in hospital and had surgery. However, the nature of their operation and, particularly, their peers' reaction to it, are not remotely similar to hypospadias.

**2** The patients, the controls, the surgeons and the authors were all from the same hospital: the Karolinska Institute, Sweden. There might be differences in other hospitals.

**3** Although parental background was investigated, parental attitudes to the hypospadias or the appendicectomy were not.

**4** The authors set out by predicting the abnormalities from psychoanalytical theory and appear to have constructed the investigations to prove them.

**5** The patients clearly did not have a good result from their surgery: 13 had a spraying stream, five had poor flow and five had residual chordee, one of whom could not have intercourse as a result (Svensson & Berg 1983).

Nonetheless, these are very detailed and important studies and their results cannot be dismissed without proper thought. If patients treated for hypospadias have psychological problems we should seek the reasons and try to correct them.

The suggestion of Berg and Berg is that the abnormalities are the consequence of the malformed penis. If we accept that the appendicectomy control group did not have comparable surgery, it is possible that the series of operations suffered by the hypospadiacs is the cause. Berg and Berg stress the fact that hypospadias surgery was started at 3 to 4 years old when the ego is particularly vulnerable. If either of these explanations is correct, single stage surgery in infancy (assuming the surgical results are excellent) should solve the psychological problems. Likewise better counselling of the parents would improve their attitudes and so produce better orientated patients.

It is also possible, as Berg and Berg considered, that the psychological disturbances are a part of a syndrome which includes hypospadias. An endocrine failure might cause both. In searching for such a cause, Berg and colleagues found low serum 5-alpha reductase levels in hypospadiacs (Berg *et al.* 1983b). Poor sperm quality has also been reported in 50% of a series of adult hypospadiacs (Zubowska *et al.* 1979). If hypospadias is more than just an example of target organ failure and is part of a more complex syndrome, the psychological abnormalities will continue to be seen.

It is tempting for surgeons to be sceptical of psychological theories when there is a clear cut anatomical problem. It does seem most likely that successful single stage surgery will give better long-term results. I think it would pay to keep an open mind and, at least, to provide proper counselling for the parents until we know the long-term results of the new techniques.

## ANOMALIES ASSOCIATED WITH HYPOSPADIAS

In spite of some conflicting reports from the past, it is now generally agreed that renal and ureteric anomalies with hypospadias are very rare. Combining three recent reports from three countries, only seven significant renal abnormalities were found in 360 patients. In three of them renal investigations would have been indicated because of anorectal agenesis (Kelly *et al.* 1984, Cerasaro *et al.* 1986, Davenport & MacKinnon 1988). In a retrospective review of 460 patients Khuri found 14 patients who required surgery for upper tract anomalies: screening of patients with proximal hypospadias or with other congenital anomalies was recommended (Khuri *et al.* 1981).

In the lower urinary tract one centre has found a very high incidence of Müllerian duct remnants, especially a prostatic utricle. Eighty-four examples were found on retrograde urethrography in 280 patients. Only 14 were of substantial size (grade II or III on their scale, see Chapter 17) and only six were symptomatic. Large utricles were always associated with scrotal or perineal hypospadias. Eight patients had other Müllerian remnants and ambiguous sex, although they presented with hypospadias (Ikoma *et al.* 1985, 1986).

Of more importance than these rare congenital anomalies are ones that may be acquired as a result of hypospadias repair. The most common of these arise from urethral obstruction which may develop from inadequate growth of the neo-urethra. The incidence of such problems is unkown even with the older repairs. The penile skin should be testosterone sensitive and so grow with the penis. Suggestions that preputial skin might be deficient in androgen receptors and so fail to grow appear to be unfounded (Coulam *et al.* 1983).

When the neo-urethra produces bladder outflow obstruction the symptoms are usually of poor stream. I have seen one case presenting with detrusor instability out of 19 adult patients with late hypospadias problems.

Vesico-ureteric reflux has been reported in 21 patients. This abnormality may occur even if the neo-urethra has not stenosed and the preoperative cystogram is normal. However, in 10 patients the reflux resolved after revision of the urethroplasty and only two patients required reimplantation of the ureters (Sharfir *et al.* 1982).

## LATE SURGICAL PROBLEMS

Even when a patient has not had a perfect result from hypospadias repair, he may not have sufficient symptoms to want further surgery. In some cases he may develop symptoms many years after a successful repair: up to 50 years has been reported (Flynn *et al.* 1980).

Symptoms are usually of stricture, fistula or chordee, and may be complicated by a stone or hair ball in the neo-urethra. Although the problem may, at first sight, appear simple, it should be assumed that all have a total inadequacy of the repair until proved otherwise. Many may be described as 'hypospadiac cripples' with a neo-urethra that is too short, too narrow and of poor material. No specific type of primary repair is particularly associated with this disastrous complication (Stecker *et al.* 1981).

Hair in the urethra may cause irritation, infection, obstruction or stones. Hair-bearing skin should not be used for urethroplasty but sometimes there is little choice. Large collections of hair, especially when complicated by a hair ball or stone, require endoscopic or even open removal (Fig. 15.1). Smaller collections of hair can be removed by instillation of thioglycolic acid. This chemical is sterile and will dissolve urethral hair in 75% of cases after 10 minutes. Patients have dysuria for up to 24 hours afterwards. It is commercially available as Immac, a depilator manufactured by the International Chemical Co. Ltd. (Bagshaw *et al.* 1980).

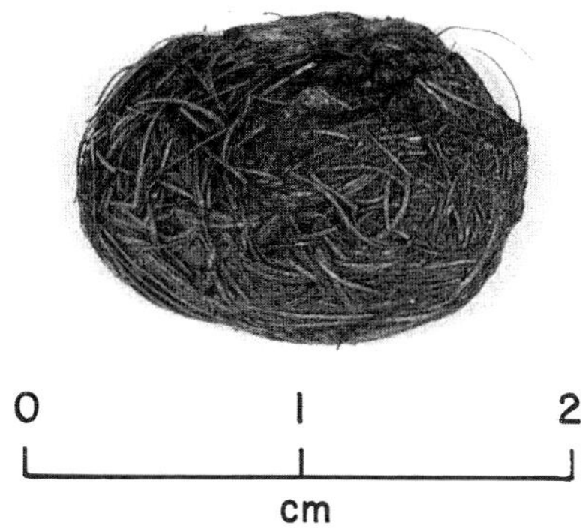


**Fig. 15.1** A tight, hard hair ball removed from a reconstructed hypospadiac urethra.

Chordee may occur with a urethra of normal calibre. Correction of the deformity by excision of the ventral chordee tissue will result in a urethra that is too short and further urethroplasty is needed. If the penis is of adequate length, the patient may be content with a dorsal Nesbitt's procedure rather than risk yet more reconstruction.

The site of chordee may be easy to identify, being opposite the neo-urethra. Occasionally, I and others have found the deformity to be more proximal (see Fig. 2.2, and Svensson & Berg 1983). In difficult cases an artificial erection will clarify the problem. This should be achieved either by intracorporeal injection of papaverine or by the infusion technique (see Chapter 2). If a tourniquet is put around the penis at scrotal level and saline injected into the corpora, the chordee may be missed.

In the majority the whole neo-urethra is hopeless. All would agree that the reconstruction of such difficult cases must include wide exposure, radical excision of the old urethra and all other tissues contributing to the chordee and reconstruction of the urethra from good skin by a meticulous technique (Stecker *et al.* 1981).

The destructive part of the operation is relatively easy. The temptation is to be too conservative. The urethra must be cut back to really good tissue: the old external meatus may have been inappropriately preserved at the original operation. Good urethra is surrounded by spongy tissue. The chordee tissue must be stripped down to the tunica albuginea (which seems alarmingly thin at times) and the completeness checked by artificial erections.

The reconstructive phase requires imagination and an ability to use all of the available techniques as the case demands. It is usual to find that all of the prepuce and much of the spare penile skin have gone. The new tissue to be brought in must be water resistant, hairless and free from the risk of contracture. Not surprisingly, no such perfect tissue exists. The choice lies between pedicled skin which will almost certainly have to be scrotal and which is hairy, grafted skin which may contract, and bladder mucosa for which we lack long-term experience in adults.

To make a new urethra from pedicled scrotal skin is simple. The material is freely available, has a good blood supply from the dartos and can be rolled into a tube in a single stage operation. The difficulties lie in destroying the hair follicles (not all of which are actively growing hairs at any given moment) and measuring the area of skin required. It has been used with success by Blandy. He recommends the preparation of a tin-foil template rolled over a 24 FG sound. The correct size of scrotal skin can then be marked out and cut. Although he uses a flap cut transversely from the scrotum, it is easier to find relatively hairless skin in the mid-line of the scrotum. The use of a circumcising incision to deglove the penis lessens the risk of fistula.

Complete reconstruction in one stage by this technique had good results at 2 to 4 years in 18 adult hypospadias cripples. Hair was a problem in only one. Sexual and urinary function were normal (Flynn *et al.* 1980).

If a free skin graft is used the operation is best done in two stages, the graft being moved to the site of the new urethra at the first stage and the tube formation at the second. Split skin and full thickness, if necessary with meshing, both have their advocates.

The use of meshed split skin is popular in Europe. A graft of 0.1 mm thickness is cut with a compressed air driven dermatome and then meshed. It is then applied to the ventrum of the penis to cover the defect from the excised urethra. The meshing allows free drainage of serum and is said to aid healing. A second operation, at which much of the graft is rolled into a neourethra, is done at least 8 weeks later. All of nine hypospadiacs are reported to have had a good result at 2 to 8 years' follow-up. Urethrograms have shown that the calibre of the urethra is maintained (Schreiter & Noll 1987).

Unmeshed split skin may also be used, even in a single stage procedure. The donor site may be the inner aspect of the arm or the buttock. The skin is cut with a dermatome, rolled into a tube and positioned on the penis to fill the urethral gap. In 11 patients on whom this technique was used, six had a good result. There were two fistulas, two short strictures treated by urethrotomy and one complete graft failure (Burbige *et al.* 1984).

The use of full thickness preputial skin grafts in children has been championed by Devine and Horton (1977). They have been widely used and generally have stood the test of time. If there is inadequate penile skin, the graft is best taken from the groin or inner aspect of the arm (Hendren & Crooks 1980, Turner-Warwick 1988). As the length of urethra to be replaced is, by definition, long, a two-stage procedure is usual. Furthermore, the absence of spongy tissue to form a good bed for the graft adds to the risk of partial graft failure. Good results over many years have been reported for this technique as a single-stage procedure (Stecker *et al.* 1981).

Bladder mucosa as a substitute for the urethra is not new but has recently been revived. The technique has been widely used in children with hypospadias but there are no long-term results. It is not suitable for the terminal few millimetres of urethra as it hypertrophies and becomes sticky when exposed to air (Ransley *et al.* 1987). Its use in adults has been mentioned and anecdotal cases reports exist but there has been no critical assessment (Turner-Warwick 1988, Elder & Duckett 1987, Vyas *et al.* 1987).

## INHERITANCE OF HYPOSPADIAS

The study of the inheritance of uncomplicated hypospadias is hampered by two factors: absence of a survey of the offspring of hypospadiacs and the lack of knowledge in patients about their ancestors. Furthermore, there is a wide spectrum in the condition and there may be several different modes of inheritance within it. Nearly all paediatric urologists will have encountered families with several cases.

Early studies suggested that the aetiology involved several factors and this view was supported by the observation that the more proximal the external urinary meatus the higher was the incidence of hypospadias in first degree relatives (Sweet *et al.* 1974).

A later view supports a dominant Mendelian inheritance. Six families have been reported with three successive generations affected. In one of them four fathers had five sons between them, all of whom were affected (Page 1979).

A prospective survey of 430 patients identified

a 21% incidence of hypospadias in another family member and 5% had three family members affected (Bauer *et al.* 1981).

All this is very interesting but does not help in the counselling of a prospective father, especially if he has no known family history. The risk factors for producing an affected son appear to be a severe degree of hypospadias and an extensive family history of affected first degree relatives. If a normal father has produced a son with hypospadias, the risk of a further son being affected is 12% (18% if it was a penoscrotal hypospadias). If the father and son both have hypospadias the risk in a subsequent son is 26% (Bauer *et al.* 1981).

## REFERENCES


Bagshaw H.A., Flynn J.T., James A.N., Johnston S.R. & Blandy J.P. (1980) The use of thioglycolic acid in hair-bearing skin inlay urethroplasty. *Br. J. Urol.* **52**, 546–8.

Bauer S.B., Retik A.B. & Colodny A.H. (1981) Genetic aspects of hypospadias. *Urol. Clin. North Am.* **8**, 559–64.

Berg G. & Berg R. (1983a) Castration complex, evidence from men operated for hypospadias. *Acta Psychiatr. Scand.* **68**, 143–53.

Berg R. & Berg G. (1983b) Penile malformation, gender identity and sexual orientation. *Acta Psychiatr. Scand.* **68**, 154–66.

Berg R., Berg G., Edman G. *et al.* (1983a) Androgens and personality in normal men and men operated for hypospadias in childhood. *Acta Psychiatr. Scand.* **68**, 167–77.

Berg R., Svensson J., Astrom G. *et al.* (1983b) Social and sexual adjustment of men operated for hypospadias during childhood: a controlled study. *J. Urol.* **125**, 313–17.

Berg R., Berg G. & Svensson J. (1982) Penile malformation and mental health. *Acta Psychiatr. Scand.* **66**, 398–416.

Burbige K.A., Hensle T.W. & Edgerton P. (1984) Extragenital split thickness skin graft for urethral reconstruction. *J. Urol.* **131**, 1137–9.

Cerasaro T.S., Brock W.A. & Kaplan G.W. (1986) Upper urinary tract anomalies with congenital hypospadias: is screening necessary? *J. Urol.* **135**, 537–8.

Coulam C.B., Razel A.J., Kelalis P.P., Svensson J. & Spelsberg T.C. (1983) Androgen receptor in human foreskin. *Am. J. Obstet. Gynecol.* **147**, 513–20.

Davenport M. & MacKinnon A.E. (1988) The value of ultrasound screening of the upper urinary tract in hypospadias. *Br. J. Urol.* **62**, 595–6.

Devine C.J. & Horton C.E. (1977) Hypospadias repair. *J. Urol.* **118**, 188–93.

Duckett J.W. (1981) The island flap technique for hypospadias repair. *Urol. Clin. North Am.* **8**, 503–16.

Elder J.S. & Duckett J.W. (1987) Urethral reconstruction following an unsuccessful one stage hypospadias repair. *World J. Urol.* **5**, 19–24.

Elder J.S., Duckett J.W. & Snyder H. McC. (1987) Onlay island flap in the repair of mid and distal penile hypospadias without chordee. *J. Urol.* **138**, 376–9.

Flynn J.T., Johnston S.R. & Blandy J.P. (1980) The late sequelae of hypospadias repair. *Br. J. Urol.* **52**, 555–9.

Hendren W.H. & Crooks K.K. (1980) Tubed free skin graft for construction of male urethra. *J. Urol.* **123**, 858–61.

Hendren W.H. & Reda E.F. (1986) Bladder mucosa graft for construction of the male urethra. *J. Ped. Surg.* **21**, 189–92.

Ikoma F., Shima H. & Yabumoto H. (1985) Classification of enlarged prostatic utricle in patients with hypospadias. *Br. J. Urol.* **57**, 334–7.

Ikoma F., Shima H., Yabumoto H. & Mori Y. (1986) Surgical treatment for enlarged prostatic utricle and vagina masculina in patients with hypospadias. *Br. J. Urol.* **58**, 423–8.

Johanson B. & Avellan L. (1980) Hypospadias. A review of 299 cases operated 1957–1969. *Scand. J. Plast. Reconstr. Surg.* **14**, 259–67.

Kelly D., Harte F.B. & Roe P. (1984) Urinary tract anomalies in patients with hypospadias. *Br. J. Urol.* **56**, 316–18.

Kenawi M.M. (1976) Sexual function hypospadiacs. *Br. J. Urol.* **47**, 883–90.

Khuri F.J., Hardy B.E. & Churchill B.M. (1981) Urologic anomalies associated with hypospadias. *Urol. Clin. North Am.* **8**, 565–71.

Marberger H. & Pauer W. (1981) Experience in hypospadias repair. *Urol. Clin. North Am.* **8**, 403–19.

Morgan R.J., Williams D.I. & Pryor J.P. (1979) Mullerian duct remnants in the male. *Br. J. Urol.* **51**, 488–92.

Page L.A. (1979) Inheritance of uncomplicated hypospadias. *Pediatrics* **63**, 788–90.

Ransley P.G., Duffy P.G., Oesch I.L., Van Oyen P. & Hoover D. (1987) The use of bladder mucosa and combined bladder mucosa/preputial skin grafts for urethral reconstruction. *J. Urol.* **138**, 1096–8.

Schreiter F. & Noll F. (1987) Meshgraft urethroplasty. *World J. Urol.* **5**, 41–6.

Sharfir R., Tsur H., Hertz M. *et al.* (1982) Vesico-ureteral reflux in boys with hypospadias. *Urology* **20**, 29–32.

Stecker J.F., Horton C.E., Devine C.J. & McCraw J.B.

(1981) Hypospadias cripples. *Urol. Clin. North Am.* **8**, 539–44.

Summerlad B.C. (1975) A long-term follow-up of hypospadias patients. *Br. J. Plast. Surg.* **28**, 324–30.

Svensson J. & Berg R. (1983) Micturition studies and sexual function in operated hypospadiacs. *Br. J. Urol.* **55**, 422–6.

Sweet R.A., Schrott H.G., Kurland R. & Culp O.S. (1974) Study of the incidence of hypospadias in Rochester, Minnesota 1940–1970. *Mayo Clin. Proc.* **49**, 50–52.

Turner-Warwick R.C. (1988) Urethral stricture surgery. In: Mundy, A.R. (ed) *Current Operative Surgery (Urology)*, Bailliere Tindall, London, pp. 160–218.

Vyas P.R., Roth D.R. & Perlmutter A.D. (1987) Experience with free grafts in urethral reconstruction. *J. Urol.* **137**, 471–4.

Zubowska J., Jankowska J., Kula K. *et al.* (1979) Clinical, hormonal and semiological data in adult men operated in childhood for hypospadias. *Endokrynologia Polska* **30**, 565–73.

# 16 *Undescended testes*

## INTRODUCTION

The incidence of undescended testis (UDT) at birth is increasing in England. In the 1950s it was 0.8% and by 1984 it had reached 3.0%. However, many of these cases are in low birth weight babies. By 9 months of age only 1.28% of infants have a UDT (Chilvers & Pike 1989). The treatment and its timing are a matter of some debate at present. The prevailing view 20 years ago was that the testes should be in the scrotum by the beginning of schooling at 5 years old. Unfortunately many UDTs were not recognised until the school medical inspection at 5 years old and orchiopexy was not done until later.

UDT and the descended testes in cases of unilateral UDT are abnormal from 1 year of age or possibly earlier. Abnormalities are seen in spermatogenesis and in the Leydig cells. The appearances deteriorate through childhood and puberty. It is, therefore, reasonable to expect that earlier treatment will produce a better long-term result.

It will be seen later that early operation may be associated with better fertility. However, there is no proof, at present, that operation in infancy has better physical or psychological results. The disadvantage of early operation is that some retractile testes will be operated on unnecessarily. It has been pointed out that since the advent of early operation the number of orchiopexies in one hospital has risen from 7.68 per year between 1950 and 1975 to 27 per year thereafter (Kumar *et al.* 1989). This increase, although of the same magnitude as the increase in incidence of UDT found by Chilvers and Pike, is attributed partly to operations on retractile testes.

There have been occasional reports of normally descended testes going up. Although surgeons are naturally sceptical, most will have heard such stories from parents. Thirteen cases have been reported from one unit where the boys were seen by the same team to have normal testes initially and subsequently to require orchiopexy. The original examination was at 1 to 9 years old (mean: 4). Orchiopexy was necessary between 5 and 12 (mean: 8). All were unilateral and 10 were associated with a hernia (Robertson *et al.* 1988). The reality of this phenomenon is supported by the failure of the 'acquired UDT' to descend in response to HCG in 80% of cases (Schiffer *et al.* 1987, Belman 1988).

The late complications that have been identified may be the inevitable result of a primary congenital anomaly or the result of delayed treatment.

## BILATERAL CRYPTORCHIDISM

### Fertility

Men with untreated bilateral UDT are, with a few poorly documented exceptions, infertile. All of 17 men investigated by biopsy or semen analysis in one infertility clinic were 'totally sterile' (Scott 1962).

Whatever the age of surgery in childhood, the UDT grows almost to normal size. Prader has given 18.6 ml ± 4 ml for normal adult size while bilateral undescended testes, regardless of age at surgery, average 16.0 ml ± 4.9 ml (Scheiber *et al.* 1981). However, size does not correlate with function, though there is a trend for smaller testes to have worse sperm counts.

After treatment the fertility rate varies between authors from 0 to 79%. There are obvious difficulties in estimating the fertility of any group of patients operated on in childhood. The problem is compounded in cryptorchidism as the patient has a relatively minor operation and then is seen no more. It is no wonder that the reported figures vary so widely.

Fertility is often poorly defined. There is no series that reports the rate of fertility in all operated children with proof of paternity. Some report the number of children born to the wives of a sample of operated patients, or the findings in patients in infertility clinics. More commonly fertility is defined in terms of semen analysis.

One of the first papers to suggest that treatment did improve fertility pointed out that the procedure of fixation of the testis to the thigh by a stitch for the immediate postoperative period might cause avascular necrosis of the testis. In their own patients with no such fixation the authors found six of 16 patients with bilateral UDT who had 14 children. A further six patients had sperm counts that were considered fertile or had initiated a pregnancy. There was no information about the other 225 bilateral cryptorchids in the series. Surgery was done between 7 and 12 years old (Gross & Jewett 1956).

Several authors have tried to trace all patients operated during a particular period. The response rate to these surveys is around 50 to 60%. It might be assumed that the ones who did not respond had some personal reason for their decision and were not, in fact, identical to the responding group. The number of cases of bilateral UDT is usually small. Paternity is between 40 and 60% but consistently lower than for unilateral cases in each survey (Levin & Sherman 1973, Atkinson *et al.* 1975, Kumar *et al.* 1989).

The effect of age at operation has been found significant. Six of nine operated before 12 years old were fathers while only three of six operated after 12 were (Kumar *et al.* 1989). These figures are small, but are supported by an older review article which estimated fertility at only 13.5% for patients operated after puberty compared to 30% when the operation was done before puberty (Bayle 1957).

Scheiber was able to review 60% of patients who had had bilateral orchiopexies 6 to 21 years earlier. Twenty-six of 36 patients had a 'pathological' semen analysis, though the term was not defined (Scheiber *et al.* 1981).

Other authors have studied patients attending infertility clinics. This method clearly selects a poor group of patients and the pool of UDT patients from which they are drawn is unknown. Where the figures are given, however, it is clear that the incidence of UDT patients is higher in the clinic population than in the population at large: in a large French series, for example, 6.25% had UDT, 60% of which were bilateral (Plante *et al.* 1982). Although many patients in these series were said to have 'fertile sperm counts', the fact they were attending an infertility clinic implies that some of them were unable to father children. In reviewing the literature, Scott states that 37% of bilateral UDT patients have a fertile sperm count (1962). It is also clear that, in this selected group of apparently infertile men, a disproportionate number of patients with azoospermia have a history of bilateral, rather than unilateral, UDT: 80% in one series (Plante *et al.* 1982).

It has been suggested that successful treatment with HCG alone (as opposed to HCG which failed, and was followed by surgery) results in a higher proportion of 'fertile' sperm counts. Eight of 11 patients with successful HCG treatment had normal sperm counts compared to three of 11 who had HCG followed by surgery. It is not recorded whether any of the men had actually fathered a child (Albescu *et al.* 1971). These differences might reflect different degrees of abnormality in the testis/pituitary axis.

A prospective follow-up is badly needed. The Children's Hospital in Basle is undertaking a prospective study and some data are already available. As might be expected, there are degrees of testicular abnormality that may be associated with maldescent. All boys undergoing orchiopexy have testicular biopsies. At follow-up in adulthood the findings are correlated with the semen analysis. In the eight boys in their report, operated between 9 and 15 years old, five had no spermatogonia in the original biopsy and were azoospermic or severely oligozoospermic at adult follow-up. Only two boys had even a reasonable number of germ cells and at follow-up had a semen count of $37\times10^6$/ml. All had a reduced volume of ejaculate with only one above 2 ml (Hadziselimovic *et al.* 1984).

There does seem to be a spectrum of testicular abnormalities. The severity may be dependent on dysgenesis from birth (or earlier) or on the age at orchiopexy or both. If it is true that untreated bilateral UDT causes infertility, surgery must improve the situation. Early surgery is better than late surgery, though how early is uncertain. The fertility rate in any cohort of men born with bilateral maldescent is impaired.

## Endocrine function

Serum testosterone and LH levels are normal both before and after surgery for bilateral cryptorchidism. The FSH levels taken as an average are also normal. However, there is wide variation and abnormally high levels have been found in some patients with poor sperm counts. Presumably these patients do not produce sufficient inhibin to switch off pituitary FSH production.

Basal LH levels are variable, being reported as high, normal or low by different authors. Poor Leydig cell function and poor spermiogenesis are indicated by the exaggerated responses that have been shown of both LH and FSH to gonadotrophin-releasing hormone (GnRH). After injection of 200 mg of GnRH there was a 7.7-fold rise in LH and 3.3-fold rise in FSH (compared to 3.3 and 2.1 for controls). The abnormally high levels, especially of FSH, were maintained at 2 hours after the injection instead of returning to normal. There was a correlation with pathological sperm count in these results (Scheiber *et al.* 1981, Bollerslev *et al.* 1986). Similar responses occur in experimental cryptorchidism in the rat (Jansz & Pomerantz 1986).

## Risk of neoplasia

There is no doubt that cryptorchidism predisposes to germ cell neoplasia. The question is, to what extent?

Whitaker's classic review of 13 089 cases from the literature gave a 9.8% incidence of UDT. The number with bilateral UDT is not recorded. The risk of neoplasia, if these figures are accepted, depends on the incidence of UDT in the population. Although the best figures available at the time, Whitaker has cast some doubt on them recently (Whitaker 1988). The widely quoted figure of a 35-fold increase in risk was based on a general incidence of UDT of 0.28% to 0.3% (Whitaker 1970, Martin & Menck 1975).

In calculating an accurate figure, the statistician has to allow for the changing incidence of both the neoplasm and UDT. The incidence of testicular neoplasms is increasing in some countries, especially Denmark, and remains rare in Negroes. The risk may differ by time and place.

Denmark has a particularly good cancer and population registry. A study of 509 consecutive patients admitted for treatment of UDT from 1949 to 1960 provides interesting data. The risk of neoplasia was compared in the study group with an expected figure in age matched men derived from the cancer registry. In the 167 men with bilateral UDT there were four cases of neoplasia (three seminoma and one embryonal carcinoma). The risk was 9.3-fold over the normal population. The number of seminomas produced a late age of diagnosis so that the high risk period was in the fourth decade of life (Giwercman *et al.* 1987).

In a careful analysis of the world literature, Chilvers and Pike have calculated that the overall increased risk of neoplasia in patients with any UDT is 5.4, but the 95% confidence limits were wide at 3.3 to 8.3. However, when they considered only patients treated at the Royal Marsden Hospital, UK, they calculated the relative risk at 5.1. The similarity of this figure to the review figure of 5.4 supports the accuracy. The relative risk for those with bilateral UDT was 11.7 which compares well with the Danish figure. About one boy in 44 with bilateral UDT will develop a neoplasm (Chilvers & Pike 1989).

An interesting piece of additional and unexpected information came out of the Danish study. Although there was no increased risk of neoplasia in the study group overall, there were two cases of bladder carcinoma which, with so young a group, gives a relative risk of 10! Such accurate figures are not available for every country.

The higher the testes in the abdomen, the greater the risk of neoplasia. Smith quotes a figure of 1 in 20 intra-abdominal testes developing malignancy, but the data are more than 40 years old (Smith 1978). Some intra-abdominal testes do not contain any germ cells and so, presumably, cannot develop a germ cell neoplasm. However, the underlying trend has been confirmed by the incidence of carcinoma *in situ* (CIS) in undescended testes at various levels in adults. CIS was found in four of 16 intra-abdominal testes compared to three of 44 inguinal testes (7%). Ten of the 16 abdominal testes contained Sertoli cells only (Ford *et al.* 1985).

Carcinoma *in situ* can be found in biopsies of the prepubertal testis taken at orchiopexy. An incidence of seven cases in 1331 biopsies has been reported (Hadziselimovic *et al.* 1984). The significance of *in situ* change at this age is unknown.

## UNILATERAL UNDESCENDED TESTIS

### Fertility

Untreated unilateral UDT is compatible with paternity though the high incidence of such cases in infertility clinics suggests that there is reduced fertility. Scott found that 60% of his patients in this group had 'infertile sperm counts' and similar figures were found in comparable papers (1962).

In treated cases the figures for fertility vary from 12% to 92%. The same difficulty with inadequate data as in bilateral UDT is apparent. From the vast mass of statistics on UDT it is difficult to draw any firm conclusions. The normally descended testis in cases of unilateral UDT does not seem to be normal, but there is no agreement on just how abnormal it is. Nor on whether the age of orchiopexy makes any difference. Nor whether the continued presence of the undescended testis in the body (either in the scrotum or in the original undescended site) worsens the damage.

After childhood orchiopexy the single undescended testis grows almost normally. It is not statistically different in size from normal testes nor from bilaterally undescended testes. There is a slight trend for normal adult testes to be bigger than unilateral UDTs which are themselves bigger than bilateral UDT (18.6 ml vs. 17.6 ml vs. 16.0 ml). As with bilateral UDT, size does not correlate with function though there is a trend for bigger testes to have better seminal profiles (Scheiber *et al.* 1981).

In terms of producing babies the incidence of infertility does not appear to be very high. About two-thirds of couples where the male partner had had unilateral UDT have children. This figure is based on a survey of about 50% of a patient group operated on between 1950 and 1960 and traced in 1975. Again, there is no reason to suppose that the untraced patients would be similar. It is not known whether the couples with no children were infertile involuntarily

(Lipshultz *et al.* 1976). Similar figures are given by other authors (Levin & Sherman 1973, Atkinson 1975). An identical survey from Scotland produced a figure of 83.9% fertility for UDT patients. An interesting feature was the observation that the father's age at the birth of the first child was the expected normal when his orchiopexy had been done before 18 years old. Those who were operated after 18 were older when their first child was born, suggesting that they had had difficulty with conception and were subfertile (Kumar *et al.* 1989).

Even in patients attending infertility clinics, sperm analyses are normal in about 75% of patients (Scott 1962, Levin & Sherman 1973).

In a full review of the world literature Chilvers and Pike concluded that 43% of reported patients with treated unilateral UDT had azoospermia or oligozoospermia. They also found that the same figure applied to patients who had not been treated. They concluded that treatment did not improve fertility (1989). Of course, as they point out, the figures are suspect as the reported patients have always been selected in some way.

An alternative explanation could be that patients with unilateral UDT have the same rate of infertility as the normal population. The high incidence of poor sperm counts reported could be due to selection bias. If this were the case, it is hardly surprising that operation does not improve fertility.

Scheiber's late follow-up of orchiopexy patients is less complete for unilateral cases of whom he only managed to review 46 of 615 cases. Orchiopexy was performed from nine to 18 years old. Semen analyses were normal in 13, doubtful in 23 and pathological in 10, though the terms were not defined (Scheiber *et al.* 1981). Low mean sperm densities have been found generally, though not outside the range that is consistent with fertility. Motility of the sperm tends to be normal.

Two interesting studies have been done on patients with unilateral treated UDT of proven fertility who were requesting vasectomy. They were persuaded to have the operation done in two stages, ligating the vas of the normally descended testis first. When semen analyses were done between the operations, only one of 16 patients had a normal sperm count. This obviously suggests that surgery had not improved the function of the UDT (Eldrup & Steven 1980, Alpert & Klein 1983).

Reports of testicular biopsies give inconsistent results. Hedinger showed that from 2 years old onwards spermatogonia counts in the descended testis were lower than those in controls and that 'compensatory hypertrophy' in this context was uncommon (Hedinger 1982). This finding was supported by Hadziselimovic who also found that a poor tubular germ cell count at the time of orchiopexy correlated with a poor spermiogram in adult life (Hadziselimovic *et al.* 1984). Conversely, Kirby found no differences in the biopsies of the scrotal testes in unilateral UDT and controls, while the undescended testes had significantly lower total tubular fertility indices (Kirby *et al.* 1985). There have been reports of histological appearances improving after orchiopexy (Levin & Sherman 1973).

A further complicating factor is the condition of the vas and the epididymis. It has recently been observed, in a retrospective study, that 88% of epididymes and 93% of vasa from undescended testes were immature. The immaturity was associated with absence of spermatogonia or a low tubular fertility index (DePalma *et al.* 1988). This possibility requires further investigation and it may be that poor transport, even on the normally descended side, is as much to blame for subfertility as poor spermatogenesis.

The balance of evidence favours the notion that the scrotal testis is not completely normal and that it cannot wholly compensate for its abnormal partner. However, fertility is near normal.

## Endocrine function

The hormonal findings are similar to those in

patients with bilateral UDT though less severe. Basal levels of LH and FSH are variable. There is an exaggerated response to gonadotrophin releasing hormone but it is not as marked as in bilateral UDT. The response is the same in experimental rats (Lipshultz *et al.* 1976, Jansz & Pomerantz 1986).

### Risk of neoplasia

Calculation of the risk of neoplasia in unilateral UDT is subject to the same difficulties and variations as in bilateral UDT.

The most recent figure quoted in the *Journal of Urology* is a 9.7-fold increased risk in all cases of cryptorchidism (Farrer *et al.* 1985). The Danish study showed that the increased risk for unilateral UDT was only 2.4 (Giwercman *et al.* 1987). For English men the relative risks have been given as 4.0 for the undescended testis and 1.7 for the scrotal testis; the overall risk was 6.8 which is about half the risk for those with bilateral UDT. About one boy in 120 with unilateral UDT will develop a neoplasm (Chilvers & Pike 1989).

Carcinoma *in situ* is uncommon in the normally descended testis. There were no cases in 400 autopsies of men from 18–50 years old after sudden death (Giwercman *et al.* 1988). It was only found once in Ford's series of 30 biopsies of the normal testis in unilateral UDT. Furthermore CIS was never found in 52 cases of successful unilateral orchiopexy (Ford *et al.* 1985). Skakkebaek's group found CIS in 2% of biopsies of men with a history of UDT, though it is not said which testes were considered; this incidence is higher than in any reports of infertile men (Giwercman *et al.* 1988).

In practice, successful orchiopexy does not completely abolish the risk of neoplasia. However, Smith has pointed out that there are few reported cases in boys having successful orchiopexy before 10 years old and none with surgery before 6 years old. In unilateral UDT, 20% of cases occur in the normal testis (Smith 1978).

## MANAGEMENT OF ADULTS WITH UNDESCENDED TESTIS

### History

It will be seen later that there is some dispute about the need for treatment at all. It is pertinent to ask the patient why he has attended as a grown up when he had no treatment as a child.

Patients who have heard of the risk of neoplasia are hardly likely to accept the view that the risk of dying from an orchiectomy is greater than the risk of dying from a testicular neoplasm. Similarly, those who wish to have a prosthesis inserted to make them look normal are requesting an operation anyway.

A difficult group are those in whom there is a chance finding of UDT at a medical for some other reason. Most of these patients know perfectly well that they have a testis missing but have chosen to have nothing done.

### Examination

The specific points for the examination are the positions of the testes and the development of the scrotum. In patients with bilateral UDT which is a part of a more fundamental failure of sexual development, there may be signs of deficient masculinisation.

### Investigation

Much has been written about the means of locating the impalpable undescended testis in childhood and adult life.

The simplest investigation is an ultrasound. Unfortunately, it is inaccurate with both false negatives and positives. In one series it failed to locate 30% of testes that were palpable in the inguinal canal and 62% of impalpable testes. There were two false positive examinations (Weiss *et al.* 1986).

CT scanning, although non-invasive, is expensive. It is good at localising testes below the inguinal ring but not above it. Some authors have regarded it as the investigation of choice with a success rate of about 85% (Lee & Glazer 1982, Ford *et al.* 1985, Leon *et al.* 1986) but the false negative rate may be as high as 44% (Reen 1985).

MRI has been used in children. In the only report to date it identified four of five impalpable testes but all were below the inguinal ring (Landa *et al.* 1987). MRI is a non-invasive and safe investigation but it is expensive and the patients find the examination very traumatic because of the noise it generates in a confined space.

The invasive investigations are spermatic venography and arteriography. Arteriography has been little used but the results have been impressive if the correct artery is found. In the largest series the success rate was 80% with no false negatives (Khademi *et al.* 1980). Venography also requires a skilful radiologist and fails if the correct vein is not found. In one series there were four such failures in 11 impalpable testes, but in one no testicular vein (or testis) was found at surgery (Pommerville *et al.* 1982). The success rate can be as high as 75% (Riebel *et al.* 1987). The presence of a pampiniform plexus usually, but not always, indicates the presence of a testis. Abrupt termination of the vein usually means that there is no testis present.

Any of these investigations may be used to look for the impalpable testis. There is no point in using them if the testis is palpable. But should they ever be used?

If the patient is going to have an operation anyway, I do not investigate. The patient is anaesthetised and a laparoscopy performed. Malone and Guiney (1984) have shown with 45 testes that the position can always be identified or predicted by this means. If a vas is seen meeting testicular vessels, especially hypoplastic vessels, with no testis there should be no germ cells; theoretically, no operation need be done. Although Malone and Guiney found that 42% of impalpable testes (in children) were intra-abdominal, I have had the same experience as Whitaker (1988), that the testis is just above or just below the internal ring.

In two groups full investigation should be done before operating. In those who have had a previous exploration at which the testis was not found, the next operation is likely to be easier if the position of the testis can be found. In patients with bilateral UDT knowledge of the position will help in the assessment of the cancer risk and the decision on orchiopexy. Groin ultrasound, followed by spermatic venography if it is negative, are the most useful investigations. Laparoscopy should be done before exploring bilateral UDT cases to confirm the findings.

## Treatment

In fit patients with unilateral UDT presenting between the end of puberty and 40 years old, the testis should be removed. Whatever precise figure is put upon the risk of neoplasia, such an operation seems more attractive.

The rare cases who present after 40 have a difficult problem. In the first few years after 40 there may be one or two patients who already have an undiagnosed testicular neoplasm or CIS in their undescended testis. An occasional patient, later in life, will develop a lymphoma or late seminoma although it has not been shown that there is an increased risk in UDT. If an older patient requests advice on his management, might it not be safer to recommend orchiectomy? A policy of observation of an impalpable testis is difficult to follow: the short-comings of investigation have already been discussed and the testis might only be found during 'observation' when it had become a substantial mass.

It has been argued that the risk of death is greater from the operation than from neoplasia except in the group from puberty to 32 years old (Farrer *et al.* 1985). This assumes, however, that should a neoplasm occur in an impalpable testis, it is found and treated promptly. The single most important factor in treatment failure in germ cell tumours is delay. The 'close observation and frequent examinations' suggested for patients over 32 must include a number of visits to the doctor, X-rays and blood tests for many years.

A policy of observation should only be followed in fully informed patients at their own request. This is only likely when the UDT has been a chance finding during examination for another reason.

In bilateral UDT presenting in adulthood, orchiectomy will almost always mean life-long testosterone replacement. I have a few young adult patients with anorchia from a variety of causes who have normal sexual function without supplements. About 5% of sexually active men undergoing castration for carcinoma of the prostate continue to have erections. Although histology has shown that the adult UDT is of no use for spermatogenesis, it is of use for androgen production (Ford *et al.* 1985).

Investigation should identify the lower testis. It should be explored and orchiopexy attempted. If it is possible to get it to the scrotum, it should be fixed with sutures and not put in a dartos pouch: the skin overlying is not always sufficiently vascularised to survive. The testis should be biopsied to exclude CIS.

If, after 6 months, it appears that the testis has survived, a decision can be made about the other side. The scrotum is seldom well enough developed to accommodate two testes and so contralateral orchiectomy will usually be chosen. If it is impossible to get either testis to the scrotum, both should be removed.

## REFERENCES


Albescu J.Z., Bergada C. & Cullen M. (1971) Male fertility in patients treated for cryptorchidism before puberty. *Fertil. Steril.* **22**, 289–33.

Alpert P.F. & Klein R.S. (1983) Spermatogenesis in the unilateral cryptorchid testis after orchiopexy. *J. Urol.* **129**, 301–2.

Atkinson P.M. (1975) A follow-up study of surgically treated cryptorchid patients. *J. Pediatr.* **10**, 115–18

Bayle H. (1957) *La Function Endocrine du Testicule.* Masson et Cie, Paris. pp. 466–90.

Belman A.B. (1988) Acquired undescended (ascended) testis: effects of human chorionic gonadotrophin. *J. Urol.* **140**, 1189–90.

Bollersev J., Rohl H., Sorensen E.K. & Bennet P. (1986) Gonadotrophin and androgen levels in patients operated upon for cryptorchidism. *Dan. Med. Bull.* **33**, 336–8.

Chilvers C. & Pike M.C. (1989) Epidemiology of undescended testis. In: Oliver R.T.D., Blandy J.P. & Hope-Stone H.F. (eds) *Urological and Genital Cancer.* Blackwell Scientific, Oxford, pp. 306–21.

DePalma L., Carter D. & Weiss R.M. (1988) Epididymal and vasal immaturity in cryptorchidism. *J. Urol.* **140**, 1194–6.

Eldrup J. & Steven K. (1980) Influence of orchiopexy for cryptorchidism on subsequent fertility. *Br. J. Surg.* **67**, 269–70.

Farrer J.H., Walker A.H. & Rajfer J. (1985) Management of the postpubertal cryptorchid testis: a statistical review. *J. Urol.* **134**, 1071–6.

Ford T.F., Parkinson M.C. & Pryor J.P. (1985) The undescended testis in adult life. *Br. J. Urol.* **57**, 181–4.

Giwercman A., Grindsted J., Hansen B., Jensen O.M. & Skakkebaek N.E. (1987) Testicular cancer risk in boys with maldescended testis: a cohort study. *J. Urol.* **138**, 1214–16.

Giwercman A., Muller J. & Skakkebaek N.E. (1988) Carcinoma *in situ* of the undescended testis. *Seminars in Urology* **6**, 110–19.

Gross R.E. & Jewett T.C. (1956) Surgical experiences from 1222 operations for undescended testis. *J.A.M.A.* **160**, 634–41.

Hadziselimovic F., Hecker E. & Hergzoz B. (1984) The value of testicular biopsy in cryptorchidism. *Urol. Res.* **12**, 171–4.

Hedinger C.E. (1982) Histopathology of the undescended testis. *Eur. J. Paediatr.* **139**, 266–71.

Jansz G.F. & Pomerantz D.K. (1986) A comparison of Leydig cell function after unilateral and bilateral cryptorchidism and efferent duct ligation. *Biol. Reprod.* **34**, 316–21.

Khademi N., Seebode J. & Falda A. (1980) Selective spermatic arteriography for localisation of the impalpable testis. *Radiology* **136**, 627–34.

Kirby R.S., Chapple C.R., Ward S.P. & Williams C. (1985) Is the scrotal testis normal in unilateral cryptorchidism? *Br. J. Urol.* **57**, 187–9.

Kumar D., Bremner D. & Brown P.W. (1989) Fertility after orchiopexy for cryptorchidism: a new approach to assessment. *Br. J. Urol.* **64**, 516–20.

Landa H.N., Geylys-Morin V., Matrey R.F. *et al.* (1987) Magnetic resonance imaging in the cryptorchid testis. *Eur. J. Pediatr.* **146**, 516–17.

Lee J.K.T. & Glazer H.S. (1982) Computed tomography in

the localisation of the nonpalpable testis. *Urol. Clin. North Am.* **9**, 397–404.

Leon M.N.G., Ferreiros J., Casanova R., Rodriguez R. & Pedrosa C.S. (1986) The value of computed tomography in the localisation of undescended testes. *Eur. J. Radiol.* **6**, 283–7.

Levin A. & Sherman J.O. (1973) The undescended testis. *Surg. Gynecol. Obstet.* **136**, 473–9.

Lipshultz L.I., Caminos-Torres R., Greenspan C.S. & Snyder P.J. (1976) Testicular function after orchiopexy for unilateral undescended testis. *N. Engl. J. Med.* **295**, 15–18.

Malone P.S. & Guiney E.J. (1984) The value of laparoscopy in localising the impalpable undescended testis. *Br. J. Urol.* **56**, 429–31.

Martin D.C. & Menck H.R. (1975) The undescended testis: management after puberty. *J. Urol.* **114**, 77–9.

Plante P., Pontonnier F. & Mansat A. (1982) Cryptorchidie et sterilite. *J. d'Urol (Paris)* **88**, 147–9.

Pommerville P., Futter N.G., McKay D.E. & Desmarais R. (1982) The role of gonadal venography in the management of the adult with non-palpable undescended testis. *Br. J. Urol.* **54**, 408–10.

Reen R.J.R. (1985) Computerised axial tomography v. spermatic venography in the localisation of cryptorchid testes. *Urology* **26**, 513–17.

Reibel T., Gonnermann D. & Willig R-P. (1987) Spermatic venography in undescended testes. *Pediatr. Radiol.* **17**, 39–44.

Robertson J.F.R., Azmy A.F. & Cochran W. (1988) Assent to ascent of the testis. *Br. J. Urol.* **61**, 146–7.

Scheiber K., Menardi G., Marberger H. & Bartsch G. (1981) Late results after surgical treatment of maldescended testes with special regard to exocrine and endocrine testicular function. *Eur. Urol.* **7**, 268–73.

Schiffer K.A., Kogan S.J., Reda E.F. & Levitt S.B. (1987) Acquired undescended testes. *Am. J. Dis. Child.* **141**, 106–7.

Scott L.S. (1962) Fertility in cryptorchidism. *Proc. Roy. Soc. Med.* **55**, 1047–50.

Smith R.B. (1978) Diagnosis and staging of testicular tumours. In: Skinner, D.G. & de Kernion, J.B. (eds) *Genitourinary Cancer.* W.B. Saunders Co., Philadelphia, pp. 448–59.

Weiss R.M., Carter A.R. & Rosenfield A.T. (1986) High resolution real-time ultrasonography in the localisation of the undescended testis. *J. Urol.* **135**, 936–8.

Whitaker R.H. (1970) Management of the undescended testis. *Br. J. Hosp. Med.* **4**, 25–37.

Whitaker R.H. (1988) Neoplasia in cryptorchid men. *Seminars in Urology* **6**, 107–9.

# 17 Problems of intersex, gender identity and micropenis

## INTRODUCTION

When a child is born with ambiguous genitalia there is a neonatal emergency. The chromosomal and phenotypic sex must be decided very quickly and a decision made about the rearing of the child. The accuracy of diagnosis now is much higher than it was 20 years ago; we therefore have the problem so often found in this book, of drawing conclusions from the long-term follow-up of patients whose original diagnosis is uncertain.

There are valid data on some specific diagnoses. There is also useful information on some broad categories of problems, especially the neoplastic potential of gonads and sexual development. We particularly lack long-term follow-up of those who are karyotypically male but whose inadequate genitalia have caused the child to be reared as a female.

## CONGENITAL ADRENAL HYPERPLASIA (CAH)

This condition may occur in males and females. There are two aspects to consider: the effects of the excessive fetal androgens on development and the acute adrenal insufficiency that becomes apparent at birth. This chapter is only concerned with the former except to note that patients will require steroid maintenance for life. The salt-losing tendency found in the 21-hydroxylase defect disappears during childhood so that salt supplements are not required. The sex chromosomes are normal.

### Female genitalia

Wherever the block in the pathway of steroid synthesis, excess androgen will be produced in the fetus. The female has virilisation of otherwise normal genitalia. The degree of virilisation is dependent on the levels of androgens and ranges from cliteromegaly alone to complete urogenital sinus.

The diagnosis should be made at birth and the infant will obviously be reared as a female. I have encountered only one patient in whom the sex was mistaken. The child was reared as a boy but always behaved as a girl and thought of herself as such. The clitoris was reduced in late childhood and an ileal vagina made after puberty. She now lives happily as a young woman.

The clitoris should be reduced early in life — it does not regress on its own even with optimum steroid control (Spence & Allen 1973). The original approach was to amputate the clitoris. Although it may not be essential for orgasm, there seem to be good theoretical reasons to retain at least a part of it. Some surgeons advocated a partial burying or relocation of the penis but Spence pointed out that the bulk of tissue so formed was rather unsatisfactory (Spence & Allen 1973).

Resection of the shaft of the clitoris and retention of the glans with its neurovascular bundle has been described with minor variations by several authors. A small but sensitive organ is retained and has a natural appearance after partial covering in its own prepuce. The skin of the shaft may be used to form the labia or part of the vagina (Spence & Allen 1973, Mollard *et al.* 1981, Bissada *et al.* 1987, Whitaker 1989).

A satisfactory single-stage procedure for feminising genitoplasty has been described. The essential features are: separation of the urogenital sinus from the urethra, preserving the 'urethral' meatus in the correct anatomical position; excision of the corpora; use of the clitoral and perineal skin to form a tube up to the vagina. The penile skin is 'button-holed' at two sites for the glans and the urethral meatus. The results were said to be good on eight patients aged from 3 months to 12 years, all vaginas calibrating to at least 30 FG. The length of follow-up was not given and it seems unlikely that any of the vaginas had been tested by intercourse (Gonzalez & Fernandes 1989).

With this reconstruction, the anterior commissure of the labia majora may be wide and prominent. The appearance is much improved by a small modification described by Reilly (J.M. Reilly, personal communication 1989). An inverted 'V' incision is made at the anterior end of the commissure, part of the skin tongue so formed is resected and the remainder is rolled into a tube which forms a hood for the clitoris. The outer edges of the 'V' are then closed (Fig. 17.1).

Although it is now accepted that this is the correct management of cliteromegaly the quality of sexual function in adult life has not been investigated. Bissada records that two adults on whom the operation was performed have married and one has had a normal child by caesarean section (Bissada *et al.* 1987).

If a vaginoplasty is needed the timing is a matter of debate. In all but the most severe cases, it seems sensible to perform the vaginoplasty in infancy at the same time as the phalloplasty. This is particularly so if the skin from the clitoral shaft is to be used for reconstruction.

Dilatation of the vagina may only be necessary while the wound is healing (Whitaker 1989) but Hendren is more cautious, suggesting that revision of the vaginoplasty is necessary at the beginning of adulthood (Hendren 1987). There

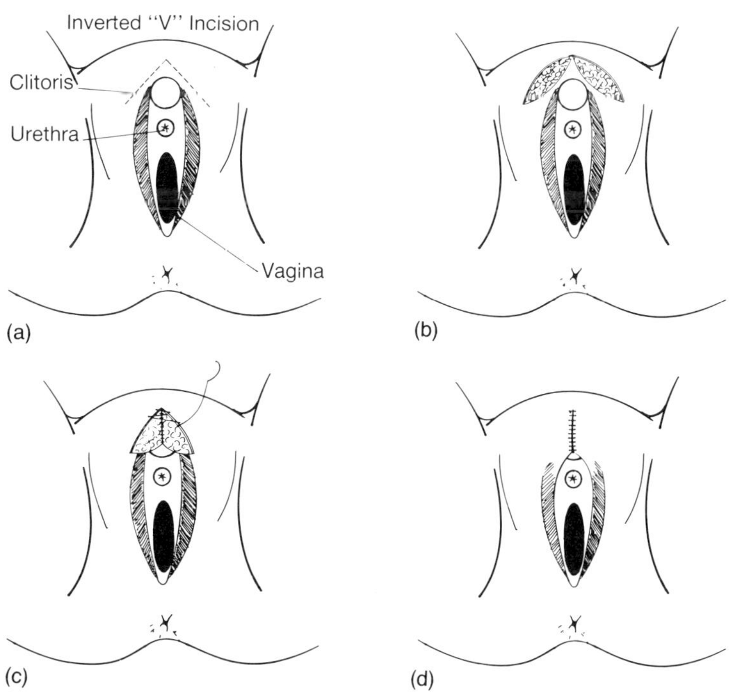


**Fig. 17.1** Reilly's modification of the operation for feminising genitoplasty. (a) An inverted 'V' incision just anterior to the commissure of the labia majora. (b) Resection of most of the tongue of skin. (c) Closure to form a hood for the clitoris. (d) Closure of the remainder of the 'V' incision. (Courtesy of J.M. Reilly.)

is no information about the sexual function of the vagina.

## Sexual development

As girls with CAH are genetically female and have normal internal gentalia they should mature normally but in some cases do not do so.

The menarche is delayed but to a very variable extent. Patients at the Johns Hopkins Hospital, USA were reported to have been delayed by a mean of nearly a year (to 13.77 compared to 12.99 years for normals). Forty percent of non-salt losers and 44% of salt losers were delayed beyond 16 years old. However, the greatest delays occurred in patients who were inadequately treated or did not comply with treatment (Klingensmith *et al.* 1977).

Even wider variation in menarche has been reported in 56 English patients with a mean of 15 years which is nearly 2 years late. The latest age of menarche was 27 and there were nine patients aged 13 to 27 who had not menstruated (and were not included in the calculation of the mean). Twenty-four patients had regular menstruation, two had become amenorrhoeic and five had oligomenorrhoea. There did not appear to be a relationship between accuracy of steroid control and any of the disorders of menstruation (Grant *et al.* 1983).

In the English and American groups it was known that at least 21 wished to become pregnant. Only 15 had been successful. Four other patients had unwanted pregnancies. The results are shown in Table 17.1.

It is interesting to note the outcome of two adult patients who must have had very mild CAH who did not start replacement therapy until 18 and 27 years old. Both started menstruating within 2 months and one had a child by caesarean section (Bissada *et al.* 1987). However, in a larger group of patients all of four patients treated after 20 years of age who wished to get pregnant were infertile due to anovulation or absence of corpora lutea (Klingensmith *et al.* 1977).

## Inheritance

None of the reported offspring of women with CAH have themselves been affected. However, there is a family pattern with several siblings being affected. 17-Hydroxylase deficiency is inherited as an autosomal recessive trait and has been linked to the HLA locus on the sixth chromosome (Levine *et al.* 1978).

As the deficiencies are manifest during early uterine growth, the possibility exists of measuring the excess levels of the appropriate steroid precursors in the amniotic fluid. To make this worthwhile, clinicians would have to know from the family history that the fetus was at risk.

Both HLA typing and measurement of 17-hydroxyprogesterone (17-OHP) in the amniotic fluid have been used to predict the outcome of at risk pregnancies (Marcus *et al.* 1979, Pollack *et al.* 1979).

Fortunately the normal levels of amniotic fluid 17-OHP and 21-deoxycortisol in normal pregnancy do not overlap with the levels found in pregnancies with CAH. Pregnancies with heterozygous carriers and homozygotes are normal. With this technique correct prenatal diagnosis of affected offspring was made in 11 pregnancies (Gueux *et al.* 1988). The finding of a DNA defect in fetal amniocytes identical to the defect in the parents will also predict an affected offspring, but experience with this technique is much more limited (Reindollar *et al.* 1988).

When prenatal diagnosis is made or suspected, there may be some doubt about the action to take. In Gueux's series seven of 11 pregnancies were terminated and four produced the predicted CAH child (Gueux *et al.* 1988). An intriguing alternative is to treat the mother with steroids that cross the placenta to suppress the fetal adrenal. Two such cases (one successful and one partially successful) have been reported. The mothers were given hydrocortisone or dexamethasone throughout pregnancy (David *et al.* 1984).

**Table 17.1** Pregnancies in congenital adrenal hyperplasia (from Klingensmith *et al.* 1977, Grant *et al.* 1983).

| *n* | Pregnancies | Delivery | Complications | Offspring |
|---|---|---|---|---|
| *Salt losers* | | | | |
| 1 | 3 | FTND | None | Normal |
| 1 | 1 | FTND | None | Normal |
| 2 | 1 | TOP | | |
| *Non-salt losers* | | | | |
| 1 | 1 | Caesarean | Eclampsia | Normal |
| 1 | 1 | Caesarean | Fetal distress | Normal |
| 2 | 1 | * | | ** |
| 3 | 2 | * | | ** |
| 1 | 3 | * | | ** |
| 1 | 1 | TOP | | |
| *Not stated* | | | | |
| 1 | 1 | TOP | | |
| 1 | 1 | * | | ** |

FTND = Full-term normal delivery.
TOP = Termination of pregnancy.
* = Only eight of these 12 pregnancies went to full term and all deliveries were by caesarean section for cephalopelvic disproportion. One delivery was vaginal but the infant was premature and weighed 1700 G; caesarean would have been necessary at full-term.
** = Eight of nine living children were normal; one had mild spastic diplegia. Of the unsuccessful pregnancies, two ended in spontaneous mid-term abortion and one in the premature stillbirth of an infant with myelomeningocele and multiple skeletal anomalies.

## Psychosexual development

If the correct gender assignment is made at birth, it would be thought that development in the female role would be normal. However, there is some evidence in animals that irreversible changes occur in the developing brain if it is exposed to excess androgens *in utero*. Evidence that these effects are present in females with CAH is incomplete.

Early reports showed that CAH females were 'tomboys' and had less interest in role rehearsal for marriage and children (Ehrhardt *et al.* 1968). Some of the girls in this study had been treated late which may have influenced the outcome. Reviewing this work and other papers Ehrhardt concluded that findings of increased male and decreased female games in girls exposed to androgens *in utero* could tentatively be accepted. She comments that the trend was in an expected direction and occurred in spite of apparent efforts by the mothers to oppose them. In terms of sexual behaviour most women were found to act in an exclusively heterosexual manner even though half had bisexual fantasies (Ehrhardt & Meyer-Bahlberg 1981).

Difficulty arises in the selection of controls. Even if it is accepted that early genital reconstruction does not affect perception of gender, constant steroid medication and hospital supervision may. A study of sex role and self-image has used diabetics and normal students as controls. The results are weakened by the inclusion of two males with 10 females in the study group. There was no difference in sex role behaviour between CAH and diabetic patients and only a marginal difference between them and normals. There was no difference in self-esteem between any of the groups (Mosely *et al.* 1989).

It seems likely that a combination of immediate diagnosis, correct medical and surgical treatment and proper counselling of parents leads to near normal development.

## CAH IN MALES

Male infants with CAH are normal at birth unless they are salt losers. In non-salt losers the diagnosis may be missed until later in childhood or even until adult life especially if there is no family history to alert the paediatrician. Untreated boys with CAH may have signs of excess androgen production such as rapid growth, hirsutism and precocious puberty. The epiphyses then close prematurely so that final stature is short. In a group of 30 men the heights ranged from 150–178.6 cm (mean 164 cm) which is significantly lower than the national mean and was also less than their fathers. The age at which treatment was begun was irrelevant (Urban *et al.* 1978).

Untreated adult males usually have oligozoospermia while those that have been treated in childhood have normal spermatogenesis even when the treatment is discontinued.

The mechanisms that cause oligozoospermia are disputed. It was originally suggested, quite logically, that excess adrenal androgens suppressed the pituitary production of LH and FSH so that the testes which were normal did not receive adequate stimulation (Prader *et al.* 1977). However, in a later series it was shown that LH and FSH, although lower than average, were not below the normal range. Spermatogenesis was unrelated to gonadotrophin levels or to treatment. Eighteen of 20 patients had either normal sperm counts or had fathered children. Three patients who had discontinued treatment remained fertile (Urban *et al.* 1978).

Even in patients who have presented late, often with primary infertility, paternity is possible. Five of Urban's 15 fertile patients did not start steroids until late childhood or adulthood; two others had never had treatment and each had fathered three children. Two patients have been reported with untreated CAH and infertility who became fertile when steroids were started (Wischusen *et al.* 1981, Mirsky & Hines 1989).

A rather frightening late presentation of CAH is with a testicular mass. Fortunately, the masses are formed of hypertrophied adrenal rests which are benign. They disappear with steroid treatment. Patients then develop normal spermatogenesis and become fertile (Prader *et al.* 1977, Cutfield *et al.* 1983).

## LATE ONSET CAH

Symptoms and signs of CAH which may be obvious to the patient (or parents) or be found on careful search, may develop after birth. In childhood the usual presentation is masculinisation in females. In adults, cases have presented up to 54 years old with a variety of symptoms including hirsutism and cliteromegaly. A past history of abnormal puberty and transient amenorrhoea may be found but the patients have usually been fertile. The autosomal recessive inheritance and the HLA linkage are the same as in the classical form of CAH (Kohn *et al.* 1982).

## MALE PSEUDOHERMAPHRODITES (MPH)

This is a complicated group of patients with wide variation in phenotype and natural history. Karyotypically they may have one or more cell lines but none are XX and some cells must be XY. There are several hormonal defects that may be responsible. When the genitalia are ambiguous at birth, the diagnosis should be made early but in patients who are now adults, it may have been delayed or incomplete. Some forms are so phenotypically female that there is no suspicion of abnormality until puberty.

## Early presentation

The management of MPH patients with ambiguous genitalia will have been decided long before adolescence (Donaghoe *et al.* 1979). The decisions on gender assignment, assuming the diagnosis is made accurately, are relatively easy. Patients with largely female genitalia and little or no gonadal source of testosterone usually have a reconstructable vagina and are reared as females. This group includes pure gonadal dysgenesis; mixed gonadal dysgenesis (MGD) patients unless there is a descended testis; 17-ketosteroid reductase deficiency and 5-alpha-reductase deficiency.

These patients require careful management at puberty. If the gonads are removed in infancy, oestrogen supplements will be required to allow adult female development.

Other patients have sufficient androgen production *in utero* to develop male characteristics. At birth they have some penile development and may have a descended testis. Even though they may have some internal female structures, they should be brought up as boys. This group includes some patients with MGD and dysgenetic MPH. The management of the gonads requires accurate diagnosis because of the risk of benign or malignant neoplasia in some groups (see below).

## Effects of puberty — delayed diagnosis

Incorrect or missed diagnosis at birth will result in inappropriate or absent development at puberty. Gender identity is established by a process of early learning and does not result only from hormonal influences (Ehrhardt & Meyer-Bahlburg 1981). Failure to mature in the anticipated manner at puberty should not lead to any weakening of that identity, but will certainly cause considerable anxiety. A possible exception to this general rule is seen in 5-alpha-reductase deficiency where apparent females develop distinctly male behaviour at puberty (Imperato-McGinley *et al.* 1979).

### *'Girls' who fail to develop*

No patients have an XX cell line and so none can develop as normal adult females. Those with pure gonadal dysgenesis (XY) appear to be normal female infants, though sometimes with some signs of Turner's syndrome. They may have a uterus and fallopian tubes but not ovaries. Ironically, they may develop an oestrogen-secreting gonadal neoplasm (see below). At puberty they do not develop secondary sexual characteristics. Some may even have sufficient testosterone production to show penile development.

Patients with oestrogen deficiency are treated with oestrogen supplements. Careful follow-up is essential, not only to monitor endocrine function but for onset of complications. Prolonged oestrogen treatment may precipitate endometrial carcinoma in patients who have a uterus and gonadal dysgenesis.

In a series of 24 patients followed for at least 5 years (mean:12.3), three developed frank malignancy or premalignant changes. The histology in these three cases, and two others from the literature, was adenocarcinoma or an unusual mixed adenosquamous type. Although this histology is normally associated with a poor prognosis, the reported patients did well. The neoplasms developed after a mean of 31 years' treatment (Cutler *et al.* 1972).

The condition of 5-alpha-reductase deficiency is particularly interesting. It is only comparatively recently that it has been discovered and defined. Groups of patients were found in isolated communities so that affected individuals were not subjected to medical interference. Testosterone production is normal but dihydrotestosterone (DHT) production is limited. Patients are thought to be girls at birth although the 'clitoris' may be a little large. There may be a vaginal opening or a urogenital sinus. Testes are present but undescended.

At puberty the secondary sexual characteristics that are dependent on testosterone develop, but those requiring DHT do not. Patients become aggressively male in behaviour. In the primitive communities in which large groups are found, the female role is completely rejected in spite of the obvious problems that are caused in the family. The penis grows, the voice breaks and the body habitus becomes conspicuously male. Acne and facial hair do not develop and the testes do not descend (Imperato-McGinley *et al.* 1979).

The nature and extent of the change in sexual identity shown by these patients have been questioned. The original authors held the view that in those that had been unambiguously raised as girls, all but one had successfully changed to male gender identity after puberty (Imperato-McGinley *et al.* 1979). Rubin later pointed out that only 13 of 19 such patients had made the change and cast doubt on the type of upbringing that they had experienced. Rubin also mentioned that all of 13 such patients reported from more 'westernised' societies who went unrecognised until well into puberty or beyond, maintained their female role in spite of disfiguring virilisation (Rubin *et al.* 1981). In most circumstances the hormonal environment does not play a large part in gender identity. Nonetheless, patients with 5-alpha-reductase deficiency do seem to find a change of identity at puberty rather easier than most groups.

A similar hormonal situation is seen in patients who are able to synthesise androgens but lack specific binding sites, especially for DHT, in the target organs. This condition is known as androgen receptor defect and, in its complete form, as the testicular feminisation syndrome. In the complete form the external genitalia are female at birth but the vagina is blind ending. At puberty patients develop as females but do not have pubic or axillary hair. In less complete forms the genitalia are ambiguous but tend to be female and at puberty there is some masculinisation (Glassberg 1985).

Patients with testicular feminisation exhibit typical female behaviour in childhood and adult life. Children play 'typical' female games. In adults there is a preference to be a housewife with no outside job (Ehrhardt & Meyer-Bahlburg 1981).

There are a series of rare conditions in which an enzyme necessary for testosterone production is absent. Some patients are identified early as they also have deficient cortisol production. Others may not be identified until puberty; for example the condition of 17-ketosteroid reductase deficiency produces infants with apparently female genitalia which become partly masculinised at puberty (Glassberg 1985).

### *'Boys' who fail to develop*

MPH infants who are born with sufficient male genitalia to be classified as males without any questions being raised are, of course, being assigned to their correct gender. They have a source of androgens and should develop normally at puberty. The diagnosis, particularly of MGD, may come to light in childhood if an exploration is made for an undescended testis — only a streak will be found.

For reasons that are unclear, patients with MGD are short but even so the diagnosis may not be suspected.

Patients with persistent Müllerian duct syndrome have bilateral undescended testes. Occasionally investigation or surgery in childhood will show the presence of a uterus and tubes.

## TRUE HERMAPHRODITES

A true hermaphrodite has both ovarian and testicular tissue. The chromosomes are variable, about half of the patients being 46XX, 20% 46XY and 30% mosaics (Bernirschke *et al.* 1972).

Although it would be expected that the chromosomal pattern would be fixed, I have one patient whose proportion of XY cells has steadily increased. When first investigated at the age of four, half his chromosomes were XX and half XY. His genitalia were ambiguous but were considered to be more male than female and he was raised as such. He was reassessed at intervals to 18 years old, having no treatment. His XY complement rose steadily to 79%. He was clearly male with good development of male primary and secondary sexual characteristics. Serum testosterone, LH and FSH were normal. His sperm count was low at $5 \times 10^5$ per ml. Those sperm that were present were normal and showed lively movement. Although of interest, no great significance can be attached to one case, especially as the chromosomes in the peripheral blood may not be the same as those in the gonads.

The condition of the genitalia at birth ranges from virtually normal female to virtually normal male so that, although a rare condition, there is a high rate of late diagnosis.

## GONADAL NEOPLASIA

One of the most influential factors in the management of patients with intersex is the risk of neoplasia in the gonads. Biopsy may be necessary to define both the type of gonad present and the neoplastic risk. The majority of neoplasms are of germ cell origin and so some germ cells must be present in the gonad, primitive and small in number though they may be (Scully 1981). Indeed the risk of neoplasia is higher with more dysplastic germ cells, or with the coexistence of ovarian and testicular tissue in the same gonad (as in true hermaphrodites).

### Gonadal dysgenesis

In gonadal dysgenesis the gonads may contain testicular tissue or be a streak or there may be one of each (Robboy *et al.* 1982). Both are at risk. The 'testis' has about a 30% incidence of gonadoblastoma which may become invasive. Dysgerminoma or seminoma may occur in the streak gonad. Non-seminomatous germ cell tumours occur rarely in dysgenetic gonads.

The risk is highest in the group with pure gonadal dysgenesis with 46XY chromosomes. They have a 20 to 30% incidence of gonadoblastoma of which about a third will progress to malignancy (Savage & Lowe 1989).

Neoplasms may occur before puberty although the risk is said to rise rapidly after puberty (Manuel *et al.* 1976). However, in a personal series Savage had two of five cases in childhood and the remainder in the 'peripubertal period' (Savage & Lowe 1989).

Gonadoblastoma is composed of Sertoli and germ cells with occasional Leydig cells. They may occur at any age from 6 months (and may possibly arise *in utero*), but are most common in the second and third decades. They are the characteristic tumours of the streak and dysgenetic gonads. There is some doubt as to whether gonadoblastoma is a neoplasm in its own right. It never metastasises as a gonadoblastoma and may undergo spontaneous regression. When metastases occur they are only of the germ cell element. It may be that the germ cell portion of the gonadoblastoma develops malignant change and then metastasises rather than the whole lesion being neoplastic from the outset. The endocrine cells may secrete active hormones, especially testosterone (Savage & Lowe 1989).

Dysgerminoma, on the other hand, is a malignant germ cell neoplasm from the start though it metastasises late. The term is, of course, normally applied to classical seminomas arising in the ovary. It is used in this context with seminoma when the nature of the gonad is uncertain, or alone when the gonad is ovarian.

### True hermaphroditism

Individuals with a Y chromosome have a high risk of gonadal malignancy. The group is small and the percentage risk is unknown. Those with a testis rather than an ovotestis are particularly at risk. Both gonadoblastoma and seminoma have been described (Savage & Lowe 1989).

A juvenile form of granulosa cell tumour has been described in the ovarian gonads (Zaloudek & Norris 1982). They probably arise from 'ovarian' mesenchyme but contain large follicular structures and may be oestrogen secreting. Although the cells have many mitoses, only about 10% are malignant. They may recur many years after removal.

### Male pseudohermaphrodites

The only group with a significant risk are those with androgen insensitivity, especially in its complete form of testicular feminisation syndrome. Tumours are rare in childhood though one case of seminoma was included in Savage's series (Savage & Lowe 1989). There seems to be a higher risk in adults and three cases were reported in siblings (O'Connell *et al.* 1973).

Gonadal biopsies in childhood have identified atypical cells which appear to precede the development of CIS in adulthood (Muller *et al.* 1984). The abnormal cells have similar electron microscopic features as seminoma cells though they are easily recognisable with the light microscope. In male phenotypes who are 45XO/46XY these features are considered to be an indication for gonadectomy (Muller *et al.* 1984, Savage & Lowe 1989).

### Management of the gonads in intersex

It would be wrong to remove all the gonads of all intersex patients. The indications for removal are inappropriate gonadal type for the sex-of-rearing and high risk of malignancy. The risk of malignancy is partly dependent on the diagnosis which may not always be certain.

In his review of the literature Savage concludes that neoplasms are present on presentation in 15% of children with mixed gonadal dysgenesis, 5% with androgen receptor defect and 1% of true hermaphrodites. As in the normal population the neoplasms are more common in undescended gonads and the higher the gonad, the higher the risk. However, unlike the normal population, they may occur at any age even though the risk is greater in young adults (Savage & Lowe 1989).

Several steps are necessary to assess the future risk of neoplasia in any individual. The first and most important is to establish the diagnosis. The highest risk is in patients with gonadal dysgenesis with lesser risks in true hermaphroditism and testicular feminisation. There is no increased risk in CAH. Gonadal biopsy may be indicated. The finding of Müllerian duct remnants suggests gonadal dysgenesis may be present.

In all cases the karyotype will have been determined. Aside from contributing to the diagnosis, knowledge of the chromosomes may help in the assessment: in true hermaphrodites the risk of neoplasia is higher when a Y chromosome is present.

The position of the gonads must be established by ultrasound, CT or laparotomy. The risk of malignancy in high gonads is so high that they should be removed. This is especially so as they are unlikely to be able to produce adequate testosterone in adult life (Kofman *et al.* 1981).

## MÜLLERIAN DUCT REMNANTS

Although not truly an intersex condition, persistence of Müllerian duct remnants may be found in children and adults. The most common reported findings are of tubular utricles and Müllerian cysts (Morgan *et al.* 1979, Ikoma *et al.* 1985, 1986). In patients with normal genitalia, symptoms are of urinary infection, urethral bleeding or incontinence (Morgan *et al.* 1979).

When especially sought for, the incidence of prostatic utricle in association with hypospadias is high, at least in the Japanese. Ikoma reported the results of retrograde urethrography in 280 patients with hypospadias and found that 77 (27.5%) had some form of utricular enlargement. However, in only 14 patients was the utricle of any size and only six were symptomatic. The incidence of utricles and their size were related to the degree of hypospadias, large utricles only occurring with scrotal or perineal hypospadias. In addition there were eight cases of vagina masculinus which presented as hypospadias even though all had a scrotal urinary meatus. All were in fact intersex cases, four with MGD, three MPH and one true hermaphrodite (Ikoma *et al.* 1985).

In the proposed classification (Fig. 17.2), utricles of grades 0 to II arise from an opening above the external sphincter. They may become infected but are unlikely to cause dribbling incontinence. Grade III utricles have an opening below the external sphincter and may, therefore, cause dribbling. I think it questionable that the grade III structures that do not arise from the veru are truely Müllerian duct remnants. They would be better regarded as a persistence of the sinovaginal bulb which, in the female, would have formed the lowest fifth of the vagina.

The cystic remnants can usually be felt on rectal examination. Tubular structures are best found on micturating cystogram. Both the IVU and the retrograde urethrogram are reported to have a failure rate of at least 25% (Morgan *et al.* 1979). In patients who dribble after a hypospadias repair it must be remembered that a baggy neo-urethra, especially at its junction with the original external meatus, is a more common finding.

There seems to be little justification to operate on symptomless abnormalities that are a chance finding. When excision is required one of several approaches may be used. Utricles are intimately related to the urethra, sphincters, bladder base, vasa and nerves of erection. They may be hazardous to remove. However, perineal, abdomino-perineal, parasacral and suprapubic approaches have all been used. If laparotomy is needed to look for other Müllerian structures, an extravesical approach is satisfactory. No complications were encountered in four cases but the lower apex of the dissection my be difficult. Ikoma recommends a transtrigonal approach which gives an excellent exposure of the utricle. Transient vesico-ureteric reflux was reported in one of four cases but none became impotent.

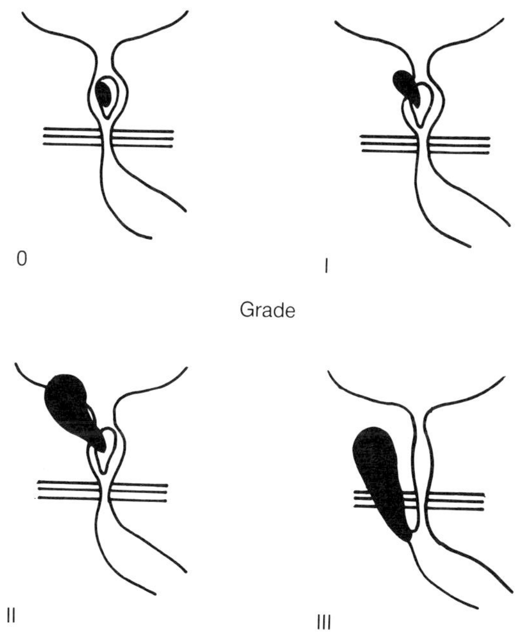


**Fig. 17.2** Classification of Müllerian remnants found in hypospadias according to Ikoma (from Ikoma *et al.* 1985, with permission).

All approaches are said to give good results and no patients are thought to have been made impotent (Morgan *et al.* 1979, Ikoma *et al.* 1986).

## THE SMALL PENIS

The author of a review on the small penis is not to be envied. He is faced with the difficulties in definition and nomenclature, with the complexities of the endocrinology, the successes and failures of medical treatment, the failure of surgeons to make the penis (at any age) longer and the ultimate worry of whether the infants are boys at all and if they are, whether they should remain so.

It is generally agreed that a small penis must have normal anatomy but be more than 2 or 2.5 standard deviations below the normal stretched length. The normal stretched length at birth is 3.5 cm with the 10th centile at 2.6 cm and the

90th at 5.1 cm. The standard deviation is variously given as 0.4 and 0.7 cm. Thus a small penis ranges from 1.75 cm to 2.7 cm depending on the paper from which normals are taken (Feldman *et al.* 1975, Flatau *et al.* 1975). Growth curves have been constructed from which the normal penile lengths can be derived at any age (Fig. 17.3 and see Schonfeld 1943).

A truly small penis is not a common finding in the neonate. In some cases it occurs as a part of a more general failure of genito-urinary development such as exstrophy or perineal hypospadias. In others it is part of an endocrine deficiency such as hypogonadotrophic hypogonadism. Many cases are due to an undefined androgen insensitivity or have no recognisable cause. The term 'micropenis' is best reserved for the small penis which is a part of a generalised endocrinopathy affecting androgen target organs (Allen 1989).

When a small penis is found, the first referral would commonly be to an endocrinologist. Indeed it has often been pointed out that micropenis may be the only sign of a major endocrinopathy. Hormonal treatment for a specific endocrinopathy may cause sufficient growth to bring the penile length back into the normal range. The urologist will never be asked to see such infants. A trial of hormonal therapy should always be made in the severe but undiagnosed case before surgical reconstruction or, especially, when gender re-assignment is contemplated.

After all of this hard work by others, the urologist may be asked to see a child with a small penis. The questions that then arise are what use will the present organ be, can it be made any bigger and, in an extreme case, should a gender re-assignment be made?

## Voiding and sexual function with a small penis

Little boys are known to be very conscious of their genitalia. A useful objective criterion is the ability to void standing up, through the

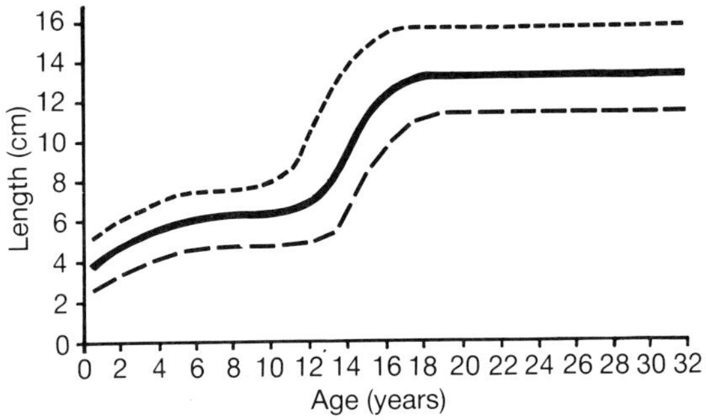


**Fig. 17.3** Growth curves for penile length from growth to maturity (from Schonfeld 1943, with permission).

opened flies. It is surprising how short a penis can be used to accomplish this task, especially if the boy is given adequate tuition and knickers and trousers with wide enough openings. My own groups of continent exstrophy males and small penis patients can all void in the approved manner.

Reilly has investigated the male role in 20 patients who had a small penis from a variety of causes (eight pre- and 12 postpubertal). Patients were included only if their penis, at the time of review, conformed to the standard definition of 'micropenis' even though some had previously had hypospadias. In spite of the very short length of penile shaft (Fig. 17.4), all were able to void with an easily directed stream through the opened fly (Reilly & Woodhouse 1989).

It is more difficult to get away with an abnormal appearance. Although the majority of my adult exstrophy patients went to ordinary schools and played ordinary games few were able to change or shower in public. The presence of a cutaneous diversion may have been as influential as the abnormal genitalia.

It is interesting to compare the pre- and postpubertal groups of micropenis patients reviewed by Reilly as they were the offspring of different generations of parents. The distribution of penile lengths is shown in Fig. 17.5. Half of the older group remembered unhappy experiences of

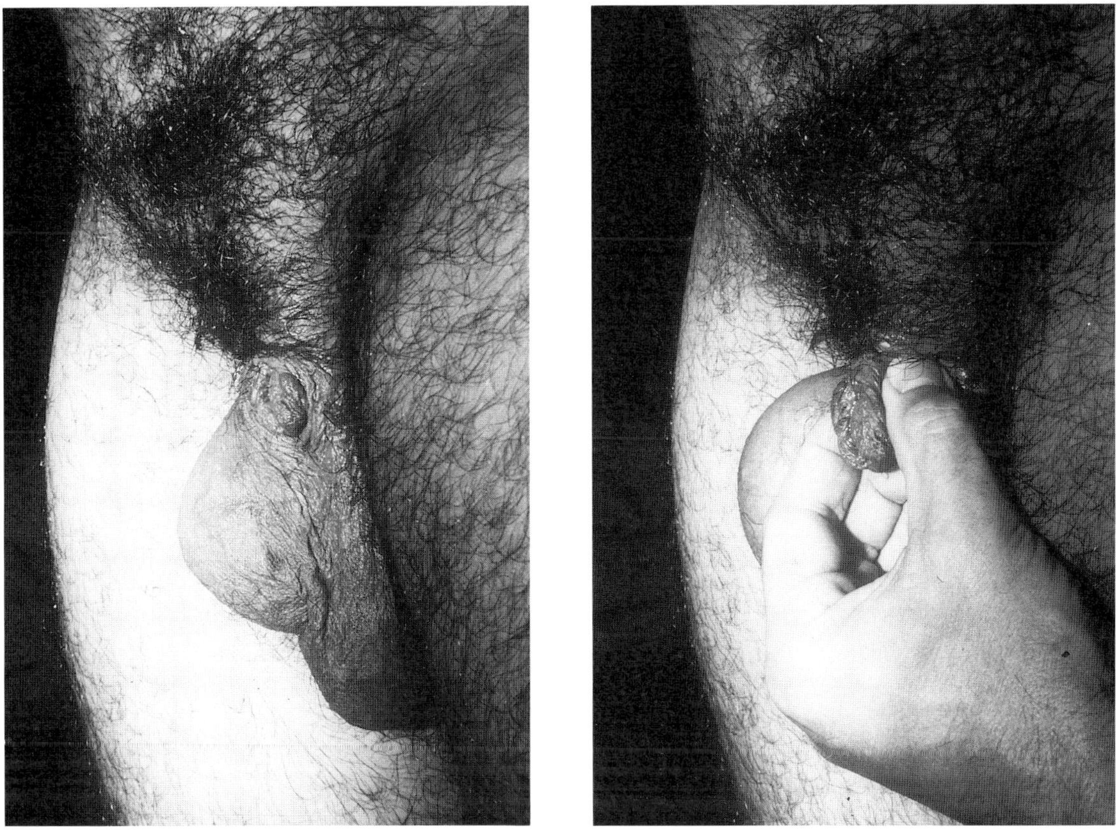

**Fig. 17.4** Clinical photographs of micropenis in an adult (a) flaccid, and (b) stretched.

teasing by their peers because of their small penis. In the younger group all eight were able to change and shower without comment from their peers. This difference is attributed to better counselling of parents. Supportive parents who encouraged 'normality' produced confident and well-adjusted children (Reilly & Woodhouse 1989).

The most surprising feature of these patients was the firmness with which they were established in the male role and the success that they had in sexual relationships. In Reilly's adult group all had heterosexual interests, erections and orgasms; 11 of 12 had ejaculates.

Three-quarters had had sexual intercourse. The mean age of sexual debut was 16.4 years (range 13.5 to 20) while the normal is 16.2. All claimed to find intercourse enjoyable though their partners' views are unknown. One patient had a wife and a mistress. The partnerships were stable and long-lasting, a situation that some patients attributed to the extra attention that had to be paid to intercourse because of the short penis. Although vaginal penetration was usual, there was an experimental attitude to positions and methods. One patient was the father of a child (Reilly & Woodhouse 1989). I have one other patient said to have male pseudohermaphroditism who has a Johnson score of nine on testicular biopsy.

There is little supportive evidence for this data from other units. However, ours is sufficiently consistent that it seems safe to conclude that even the possession of the very small penis illustrated in Fig. 17.4 is compatible with a normal male role, especially with proper parental support. Therefore, a very small penis should not, on its own, be an indication for re-assignment to the female gender.

Males may, occasionally, be born without a penis or lose it as a result of trauma (surgical or otherwise) early in life. Many congenital cases have a small perineal skin tag between the anus and the scrotum which has been shown in at least one case, to contain cavernous tissue (Beasley *et al.* 1987). Traumatic cases are likely to retain the deep part of the corpora and some peri-urethral erectile tissue. There is no guidance in the literature to help with the long-term management, in these rare cases. The choice lies between gender re-assignment, penile reconstruction or perseverance in the male role without surgery. In traumatic cases, unless occurring in the first few days of life such as with ritual circumcision, gender re-assignment may be too late.

I have one patient whose penis was amputated bit by bit in 11 operations (elsewhere) for epispadias. He ended up continent and with normal testes but no penis. A short segment of the deep part of the left corpus can just be felt in perineum. He is now 23, happily living with his girlfriend and having mutually satisfactory sexual relations with orgasm and limited ejaculation.

It is very dangerous to draw conclusions from single cases. However, observations with this man and with patients with a very small penis suggest that male sexual satisfaction is possible with less of a penis than one might think.

## Medical treatment of the small penis

It cannot be emphasised too strongly that a small penis may be the only presenting sign of a specific endocrine anomaly (among many others, Walsh *et al.* 1978, Salisbury *et al.* 1984). Correct treatment may restore the child and his penis to normality.

There then remain a group of boys with a small penis who are either of undefined diagnosis or who lack definitive treatment. The role of hormone treatment is uncertain. If there is good volume of erectile tissue and no androgen insensitivity, the penis will grow with testosterone or HCG treatment. Both may be given by injection but testosterone may also be applied as a cream. Accelerated linear growth and osseous maturation occur with therapy but return to normal afterwards (Guthrie *et al.* 1973, Klugo & Cerny 1978, Burstein *et al.* 1979). Young boys respond better than older boys but there is no correlation with the initial length of the penis. Topical and intramuscular testosterone have also been used to enlarge the small penis with hypospadias to make later urethroplasty easier. The results were more consistent with i.m. supplements and the side-effects were minimal. In one reported series it is interesting to note that the growth was referred to as 'temporary' (Tsur *et al.* 1983, Gearhart & Jeffs 1987).

There is no doubt that early treatment has a role in defining responsiveness of the genitalia to testosterone. The resulting growth encourages the parents to persevere with upbringing in the male gender. From the young boy's point of view, the improved growth usually brings the penis into the normal range of size; as there is very little growth of the normal penis from birth to 6 years old (Burstein *et al.* 1979), the appearance will be similar to that of the peer group.

The late results of this treatment are much less clear. The follow-up in most series is short. It would seem from our own patients that the position on the growth curve is not maintained.

Reilly's series of 12 postpubertal boys included patients with a variety of diagnoses: four hypogonadal hypogonadism, three with MGD, three idiopathic and two male pseudohermaphrodites. Eleven of 12 had had courses of hCG or testosterone in childhood and 10 had responded (the non-responder had hypogonadal hypoganadism). The treatment was similar to that given to the prepubertal group in the same series. Although treated boys are close to the 10th centile before puberty, they are well below it in adulthood, although some further growth did occur at puberty (Fig. 17.5). The effect of hormonal treatment is not carried through puberty; indeed it may be that the treatment only did that which puberty would do anyway.

Puberty was only delayed in two patients, both of whom had hypogonadal hypogonadism. Three patients had clinical and biochemical testosterone deficiency after puberty and had oral supplements. All three have a markedly eunochoid appearance (Reilly & Woodhouse 1989).

Late treatment of a 12 and 17 year old boy have been reported. The responses were poor (Klugo & Cerny 1978). It is not known whether retreatment of those treated in infancy would be helpful, but it seems unlikely that drugs would provide better stimulation than the hormone surge of puberty.

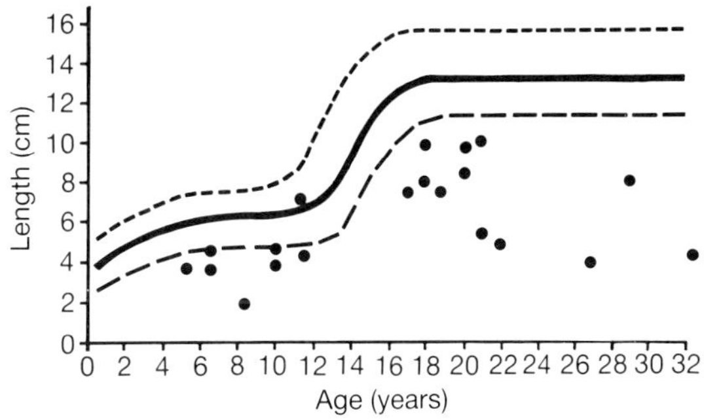


**Fig. 17.5** Growth curves for penile length as in Fig. 17.3 with the penile lengths of the patients reviewed by Reilly & Woodhouse represented by the dots (from Reilly & Woodhouse 1989, with permission).

## Surgical treatment of the small penis

Small penis is not a condition that lends itself to surgical correction. If the penis is, in fact, present and normal but buried, it may be unburied by a variety of techniques. Surgery makes the best use of the available penis by removing the surrounding fat and suturing the penile skin to the pubis. Kinks and webs in the corpora are released. Good results at follow-up to 1 year have been reported (Maizels *et al.* 1986). Although there is no long-term follow-up, it is reasonable to expect normal development of the essentially normal penis.

It may even be that surgery is not essential for the buried penis anyway: Brown has stated that the condition resolves at puberty (1962). I have encountered two cases in which an allegedly 'micropenis' has grown to normal size at puberty.

No operation has yet been devised to make the corpora of the truly small penis longer. Theoretically the techniques used for female to male gender re-assignment could be used. They would certainly not appeal for the infant as the phallus created would not grow. They seem to be also of limited appeal for the grown-up who will have his small but sexually sensitive penis replaced by a large but insensitive and inert object.

There are some special problems that can be corrected. If there is associated hypospadias the chordee can be corrected and a urethroplasty done. The epispadiac penis can be improved by the operations described in Chapter 13.

Thereafter a decision must be made, as early as possible, about gender re-assignment. In the light of our findings that sexual function is good in uncomplicated cases, I certainly feel that small penis alone should not be an indication for re-assignment.

Male to female gender re-assignment has often been suggested as a management for grossly inadequate male genitalia. The indication is especially strong if the genotype is anything other than 46XY.

There is no doubt that very acceptable girls can be made. They are likely to require a vaginoplasty after puberty. McLorie has recommended this management for patients with isolated small penis if it does not achieve 2 cm of stretched length 1 month after administration of 50 mg of testosterone i.m. Three cases are reported with two year follow-up (McLorie *et al.* 1989).

The same is also suggested for all cases of cloacal exstrophy. The recommendation is based on a series of 25 patients, seven of whom were not converted to females because of parental refusal. Three of the seven have reached puberty. Two have spent long periods in psychiatric and correctional institutions for sexual problems and the third has not been able to function sexually (McLorie *et al.* 1989).

This is a problem that affects a very small number of patients but more long-term information must be collected. If gender reassignment is to be made the decision must be made in the first few weeks of life. As the surgery is irreversible, it is essential that it is done only after the most careful thought and on the most accurate evidence.

## REFERENCES


Allen T.D. (1989) Micro penis — clinical classification. *Dial. Ped. Urol.* **12**, 3–4.

Beasley S.W., Hutson J.M., Kelly J.H. & Howat A.J. (1987) Re: Testicular function in 12 cases of penile agenesis (letter) *J. Urol.* **317**, 137.

Bernirschke K., Naftolin F., Gittes R. *et al.* (1972) True hermaphroditism and chimerism. A case report. *Am. J. Obstet. Gynecol.* **113**, 449–51.

Bissada N.K., Sakati N., Woodhouse N.J.Y. & Morcos R.R. (1987) One stage complete reconstruction for patients with congenital adrenal hyperplasia. *J. Urol.* **137**, 703–5.

Brown J.J.M. (1962) Surgery of childhood. Edward Arnold, London, pp. 1159–81.

Burstein S., Grumbach M.M. & Kaplan S.L. (1979) Early determination of androgen responsiveness is important in the management of microphallus. *Lancet* **ii**, 983–6.

Cutfield R.G., Bateman J.M. & Odell W.D. (1983) Infertility caused by bilateral testicular masses secondary to congenital adrenal hyperplasia (21-hydroxylase deficiency). *Fertil. Steril.* **40**, 809–14.

Cutler B.S., Forbes A.P., Ingersoll F.M. & Scully R.E. (1972) Endometrial carcinoma after stilbestrol therapy in gonadal dysgenesis. *N. Engl. J. Med.* **287**, 628–31.

David M. & Forest M.G. (1984) Prenatal treatment of congenital adrenal hyperplasia resulting from 21-hydroxylase deficiency. *J. Ped.* **105**, 799–803.

Donahoe P.K., Crawford J.D. & Hendren W.H. (1979) Mixed gonadal dysgenesis: pathogenesis and management. *J. Pediatr. Surg.* **14**, 287–300.

Ehrhardt A.A., Evers K. & Money J. (1968) Influence of androgens and some aspects of sexually dimorphic behaviour in women with the late treated adrenogenital syndrome. (See also early treated disease in the following article.) *Johns Hopkins Med. J.* **123**, 115–22, 123–67.

Ehrhardt A.A. & Meyer-Bahlburg H.F.L. (1981) Effects of prenatal sex hormones on gender related behaviour. *Science* **211**, 1312–18.

Feldman K.W. & Smith D.W. (1975) Fetal phallic growth and penile standards for newborn male infants. *J. Pediatr.* **86**, 395–8.

Flatau E., Josefsberg Z., Reisner S.H., Bialik O. & Laron Z. (1975) Penile size in the new born infant. *J. Pediatr.* **87**, 663–4.

Gearhart J.P. & Jeffs R.D. (1987) The use of parenteral testosterone therapy in genital reconstructive surgery. *J. Urol.* **138**, 1077–8.

Glassberg K.I. (1985) Intersex disorders. In: Whitfield H.N. & Hendry W.F. (eds) *Textbook of Genitourinary Surgery*, Vol. I. Churchill Livingstone, Edinburgh, pp. 241–63.

Gonzalez R. & Fernandes E.T. (1989) Single-stage feminization genitoplasty. *J. Urol.* **143**, 776–8.

Grant D., Muram D. & Dewhurst J. (1983) Menstrual and fertility patterns in patients with congenital adrenal hyperplasia. *Pediatr. Adol. Gynecol.* **1**, 97–103.

Gueux B., Fiet J., Couillin P. *et al.* (1988) Prenatal diagnosis of 21-hydroxylase deficiency congenital adrenal hyperplasia by simultaneous radioimmunoassay of 21-deoxycortisol and 17-hydroxyprogesterone in amniotic fluid. *J. Clin. Endocrin. Metab.* **66**, 534–7.

Guthrie R.D., Smith D.W. & Graham C.B. (1973) Testosterone treatment for micropenis during early childhood. *J. Pediatr.* **83**, 247–52.

Hendren W.H. (1987) Editorial comment. *J. Urol.* **137**, 705.

Ikoma F., Shima H. & Yabumoto H. (1985) Classification of enlarged prostatic utricle in patients with hypospadias. *Br. J. Urol.* **57**, 334–7.

Ikoma F., Shima H., Yabumoto H. & Mori Y. (1986) Surgical treatment for enlarged prostatic utricle and vagina masculina in patients with hypospadias. *Br. J. Urol.* **58**, 423–8.

Imperato-McGinley J., Peterson R.E., Gautier T. & Sturla E. (1979) Male pseudo hermaphroditism secondary to 5-alpha-reductase deficiency. *J. Steroid Biochem.* **11**, 637–42.

Klingensmith G.J., Jones H.W. & Blizzard R.M. (1977) Glucocorticoid treatment of girls with congenital adrenal hyperplasia: effects on height, sexual maturation and fertility. *J. Pediatr.* **90**, 996–1004.

Klugo R.C. & Cerny J.C. (1978) Response of the micropenis to topical testosterone and gonadotrophin. *J. Urol.* **119**, 667–8.

Kofman S., Palacios G.P., Medina M., *et al.* (1981) Clinical and endocrine spectrum in patients with 45XO/46XY karyotype. *Hum. Gen.* **58**, 373–6.

Kohn B., Levine L.S., Pollack M.S. *et al.* (1982) Late onset steroid 21-hydroxylase deficiency. *J. Clin. Endocrinol. Metab.* **55**, 817–27.

Levine L.S., Zachman M., New M.I. *et al.* (1978) Genetic mapping of the 21 hydroxylase deficiency gene within the HLA linkage group. *N. Engl. J. Med.* **299**, 911–15.

McLorie G.A., Khoury A.E. & Husmann D.A. (1989) Surgery for micropenis in childhood. *Dial. Ped. Urol.* **12**, 6–7.

Maizels M., Zaontz M., Donovan J., Bushnick P.N. & Firlit C.F. (1986) Surgical correction of the buried penis. *J. Urol.* **136**, 268–71.

Manuel M., Katayama K.P. & Jones H.W. (1976) The age of occurrence of gonadal tumours in intersex patients with a Y chromosome. *Am. J. Obstet. Gynecol.* **124**, 293–300.

Marcus E.S., Holcombe J.H., Tulchinsky D., Rich R.R. & Riccardi V.M. (1979) Prenatal diagnosis of congenital adrenal hyperplasia. *Am. J. Med. Gen.* **4**, 201–4.

Mirsky H.A. & Hines J.H. (1989) Infertility in a man with 21-hydroxylase deficient congenital adrenal hyperplasia. *J. Urol.* **142**, 111–13.

Mollard P., Juskiewenski S. & Sarkissian J. (1981) Clitero-plasty in intersex: a new technique. *Br. J. Urol.* **53**, 371–3

Morgan R.J., Williams D.I. & Pryor J.P. (1979) Mullerian duct remnants in the male. *Br. J. Urol.* **51**, 488–92.

Mosely M., Bidder R. & Hughes I. (1989) Sex role behaviour and self image in young patients with congenital adrenal hyperplasia. *Br. J. Sexual Med.* **16**, 72–5.

Muller J., Skakkebaek N.E., Neilson O.H. & Graem N. (1984) Cryptorchidism and testis cancer: atypical germ cells followed by carcinoma *in situ* in adult age. *Cancer* **54**, 629–34.

O'Connell M.J., Ramsey H.E., Whang-Peng J. & Wiernik P.H. (1973) Testicular feminisation syndrome in 3 siblings: emphasis on gonadal neoplasia. *Am. J. Med. Sci.* **265**, 321–33.

Pollack M.S., Maurer D., Levine L.S. *et al.* (1979) Prenatal diagnosis of congenital adrenal hyperplasia (21-hydroxylase deficiency) by HLA typing. *Lancet* **i**, 1107–10.

Prader A., Zachman M. & Illig R. (1977) Normal spermatogenesis in adult males with congenital adrenal hyperplasia after discontinuation of therapy. In: Lee P.A., Plotnick L.P., Kowarski A.A. & Migeon C.J. (eds) *Congenital Adrenal Hyperplasia*, 1983. University Press, Baltimore, pp. 397–401.

Reilly J.M. & Woodhouse C.R.J. (1989) Small penis and male sexual role. *J. Urol.* **142**, 569–71.

Reindollar R.H., Lewis J.B., White P.C. *et al.* (1988) Prenatal diagnosis of 21-hydroxylase deficiency by the complementary DNA probe for cytochrome P-450 $_{c\text{-}21OH}$. *Am. J. Obstet. Gynecol.* **158**, 545–7.

Robboy S.J., Miller T., Donahoe P.K. *et al.* (1982) Dysgenesis of testicular and streak gonads in the syndrome of mixed gonadal dysgenesis: perspective derived from a clinopathologic analysis of 21 cases. *Hum. Path.* **13**, 700–16.

Rubin R.T., Reinisch J.M. & Haskett R.F. (1981) Postnatal gonadal steroid effects on human behaviour. *Science* **211**, 1318–24.

Salisbury D.M., Leonard J.V., Dezateux C.A. & Savage M.O. (1984) Micropenis: an important early sign of congenital hypopituitarism. *Br. Med. J.* **288**, 621–2.

Savage M.O. & Lowe D.G. (1990) Gonadal neoplasia and abnormal sexual differentiation. *Clin. Endocrinol.* **32**, 519–33.

Schonfeld W.A. (1943) Primary and secondary sexual characteristics. *Am. J. Dis. Child.* **65**, 535–49.

Scully R.E. (1981) Gonadoblastoma: a review of 74 cases. *Cancer* **25**, 1340–56.

Spence H.M. & Allen T.D. (1973) Genital reconstruction in the female with the adrenogenital syndrome. *Br. J. Urol.* **45**, 126–30.

Tsur H., Shafir R., Shachar J. & Eshkol A. (1983) Microphallic hypospadias: testosterone therapy prior to surgical repair. *Br. J. Plast. Surg.* **36**, 398–400.

Urban M.D., Lee P.A., Migeon C.J. (1978) Adult height and fertility in men with congenital virilising adrenal hyperplasia. *N. Engl. J. Med.* **299**, 1392–6.

Walsh P.C., Wilson J.D., Allen T.D. *et al.* (1978) Clinical and endocrinological evaluation of patients with congenital microphallus. *J. Urol.* **120**, 90–5.

Whitaker R.H. (1989) Surgery for virilising congenital adrenal hyperplasia. In: Gingell J.C. & Abrams A. (eds) *Controversies and Innovations in Urological Surgery.* Springer Verlag, London, pp. 480-3.

Wischusen J., Baker H.W.G. & Hudson B. (1981) Reversible male infertility due to congenital adrenal hyperplasia. *Clin. Endocrinol.* **14**, 571–3.

Zaloudek C. & Norris H.J. (1982) Granulosa cell tumours of the ovary in children: a clinical and pathologic review of 32 cases. *Am. J. Surg. Path.* **6**, 503–12.

# 18 Neoplastic disease

## INTRODUCTION

The last two decades have seen startling advances in the management of neoplasia in children. Cures have become commonplace. There are many children who have grown up normally but now have the consequences of their treatment to contend with. There may be frank complications or 'social' problems such as a cutaneous urinary diversion and infertility. The thrust of research in some neoplasias has moved from improving survival to lessening the morbidity of treatment.

## WILM'S TUMOUR

Wilm's tumour is the most common solid neoplasm of childhood. The survival rates have been improving for many years and have advanced especially through the work of the American National Wilm's Tumor Study Group (NWTSG), the United Kingdom Children's Cancer Study Group (UKCCSG) and the Société Internationale d'Oncologie de Pédicetrie (SIOP). However, even before these major groups existed, advances had been made so that the 3-year survival of children at Great Ormond Street, UK had risen from 14% in 1944 to 50% in 1959 (Plowman 1989).

Successful treatment depends on full staging and combined care by surgeons, radiotherapists and oncologists. The best results are seen when children are treated in special centres (Kramer *et al.* 1984). Surgery remains the first line of treatment and in a series of patients treated in the early 1960s there were no survivors (regardless of stage) amongst those who did not have a radical nephrectomy. This series also showed the value of adjuvant radiotherapy. However, the 2 year relapse rate was 66% and the survival amongst relapsers was only 11% at 3 years (Ledlie *et al.* 1970).

Surgery now has a mortality of 1–2%. Wide local extension including the inferior vena cava or the diaphragm can be managed with preoperative chemotherapy with some cures at up to 15 years' follow-up (Kogan *et al.* 1986). Partial nephrectomy is reserved for the 5% of patients with bilateral disease when the side with the smaller lesion can often be managed by conservative surgery.

The dose of radiotherapy has been reduced in recent trials. In the 1960s however, up to 40 Gy was given to large fields. There was a high late complication rate from scoliosis, nephritis and pulmonary fibrosis. From the first NWTSG trial onwards the indications, doses and fields have been steadily reduced (to only 10 Gy in some cases). It is now used where there is tumour spillage or incomplete local resection (stage III), for metastatic disease (stage IV) and in patients with unfavourable histology.

Vincristine, adriamycin and actinomycin-D are the most active drugs. In stage I disease adjuvant vincristine and actinomycin are given for 6 months (or even vincristine alone). Stage II patients require 15 months of the same drugs. In stage III patients with operable local disease all three are given for 15 months. Metastases may respond to the triple-drug regime supplemented with radiotherapy. The addition of cyclophosphamide may be helpful.

Aside from the improved survival rates, the trials have shown that less treatment is needed than was previously thought. It is salutary to note that patients treated outside the protocols, although having the same survival, may have excessive treatment in up to 50% of cases (Pritchard *et al.* 1989).

In the UK, overall survival amongst Great Ormond Street patients in all stages is 83% (Plowman 1989). In stage I and II patients in the NWTSG trials it is 90% (D'Angio *et al.* 1980). The UKCCSG reports 95% 3-year survival in stages I and II, 82% in stage III, 59% in stage IV and 67% in stage V (bilateral disease) (Gough 1989).

Three-year survival is usually taken to be a cure but three relapses at 5 years were recorded amongst 90 long-term survivors in one series (Birch *et al.* 1988). The late deaths at up to 11 years reported in one early series were all due to the complications of treatment and reflected the high doses of radiotherapy that were given (Cassady *et al.* 1973). Of relapses 83% are in the lung, alone or with another site (Lemerle *et al.* 1983). The chance of successful salvage is related to the original staging and not to the nature of the relapse; presumably because lower stage patients will have more treatment options remaining. Relapse is treatable in 70% of stage I patients, 50% of stage II and 10% of stage III and IV. There are no survivors when relapse occurs in bone (Gough 1989). Radiation is useful for relapse and the second-line drugs are ifosfamide and etoposide.

The treatment of Wilm's tumour is completed and the outcome known in childhood (except for a few late presenters). The adult urologist will deal with the long-term consequences of the chemotherapy and radiation. The loss of a kidney alone is not a problem. The 'urological' effects of radiation, especially at the doses used in the 1960s, may be severe. The chemotherapy, with the exception of cyclophosphamide, leaves its marks elsewhere. The urological consequences are dealt with below.

Second malignancies, although uncommon, are particularly associated with Wilm's tumour. Those with bilateral tumours, associated congenital anomalies and the rhabdoid histological variant are at higher risk (Meadows 1985).

### Pregnancy after Wilm's tumour

The success with which Wilm's tumour is treated is reflected in the large number of pregnancies in survivors. The main data come from a multicentre review of 246 pregnancies. An attempt was made to trace 302 eligible patients who had been cured of Wilm's tumour over a 48 year period. In 237 patients who were found, 118 reported 246 pregnancies. It is not recorded whether the other 119 patients were infertile. There were two sets of twins, 32 induced and 21 spontaneous abortions.

In women the most important factor was abdominal radiation. Sixty women had 114 singleton pregnancies, 30% of which had an adverse outcome defined as fetal or neonatal death or birth weight below 2500 g. All the 13 pregnancies in the five non-irradiated women had a normal outcome. Chemotherapy did not affect the outcome of pregnancy.

The adverse events were usually before the 37th week of pregnancy (including all the fetal deaths). Neonatal death occurred in six of the 22 low birth weight infants. The perinatal mortality was 149 per 1000 which was significantly higher than the expected level of 19 per 1000.

All the male patients with Wilm's tumour received abdominal radiation. The 34 men sired 64 pregnancies. There were two low birth weight infants and the rest were normal.

The 8.5% spontaneous abortion rate and the 2% incidence of major congenital anomalies in the offspring are unremarkable. The offspring were aged 1 month to 38 years (mean: 6 years) at the time of the report; two had died in accidents, the remainder were alive and well with no cases of Wilm's tumour (Li *et al.* 1987).

Although there is a genetic influence in the aetiology of Wilm's tumour, more than one case within a family is rare. In the SIOP study of 1040 cases, two members in each of five families were affected. These 10 cases had the same demographic features as the main group. It was concluded that the number of hereditary cases was very small (Pastore *et al.* 1988). If there is a family history it may be worthwhile to look for an abnormal chromosome 11 in the woman contemplating pregnancy. This anomaly has been associated with hereditary cases (Mulvihill & Byrne 1985).

### Adult Wilm's tumour

Wilm's tumour in adults is rare with under 200 cases reported in the world literature, mostly in series of only a few cases. It can occur at any age but about 75% of cases are in patients under 30 years old. The Armed Forces Institute of Pathology (AFIP) has records of 4798 cases of renal parenchymal carcinoma of which 109 (2%) occurred in patients in the second decade of life. Of these 109 cases 50% were Wilm's tumour. Thus, when a renal tumour occurs in an adolescent, Wilm's tumour should be suspected (Hartman *et al.* 1982).

Presentation is most commonly seen at a late stage with haematuria and pain (Byrd *et al.* 1982). On IVU, ultrasound and angiogram it is not possible to distinguish Wilm's tumour from adenocarcinoma (Hartman *et al.* 1982).

Histology is the same as in children, though there has been some dispute about the incidence of unfavourable factors: the AFIP series reported no anaplasia or sarcomatous stroma while others have suggested the same incidence of unfavourable features (Hartman *et al.* 1982, Plowman 1989).

It has been said that the prognosis is poor, but it may not be as bad as has been suggested. The 3-year survival was 24% of 31 patients in the commonly quoted paper. Three-year survival was 48% in stages I and II and 11% in stages III and IV. Many of the tumours were treated in the era before combination chemotherapy and were of large size. The results were best in the later patients, especially those treated approximately according to the NWTSG protocols, in whom there was a 70% 2-year survival. Unlike children, adults continue to have relapses at least until 4 years after treatment (Byrd *et al.* 1982).

The recommended treatment now is by NWTSG protocol but adding radiotherapy to all stages (Mesrobian 1988). The NWTSG–4 protocols are aimed at reducing toxicity of chemotherapy. Adriamycin is reserved for advanced stage and unfavourable histology. As adult onset is a poor prognostic factor it seems reasonable to use actinomycin-D, vincristine and adriamycin in all cases (Plowman 1989). The dose of radiotherapy is 45 Gy in 25 fractions. The success of these recommendations has yet to be proved. In a recent series of adults treated according to these principles, four of five patients progressed while on chemotherapy and died quickly. The fifth patient died at just over 7 years (Slevin *et al.* 1987).

## RENAL ADENOCARCINOMA IN CHILDREN

Adenocarcinoma is the most common renal neoplasm in adults but forms only 2.5% in children (quoted by Malpas 1985). In the AFIP series of 109 renal parenchymal tumours presenting between 10 and 20 years old, 50% were adenocarcinomas.

All the patients presented with one or more of the classic triad of pain, haematuria and a mass. The histological features were similar to those in adults though there was a trend to less good differentiation (Hartman *et al.* 1982).

From the little information available, the tumour appears to behave in the same manner as in adults. The only curative treatment is radical nephrectomy. Neither chemotherapy nor radiotherapy has been shown to influence the course of the disease.

## RHABDOMYOSARCOMA

Although rhabdomyosarcoma is the most common soft tissue sarcoma in childhood, it is still a very rare tumour. About 50 new cases a year are seen in the UK. The prognosis varies according to site of origin and histology. The genito-urinary tract is the most common site.

The relationship of prognosis to site of origin may be due to early diagnosis. Tumours occurring at a superficial site such as paratestis or vagina produce symptoms when small and have an excellent prognosis. Deeper tumours occurring at a functionally important site such as bladder base or prostate produce urological symptoms when small and have a good prognosis. Extravesical pelvic tumours usually present as a mass and have a poor prognosis (Raney *et al.* 1986).

Good data on management can only come from research groups such as the Intergroup Rhabdomyosarcoma Study (IRS), the Children's Solid Tumour Group (CSTG) and SIOP.

A particular difficulty with this disease is that surgery can cure some patients but only with considerable mutilation. Combination treatment may have better results and cause less mutilation. However, efforts to reduce the toxicity of combined regimes has, on occasion, led to a lower cure rate.

### Paratesticular rhabdomyosarcoma

The paratestis is a favourable site for rhabdomyosarcoma. The overall 5-year survival in the CSTG series was 81%. The deaths occurred at a steady rate until 4 to 5 years, after which they were uncommon. Relapse occurred equally often locally and with metastases. Only 15% of relapsers were salvaged (Kingston *et al.* 1983).

The IRS studies have been much larger and have accrued 2500 patients with all types of rhabdomyosarcoma between them. The overall survival in the paratestis patients was 89% at 3 years; only three patients in stage I and II relapsed. It has been the practice of this group to perform a staging retroperitoneal lymph node dissection (RPLND) and decide treatment on the result. This procedure destroys the sympathetic chain and leaves the patients infertile from ejaculatory failure. Data from the SIOP study show that RPLND is not necessary because modern imaging can stage the patients sufficiently (Raney 1989). In the current SIOP series all of 46 patients are still alive with 34 patients followed for more than 3 years (Olive-Sommerlet 1989). The CSTG results were also achieved without RPLND.

Current treatment consists of radical orchiectomy, irradiation of involved nodes and combination chemotherapy. The agents commonly used include actinomycin-D, vincristine, cyclophosphamide and ifosfamide. It is not necessary to irradiate the scrotum. If the scrotum is contaminated, hemiscrotectomy is performed.

### Bladder and prostate rhabdomyosarcoma

Rhabdomyosarcoma in the bladder and prostate has a less good prognosis. Surgery alone can cure some cases as was shown by a series in 1969: eight of 13 bladder tumours and one of nine prostate cases achieved long-term survival (Claireux & Williams 1969). However, the patients paid a high price for cure with a urinary diversion and impotence. Less than radical cystectomy was incompatible with survival (Tefft & Jaffe 1973).

Unfortunately, an approach using chemotherapy and radiotherapy as the primary treatment was not very successful. Some patients were salvaged by later pelvic exenteration. Furthermore, the combination of cyclophosphamide and radiotherapy sometimes damaged the bladder so that only 38% of patients ended up with a functioning bladder (Hays *et al.* 1982).

Current regimes use intensive chemotherapy with vincristine, adriamycin, cyclophosphamide, cisplatinum and actinomycin-D. Incomplete response is an indication for radiotherapy. Surgery, which should be used early, is reserved for incomplete responders (Gough 1989, Plowman 1989). This very aggressive regime can raise the long-term survival rate to 90%. However, up to 40% may still need exenterative surgery and the long-term morbidity in survivors will be high.

### Extravesical rhabdomyosarcoma

These rare tumours usually present with a mass which is likely to be large and not resectable. Before the era of combination therapy there were few survivors. Even with combination treatment the results are poor as they are poorly responsive. In one series only three of eight children survived between 1 and 8 years in spite of intensive combined treatment (Raney *et al.* 1986).

## TESTICULAR NEOPLASMS

Testicular neoplasms in children are very rare. The majority are germ cell tumours. In the registry of the Urology Section of the American Academy of Pediatrics set up in 1980, 269 tumours were reported up to 1987. Of these 216 were of germ cell origin; the only other group of any size were the stromal tumours which accounted for another 22 cases.

There were 176 yolk sac tumours. Most presented in stage I. Patients were treated according to the will of the physician rather than by specific protocol. Thus there is no controlled trial but some observations can be made on the regimes that were used because survival was good in all of them. It is clear that many patients were overtreated. In stage I, radical orchiectomy alone was sufficient to produce a 90% survival rate at 2 years. When metastases occurred they did so within 14 months of presentation. Retroperitoneal node dissection, radiotherapy and chemotherapy had high complication rates (including a chemotherapy death) and did not appear to contribute anything to survival. Alphafetoprotein was a useful marker of relapse.

In patients with metastases (either at presentation or relapse) chemotherapy successfully salvaged 58% of patients. The most useful drugs appeared to be vincristine and actinomycin-D (Kaplan *et al.* 1988).

Of the stromal tumours, those arising from Leydig cells (presenting with precocious puberty) were benign. Non-Leydig cell tumours were usually benign though occasional late metastases have been reported (Kaplan *et al.* 1986).

## UROTHELIAL TUMOURS

Urothelial tumours are very rare in children but occasional cases are seen in adolescents. The general view is that they have a good prognosis. Almost all the reported cases presented with low grade and stage. In two series of cases presenting at under 21 and 30 years of age respectively, totalling 36 patients, the recurrence rate was identical at 8% (Benson *et al.* 1983, Fitzpatrick & Reda 1986). Transitional cell carcinoma in the young should be treated in the same manner as in older patients and will do well by virtue of its low grade and stage.

## CONSEQUENCES OF CURE: THE EFFECTS OF RADIOTHERAPY AND CHEMOTHERAPY

Aside from the specific consequences of the individual neoplasms, there are general effects from treatment with radiotherapy, chemotherapy and, especially, from both combined.

Radiotherapy damages the spine causing retarded growth, kyphosis and scoliosis. The effect is directly proportional to the dose and inversely to the age at treatment. The liver also suffers from radiation damage, but a particular focal hepatopathy occurs when radiotherapy is combined with actinomycin or adriamycin. The appearances suggest metastatic disease so that, unless a biopsy is done, inappropriate treatment may be given (D'Angio 1982). The gastrointestinal tract, the lungs and the endocrine system may also be affected.

Adriamycin causes cardiomyopathy and may damage the liver and gastrointestinal tract. The cardiomyopathy is the most serious complication and causes heart failure in 30% of patients. It is most commonly seen when the dose exceeds 550 mg/m$^2$. Young children and those having chest radiotherapy are particularly at risk. It is an early complication (within the first 230 days) so that cases should be identified before adolescence. A similar cardiomyopathy may also be seen, occasionally, after treatment with cyclophosphamide in doses between 120 and 240 mg/kg (Von Hoff *et al.* 1982).

Vincristine is well known as a cause of peripheral neuropathies. All children receiving 4 mg total dose have depression of the ankle jerk. More serious motor neuropathies, including bladder atonia, are seen in about 33% of patients. The condition is always symmetrical. Although it becomes apparent during or soon after treatment, the late effects may be seen in adolescence as it is not always reversible (Weiss *et al.* 1974).

Cyclophosphamide causes haemorrhagic cystitis identical to that caused by radiotherapy (though it may be largely prevented by the concurrent administration of Mesna). This complication is associated with the later development of transitional cell or squamous cell bladder carcinoma. Occasionally bladder carcinoma may develop without preceding haemorrhagic cystitis (Kyle 1982).

Patients who have been cured of one cancer are at risk of developing another. A cured child has a 10 times greater incidence of malignancy at 20 year follow-up than an age-matched peer (Meadows *et al.* 1980).

Radiation is associated with the development of acute myeloid leukaemia and soft tissue and bone sarcomas. For bone sarcomas there is a dose–response relationship: the relative risk being eight for doses of 10 to 20 Gy and 30 for doses of 50 Gy or more (Meadows 1985). Osteochondroma and acute leukaemia may occur up to 26 years after treatment for Wilm's tumour (Byrd & Levine 1984). The effects may be different when the radiation is given to children as opposed to adults. However, it is comforting to note that in a recent review Hoffman concluded that there was no association between pelvic irradiation and subsequent urothelial malignancy (Hoffman *et al.* 1985).

Amongst the chemotherapeutic agents actinomycin-D, adriamycin and combination treatment for Hodgkin's disease have been particularly implicated. In this instance the effects of radiotherapy and chemotherapy may not be additive: children given radiotherapy and actinomycin have a seven-fold *less* incidence of second malignancy than those having radiation alone (D'Angio 1982).

Cyclophosphamide is associated with the development of acute nonlymphocytic leukaemia, bone tumours and solid cancers in an irradiation field (Meadows 1985).

## Renal injuries

### *Renal artery stenosis*

*Pathology.* Radiation usually affects small blood vessels and so it is hardly surprising that the renal artery is seldom damaged. The mechanism of damage is not known. Suggestions include peri-arterial fibrosis, damage to the microvascular circulation in the arterial wall and acceleration of atherosclerosis (Asscher *et al.* 1961, Rubin & Casarett 1968, Johnson *et al.* 1969).

*Presentation and incidence.* Ten patients are reported to have developed renal artery stenosis after abdominal radiation with or without cytotoxic chemotherapy. All presented with hypertension though two cases had bilateral stenoses and also developed renal failure. Diagnosis was made 4 to 12 years after treatment with 15 to 51 Gy (Salvi *et al.* 1983, Minton *et al.* 1986). Radiation seems likely to have been the cause as seven were children and one of the adults had several vascular abnormalities in the radiation field. As more children with cancer survive, the problem may become more common; in adults the condition may pass unrecognised.

Although hypertension is rare, measurement of blood pressure should be part of the follow-up regime after abdominal radiation. When hypertension is found, renal artery stenosis should be considered as a cause.

*Management.* The management of renal artery stenosis in the general population is a matter of some debate. Surgery is indicated mainly for those who have isolated renal artery lesions with little or no generalised arteriopathy.

Young patients whose cancers are cured should be candidates for surgery. The only child in the reported series who was treated medically ultimately died (McGill *et al.* 1979). Renal artery reconstruction or bypass would have been conventional until recently although three of the 10 reported patients had nephrectomies perhaps because of the surrounding radiation damage (Salvi *et al.* 1983).

The newer technique of transluminal balloon angioplasty seems ideally suited to the management of this group of patients. A successful case has been reported but with only 6 weeks' follow-up. There has also been a report of failure (Tegtmeyer *et al.* 1984, Minton *et al.* 1986).

### *Radiation nephritis*

*Pathology.* The pathogenesis of radiation nephritis is uncertain but there are three main theories: injury to the endothelial cells of the glomeruli, to the large parenchymal vessels or to the renal tubules (Williams 1986).

In humans the histological changes are non-specific and irregular. The basement membrane is thickened, the capillary endothelial cells are proliferated and the capillaries are partly occluded by thrombus. These changes reduce the glomerular blood flow and the glomerular filtration (Krochak & Baker 1986).

*Presentation and incidence.* Renal damage has been recognised as a limiting factor in abdominal radiation for many years and so the condition now is uncommon. The kidneys can tolerate less than 20 Gy. The suggestion that higher doses could be tolerated if about one-third to a half of the total renal parenchyma was shielded were not borne out with long-term follow-up (Kunkler *et al.* 1952, Rubin & Casarett 1968). Thirty-one of 84 patients who received 20 Gy to the left kidney alone had renal damage when followed for up to 20 years: five had renal failure, 12 had impaired function and 14 had hypertension (Thompson *et al.* 1971).

Two clinical syndromes of radiation nephritis are recognised. Acute nephritis occurs between 6 and 12 months after irradiation. Chronic nephritis occurs from 12 months onwards. Cases have been reported up to 19 years after irradiation. It may follow acute radiation nephritis or may appear *de novo*. The clinical features are the same as those of acute or chronic renal failure from any other cause (Krochak & Baker 1986).

Hypertension, although rare, may occur without nephritis at any time from 18 months onwards. In some patients it follows a malignant course with encephalopathy and retinopathy; renal failure may be an end result. The long-term outlook is also affected by late deterioration of nephrons that survive the original radiation injury (see Chapter 3).

*Treatment.* The treatment of these conditions is the same as if the cause is other than radiation. Acute renal failure is usually treated by dialysis until spontaneous recovery has occurred. Chronic renal failure is treated by dialysis or transplantation. Hypertension is treated medically unless there is clear evidence that damage to one kidney is driving it. Nephrectomy should only be offered if medical control is difficult.

## Ureteric injuries

*Obstruction*

Ureteric obstruction occurs almost exclusively in women irradiated for carcinoma of the cervix or uterine body and is rare after other pelvic irradiation (Blandy & Tiptaft 1985). Radiotherapy is a rare cause of retroperitoneal fibrosis (RPF). Patients with RPF may present with backache, hypertension, renal failure or, very occasionally, pyonephrosis.

*Ureterovaginal fistula*

This complication is rarely seen with radiation alone but occurs when the irradiated ureter is also damaged by surgery (Schellhammer *et al.* 1986).

## Injuries to the bladder by radiotherapy and cyclophosphamide

The bladder is always damaged by pelvic radiation and it says much for its resilience that significant complications occur in only 5 to 15% of patients (Schellhammer *et al.* 1986). It may be that all patients suffer some symptoms and that only the serious ones are recorded.

*Pathology*

The earliest visible change is mucosal hyperaemia. Late changes consist of sclerosing endarteritis, fibrosis and tissue atrophy (Upton *et al.* 1966, Anderson 1984). The timing of these changes is particularly interesting. The bladder normally has a very slow rate of proliferation. Before damage can occur, the proliferative rate must increase in response to the injury. When the injury is surgical or chemical (such as from cyclophosphamide), the response is rapid. The proliferative response to radiation is slow and so symptoms are delayed (Stewart 1986).

The eventual result of radiation injury is reduced capacity and compliance. The mucosa is diffusely vascular though often with large areas of pallor. It is liable to infection and ulceration. Further injuries (including mucosal biopsy) heal slowly (Anderson 1984, Schellhammer *et al.* 1986). There is a cumulative incidence of symptoms which reaches a peak at two years after treatment (Orton & Wolf-Rosenblum 1986, Schellhammer *et al.* 1986).

*Haemorrhagic cystitis: incidence and presentation*

Frequency and dysuria with or without bleeding occur during or immediately after radiation therapy in most patients (Bleehan 1976). Assuming the urine is sterile, there is no very effective treatment and the condition is usually self-limiting.

Late haemorrhagic cystitis may occur at any time, often years after apparently successful treatment. Such late presentation always raises the possibility of recurrent cancer and so full investigation, including cystoscopy, is essential. Biopsy of the bladder should be avoided if possible because of the risk of delayed healing and of fistula (VillaSanta 1972).

This complication has been reported in 2 to 9% of patients receiving radical radiotherapy to the pelvis (Ram 1970, VillaSanta 1972, Pillay *et al.* 1984). The lowest dose at which it can occur is not known. Combination of irradiation with systemic cyclophosphamide greatly increases the incidence of serious bleeding, to 18% in one series of children (Jayalakshmamma & Pinkel 1976).

*Treatment*

Severe haemorrhagic cystitis is difficult to treat. Not only are the patients bleeding heavily and so receiving large volumes of anticoagulated blood as transfusion, but they are often in poor health and may have thrombocytopenia. There is a tendency for the clinician to start with 'simple treatments' for fear of causing irreversible damage to the bladder. The patient, meanwhile, slips past the point where any treatment can save him or her.

The best treatment is uncertain as there have been no controlled trials. It seems that some of the treatments work for some of the time and the clinician must be prepared to change treatments quickly in the face of failure. My own experience is that clinicians undertreat acute haemorrhagic cystitis in the hope that it will stop by itself: aggressive measures should be started early in this dangerous condition.

*Surgical treatments.* For all severe cases the blood clot must be evacuated and for this general anaesthetic, a large cystoscope and several Elik's evacuators are usually necessary. The bleeding is unlikely to stop so long as the bladder is full of clot. If a particular bleeding point springs into view, it should be diathermied gently. Too much diathermy may worsen the problem by producing an indolent ulcer. Good results have been reported for diathermy alone (Lapides 1970, Pillay *et al.* 1984), but such good fortune seems rare.

The application of pressure to bleeding has an honourable surgical tradition. In the bladder 6 hours of hydrostatic distension under epidural anaesthesia has been used (Holstein *et al.* 1973, Anderson *et al.* 1976). Bleeding was controlled in five of six patients in one series (Holstein *et al.* 1973). However, although forced distension may stop mucosal bleeding, it actually causes acute interstitial and sub-mucosal bleeding (Mehrotra 1953). In the long-term it leads to bladder contraction especially after radiotherapy (Anderson *et al.* 1976). There is also a risk of bladder perforation which might prove fatal.

The last surgical resort is urinary diversion. As the patients are usually so ill, cutaneous ureterostomy or percutaneous nephrostomy is safer than a more elaborate operation. It is not clear why diversion of the urine away from the bladder should stop bleeding, but it worked for 12 of 14 reported patients (Pomer *et al.* 1983).

*Intra-vesical treatments.* Of all the treatments available, intravesical formalin is probably the best. Its poor reputation may arise from its improper use. Bladder contraction, ureteric fibrosis, anuria, incontinence and death from acute tubular necrosis are reported complications (Shah & Albert 1973, Fair 1974, Shrom *et al.* 1976, Rao *et al.* 1978). In all of these cases the regime and precautions described by Fair had not been followed (Fair 1974).

Formalin is a 37–41% solution of formaldehyde. The dose of *formalin* used is the smallest concentration for the shortest time that will stop the bleeding. One to 10% for 10 to 30 minutes have been tried. As the control of bleeding was achieved in all of 14 patients treated by Fair with one or two instillations of 1% for 10 minutes, this seems to be the regime to use first. If this fails to stop the bleeding, the concentration should be increased to 2%. Thereafter it is better to increase the exposure time rather than the concentration unless the bleeding is life-threatening. At 3-year follow-up no patient had bladder contraction in Fair's series (Shah & Albert 1973, Fair 1974, Shrom *et al.* 1976).

Silver nitrate or alum may also be used for bladder washout or irrigation. Silver nitrate is used as a 1% solution for washing out and 0.5% for irrigation for 2 to 4 days thereafter. This regime is said to be less toxic and was successful in seven of eight children (Mahesh *et al.* 1976). Unfortunately the solution has to be made up in the hospital pharmacy for each patient, it is very expensive and has a short shelf-life.

Alum 1% is a solution of aluminium ammonium sulphate or aluminium potassium sulphate. It can be used as an irrigation without preliminary washout and without anaesthetic. It is particularly good for unfit patients or when the bleeding is not immediately life-threatening (Ostroff & Chenault 1982, Kennedy *et al.* 1984). Although reasonably safe, two of eight cases in one series were complicated by paralytic ileus (Kennedy *et al.* 1984). The long-term effect on the bladder is not known.

Hyperbaric oxygen has been used as an adjunct to formalin or alum instillations and also on its own. As the basic bladder lesion is anoxia, it does seem to be a logical treatment and was successful in all of four reported cases (Schoenrock & Cianci 1986). It is only feasible if the hospital happens to have a hyperbaric oxygen chamber and the length of the 60×2 hour treatments rather limits its usefulness.

*Oral treatment.* Sodium pentosan polysulphate 100 mg t.d.s. sublingually is said to improve bladder epithelial defence mechanisms. It replaces native epithelial polysaccharide to provide an active barrier to the adherence of harmful bacteria, protein and ions. The importance of this mucus coat as a defence 'from being too much grated upon by the acrimony of the urine' was known 300 years ago (Snape 1683).

All of five patients in the only reported series responded after 4 to 7 weeks therapy but all had had other treatments as well (Parsons 1986). The drug was not available in the USA at the time of the report. Although it is available in the UK experience in radiation cystitis is limited. In my own patients seven of eight patients (including one who had cyclophosphamide for childhood leukaemia) have responded by cessation of bleeding and improved voiding frequency. Four have been able to discontinue treatment. For patients with slow bleeding that docs not cause clot retention it seems worth trying.

## Gonadal injuries

The importance of fertility after treatment for cancer has been recognised for many years. In 1973 the Royal Marsden Hospital advocated particular treatment protocols for testicular neoplasms specifically because sexual function and fertility could be preserved without compromising the cure rate (Smithers *et al.* 1973).

Successful treatment for cancers in young people, especially cervical and testicular carcinoma and leukaemias in childhood, will leave an increasing number of patients of childbearing age. If possible their treatment should be so arranged that they are able to have intercourse and have children.

### *Effects of radiotherapy*

Gonadal injury is almost invariable with direct radiation. In the adult rat testis a dose and time-response is seen for Leydig cell and spermatogenic function. A single dose of 10 Gy has been shown to halve testicular weight in 2 weeks but between 2 and 3 Gy will do the same in 8 weeks.

Leydig cell function is not affected by doses of 1 or 2 Gy. Doses of 5 Gy and above raise the serum LH at 8 weeks but it takes 10 Gy to depress the serum testosterone level (elevated LH level with normal testosterone is taken to mean that extrapituitary drive is required to stimulate the damaged Leydig cells). No dose of irradiation makes any difference at 2 weeks.

Sertoli cell function, as measured by serum FSH levels, is impaired by a single dose of 10 Gy after 2 weeks but even 2 Gy can produce some impairment after 10 weeks. Five Gy virtually abolishes spermatogenesis and there is little recovery with time (Delic *et al.* 1986).

Translating these findings into humans is difficult but it is clear that the testes are very sensitive to radiation. In addition there is the worry that fertility may be preserved but the sperm may carry chromosomal anomalies.

It seems likely that radiation damage would be worse when applied in childhood. Leiper has investigated 13 boys 3 to 9 years after direct testicular irradiation for acute lymphoblastic leukaemia. Eleven received 24 Gy and the other two had 15 and 36 Gy respectively. All had intensive cytotoxic chemotherapy and cranial irradiation as well. Five boys had complete failure of virilisation and three had arrested pubertal development. The younger the age of treatment, the worse was the effect on pubertal development. The five boys who showed normal progression included the one who had only had 15 Gy.

The gross degree of Leydig cell dysfunction that was shown might be reversible, especially if the irradiation was given late in childhood. However, even when puberty did progress, the serum LH levels were high indicating poor Leydig cell function. The damage was attributed to the testicular irradiation and not to the other treatments (Leiper *et al.* 1986).

In adults the effect of radiation on spermatogenesis is as important as endocrine function. It has been established that irradiation causes oligozoospermia but levels usually return to normal after 2 to 3 years (Sandeman 1966, Maguire 1979). In patients receiving 26 to 40 Gy for testicular neoplasms there is spillage on to the remaining testis of up to 3 Gy. This was shown to lower the sperm count in only one of seven patients and the children that were born subsequently were all normal (Sandeman 1966). However, in children the effects are more severe. When studied as adults 10 of 17 men who had been irradiated in childhood for Wilm's tumour had azoospermia or severe oligozoospermia. These patients only had scatter irradiation to the scrotum, estimated at less than 10 Gy (Shalet 1985).

In an experimental study on humans the standard seminal analysis and a sperm function test were done before and after irradiation. Seven of 11 men had sperm concentrations of less than 20 million per ml and five had less than 50% motility before any treatment at all. Furthermore, sperm of all the patients had very poor ability to penetrate the zona pellucida-free hamster egg, indicating poor sperm function. After 0.5 to 5 Gy 75% were azoospermic at 3 months but recovery began at 12 months and none were azoospermic at 36 months. Sperm function, however, remained poor with only five of seven patients with normal counts achieving even moderate hamster egg penetration (Martin *et al.* 1985).

In terms of paternity, it is interesting to see that in the Marsden patients, 34 of 74 men fathered 52 normal children after surgical and radiation therapy. One fathered a child during treatment and another 5 months after treatment ended (Smithers *et al.* 1973). The findings of an M.D. Anderson survey were more in keeping with the experimental results: only 11 of 84 men had children (Schrover *et al.* 1986).

Although clinicians are rightly concerned about chromosomal damage, in practice the risk to offspring may not be high. In another Marsden group 40 children conceived after radiotherapy for testicular neoplasms had no greater incidence of congenital malformations than 30 conceived after chemotherapy and 57 controls (Senturia *et al.* 1985).

High dose abdominal radiation in childhood always causes ovarian failure. Doses up to 10 Gy only do so in about 20% of patients (Shalet 1985).

### *Effects of chemotherapy*

Testicular atrophy from chemotherapy has been recognised since the introduction of nitrogen mustard more than 40 years ago. Chlorambucil, busulphan, cyclophosphamide, adriamycin and several combinations have been shown to cause gonadal toxicity in animals and humans (Chapman 1982). Fortunately, it seems that the prepubertal gonad, especially the ovary, is relatively resistant to the effects of chemotherapy except alkylating agents such as cyclophosphamide. All patients investigated by semen analysis after MOPP therapy in childhood were azoospermic (Whitehead *et al.* 1982). Many patients with severe testicular damage may continue to have normal FSH and LH until adulthood (Shalet 1985).

One study has followed children treated with cyclophosphamide for nephrotic syndrome for a mean of 12.8 years. Of 30 patients, four were azoospermic, nine oligozoospermic and 17 were normal. It is interesting that four of the normospermic patients had been oligozoospermic or, in one case, azoospermic, when assessed between 5.5 and 9 years earlier, showing that late recovery is possible. All had developed normal puberty and had normal sexual function. There was a strong inverse correlation between sperm density and the total dose of cyclophosphamide and duration of treatment. All those who had had 10 G or less were normospermic; all but three who had had more than 20 G were oligozoospermic or azoospermic (Watson *et al.* 1985).

Around puberty, the gonads are particularly vulnerable. In adolescent boys, combination chemotherapy with nitrogen mustard, vincristine, procarbazine and prednisolone produces eunuchoidism (D'Angio 1982). In girls up to 30 years old, combination chemotherapy including alkylating agents almost always produces ovarian failure though usually reversible; after 30 it is seldom reversible (Chapman 1982). Cyclophosphamide is the drug most likely to cause ovarian damage. Once again the gonadotrophins may remain normal in childhood in spite of severe ovarian damage (Shalet 1985).

The offspring of treated patients seem to be normal. The suggestion that there was an increased incidence of spontaneous abortions and minor congenital anomalies has not been sustained (Chapman 1982).

## REFERENCES


Anderson J.D., England H.R., Molland, E.A. & Blandy J.P. (1976) The effects of overstretching on the structure and function of the bladder in relation to Helmsteins distension therapy. *Br.J.Urol.* **47**, 835–40.

Anderson R.E. (1984) Radiation injury. In: Kissane J.M. (ed) *Anderson's Pathology* (8th edn). C.V. Mosby, St Louis, pp. 239–77.

Asscher A.W., Wilson C & Anson S.G. (1961) Sensitisation of blood vessels to hypertensive damage by x-irradiation. *Lancet* **i**, 580–3.

Benson R.C., Tomera K.M. & Kelalis P.P. (1983) Transitional cell carcinoma of the bladder in children and adolescence. *J. Urol.* **130**, 54–5.

Birch J.M., Marsden H.B., Morris Jones P.H., Pearson D. & Blair V. (1988) Improvements in survival from childhood cancer: results of a population based survey over 30 years. *Br. Med. J.* **296**, 1372–6.

Blandy J.P. & Tiptaft R.C. (1985) Benign and malignant retroperitoneal fibrosis. In: Whitfield H.N. & Hendry W.F. (eds) *Textbook of Genito-Urinary Surgery*, Vol. 1. Churchill Livingstone, Edinburgh, pp. 319–28.

Bleehan N.M. (1976) Radiotherapy. In: Williams D.I. & Chisholm G.D. (eds) *Scientific Foundations of Urology*, 1st edn, Vol. 2. William Heinnemann, London, pp. 235–42.

Byrd R.L., Evans A.E. & D'Angio G.J. (1982) Adult Wilm's tumor: effect of combined therapy on survival. *J. Urol.* **127**, 648–51.

Byrd R.L. & Levine A.S. (1984) Late effects of treatment of Wilm's tumor. In: Pochedly C. & Baum E.S. (eds) *Wilm's Tumor: Clinical and Biological Manifestations*. Elsevier Science Publishing Co., New York, pp. 347–67.

Cassady J.R., Tefft M., Miller R.M. *et al.* (1973) Considerations in the radiation therapy of Wilm's tumor. *Cancer* **32**, 598–608.

Chapman R.M. (1982) Effect of cytotoxic therapy on sexuality and gonadal function. *Sem. Oncol.* **9**, 84–94.

Claireux A.E. & Williams D.I. (1969) Tumours in childhood. In: Taylor S. (ed) *Recent Advances in Surgery*. J. & A. Churchill, London, pp. 48–83.

D'Angio G.J. (1982) The child cured of cancer. *Sem. Oncol.* **9**, 143–9.

D'Angio G.J., Beckwith J.B., Breslow N.E. *et al.* (1980) Wilm's tumor: an update. *Cancer* **45**, 1791–8.

Delic J.I., Hendry J.H., Morris I.D. & Shalet S.M. (1986) Dose and time relationships in the endocrine response of the irradiated adult rat testis. *J. Androl.* **7**, 32–41.

Fair W.R. (1974) Formalin in the treatment of massive bladder haemorrhage: techniques, results and complications. *Urology* **3**, 573–6.

Fitzpatrick J.M. & Reda M. (1986) Bladder carcinoma in patients 40 years old or less. *J. Urol.* **135**, 53–4.

Gough D.C.S. (1989) Wilm's tumour and genito-urinary rhabdomyosarcoma. *Br. J. Urol.* **63**, 109–16.

Hartman D.S., Davis C.J., Madewell J.E. & Friedman A.C. (1982) Primary malignant renal tumors in the second decade of life: Wilm's tumor versus renal cell carcinoma. *J. Urol.* **127**, 888–91.

Hays D.M., Raney R.B., Lawrence W. *et al.* (1982) Bladder and prostatic tumors in the Intergroup Rhabdomyosarcoma Study (IRS-1). Results of therapy. *Cancer* **50**, 1472–82.

Hoffman M., Roberts W.S. & Cavanagh, D. (1985) Second pelvic malignancies following radiation therapy for cervical cancer. *Obstet. Gynaec. Surv.* **40**, 611–17.

Holstein P., Jacobsen K., Pedersen F.J. & Sorensen J.S. (1973) Intravesical hydrostatic pressure treatment: new method for control of bleeding from the bladder mucosa. *J. Urol.* **109**, 234–6.

Jayalakshmamma B.J. & Pinkel D. (1976) Urinary bladder toxicity following pelvic irradiation and simultaneous cyclophosphamide therapy. *Cancer*, **38**, 701–7.

Johnson A.G., Lane B., Harding-Rains A.J., O'Connell D. & Ramsey W. (1969) Large artery damage after x-radiation. *Br. J. Radiol.* **42**, 937–9.

Kaplan G.W., Cromie W.J., Kelalis P.P., Silber I. & Tank E.S. (1986) Gonadal stromal tumors: a report of the prepubertal testicular tumor registry. *J. Urol.* **136**, 300–2.

Kaplan G.W., Cromie W.J., Kelalis P.P., Silber I. & Tank E.S. (1988) Prepubertal yolk sac testicular tumors: a report of the testicular tumor registry. *J. Urol.* **140**, 1109–12.

Kennedy C.L., Snell M.E. & Witherow R.O. (1984) Use of alum to control intractable vesical haemorrhage. *Br. J. Urol.* **56**, 673–5.

Kingston J.E., McElwain T.J. & Malpas J.S. (1983) Childhood rhabdomyosarcoma: experience of the children's Solid Tumour Group. *Br. J. Cancer* **48**, 195–207.

Kogan S.J., Marans H., Santorineau M. *et al.* (1986) Successful treatment of renal vein and venacaval extension of nephroblastoma by preoperative chemotherapy. *J. Urol.* **136**, 312–17.

Kramer S., Meadows A.T., Pastore G. *et al.* (1984) Influence of place of treatment on diagnosis, treatment and survival in 3 solid pediatric tumors. *J. Clin. Oncol.* **2**, 917–23.

Krochak R.J. & Baker D.G. (1986) Radiation nephritis — clinical manifestations and pathophysiologic mechanisms. *Urology* **27**, 389–93.

Kunkler P.B., Farr R.F. & Luxton, R.W. (1952) The limit of renal tolerance to X-rays. *Br. J. Radiol.* **25**, 190–201.

Kyle R.A. (1982) Second malignancies associated with chemotherapeutic agents. *Sem. Oncol.* **9**, 131–42.

Lapides J. (1970) Treatment of delayed intractable hemorrhagic cystitis following radiation or chemotherapy. *J. Urol.* **104**, 707–8.

Ledlie E.M., Mynors L.S., Draper G.J. *et al.* (1970) Natural history and treatment of Wilm's tumour. An analysis of 335 cases in England and Wales 1962–1966. *Br. Med. J.* **iv**, 195–200.

Leiper A.D., Grant D.B. & Chessells, A.M. (1986) Gonadal function after testicular irradiation for acute lymphoblastic leukaemia. *Arch. Dis. Child.* **61**, 53–6.

Lemerle J., Voute P.A., Tournade M.F. *et al.* (1983) Effectiveness of preoperative chemotherapy in Wilm's tumor: results of the SIOP clinical trial. *J. Clin. Oncol.* **1**, 604–10.

Li F.P., Gimbrere K., Gelber R.D. *et al.* (1987) Outcome of pregnancy in survivors of Wilm's tumor. *J. Am. Med. Assoc.* **257**, 216–19.

McGill C.W., Holder T.M., Smith T.H. & Ashcraft, K.W. (1979) Post radiation renovascular hypertension. *J. Paed. Surg.* **14**, 831–3.

Maguire L.C. (1979) Fertility and cancer therapy. *Postgrad. Med.* **65**, 293–9.

Mahesh A.P., Wrenn E.L., Jayalakshmamma B.J. *et al.* (1976) Silver nitrate irrigation to control bladder haemorrhage in children receiving cancer therapy. *J. Urol.* **116**, 85–6.

Malpas J.S. (1985) Childhood tumours. In: Whitfield H.N. & Hendry W.F. (eds) *Textbook of Genito-Urinary Surgery*, Vol. 2. Churchill Livingstone, Edinburgh, pp. 936–944.

Martin R.H., Rademaker A., Barnes M. *et al.* (1985) A prospective serial study of the effects of radiotherapy on semen parameters and hamster egg penetration rates. *Clin. Invest. Med.* **8**, 239–43.

Meadows A.T. (1985) Second malignant neoplasms. *Clin. Oncol.* **4**, 247–62.

Meadows A.T., Krejmas N.L. & Belasco J.B. (1980) The medical cost of cure: sequelae in survivors of childhood cancer. In:van Eys J. & Sullivan M.P. (eds) *Status of the Curability of Childhood Cancers*. Raven Press, New York, pp. 263–75.

Mehrotra R.M.L. (1953) An experimental study of the vesical circulation during distension and in cystitis. *J. Path. Bact.* **66**, 76–89.

Mesrobian H-G.J. (1988) Wilm's tumor: past, present, future. *J. Urol.* **140**, 231–8.

Minton M.J., McIvor F.P., Cappuccio F.P., MacGregor G.A. & Newlands E.S. (1986) Case report: renovascular hypertension following radiotherapy and chemotherapy treated by transluminal angioplasty. *Clin. Radiol.* **37**, 399–401.

Mulvihill J.J. & Byrne J. (1985) Offspring of long term survivors of childhood cancer. *Clin. Oncol.* **4**, 333–43.

Olive-Sommerlet D. (1989) International Society of Pediatric Oncology protocol. *Dial. Ped. Urol.* **12**, 4–5.

Orton C.G. & Wolf-Rosenblum S. (1986) Dose dependence of complication rates in cervix cancer radiotherapy. *Int. J. Radiation Oncol. Biol. Phys.* **12**, 37–44.

Ostroff E.B. & Chenault O.W. (1982) Alum irrigation for the control of massive bladder haemorrhage. *J. Urol.* **128**, 929–30.

Parsons C.L. (1986) Successful management of radiation cystitis with sodium pentasanpolysulphate. *J. Urol.* **136**, 813–14.

Pastore G., Carli M., Lemerle J. *et al.* (1988) Epidemiological features of Wilm's tumour: results of studies by SIOP. *Med. Ped. Oncol.* **16**, 7–11.

Pillay P.K., Teh M., Chua E.J. *et al.* (1984) Haemorrhagic chronic radiation cystitis — following treatment of pelvic malignancies. *Ann. Acad. Med.* **63**, 634–8.

Plowman P.N. (1989) Multimodality approach to paediatric urological tumours. In: Oliver R.T.D. (ed) *Urological and Genital Cancer.* Blackwell Scientific Publications, Oxford, pp. 272–88.

Pomer S., Karcher G. & Simon W. (1983) Cutaneous ureterostomy as last resort treatment of intractable haemorrhagic cystitis following radiation. *Br. J. Urol.* **55**, 392–4.

Pritchard J., Stiller C.A. & Lennox E.L. (1989) Over treatment of children with Wilm's tumour outside paediatric oncology centres. *Br. Med. J.* **299**, 835–6.

Ram M.D. (1970) Complications of radiotherapy for carcinoma of the bladder. *Proc. Roy. Soc. Med.* **63**, 93–5.

Raney R.B. (1989) Intergroup rhabdomyosarcoma study. *Dial. Ped. Urol.* **12**, 2–4.

Raney R.B., Carey A., Snyder H. McC. *et al.* (1986) Primary site as a prognostic variable for children with pelvic soft tissue sarcoma. *J. Urol.* **136**, 874–8.

Rao M.S., Bapna B.C., Chugh K.S. *et al.* (1978). Fatal complication of intravesical formalin during control of intractable haemorrhage from radiation cystitis. *Urology* **11**, 588–90.

Rubin P. & Casarett G.W. (1968) Concepts of clinical radiation pathology. In: Dalrymple G., Gaulden M. & Kallomorgen G. (eds) *Medical Radiation Biology.* W.B. Saunders, Philadelphia, pp. 160–89.

Salvi S., Gamboa J.N., Green D.M. *et al.* (1983) Renal artery stenosis and hypertension after irradiation for Hodgkin's disease. *Urology* **21**, 611–15.

Sandeman T.F. (1966) The effects of X-irradiation on male human fertility. *Br. J. Radiol.* **39**, 901–7.

Schellhammer P.F., Jordan G.H. & El-Mahdi A.M. (1986) Pelvic complications after interstitial and external beam irradiation of urologic and gynecologic malignancies. *World J. Surg.* **10**, 259–68.

Schoenrock G.J. & Cianci P. (1986) Treatment of radiation cystitis with hyperbaric oxygen. *Urology* **27**, 271–2.

Schrover L.R., Gonzales M. & von Eschenbach A.C. (1986) Sexual and marital relationships after radiotherapy for seminoma. *Urology* **27**, 117–23.

Senturia Y.D., Peckham C.S. & Peckham M.J. (1985) Children fathered by men treated for testicular cancer. *Lancet* **ii**, 766–9.

Shah B.C. & Albert D.J. (1973) Intravesical instillation of formalin for the management of intractable haematuria. *J. Urol.* **110**, 519–20.

Shalet S.M. (1985) The effects of cancer treatment on growth and sexual development. *Clin. Oncol.* **4**, 223–38.

Shrom S.H., Donaldson M.H., Duckett J.W. & Wein, A.J. (1976) Formalin treatment for intractable haemorrhagic cystitis. *Cancer* **38**, 1785–9.

Slevin J., McWilliam L.J. & Parson D. (1987) Adult nephroblastoma: 5 cases treated by surgery, radiotherapy and chemotherapy. *Clin. Radiol.* **38**, 483–6.

Smithers D.W., Wallace D.M. & Austin D.E. (1973) Fertility after unilateral orchidectomy and radiotherapy for patients with malignant tumours of the testis. *Br. Med. J.* **iv**, 77–9.

Snape A. (1683) The Anatomy of an Horse. M. Flesher, London pp. 40–1.

Stewart F.A. (1986) Mechanism of bladder damage and repair. *Br. J. Cancer* **53** (Supplement VII), 280–91.

Tefft M. & Jaffe M. (1973) Sarcoma of the bladder and prostate in children. *Cancer* **32**, 1161–77.

Tegtmeyer C.J., Kellum C.D. & Ayers C. (1984) Percutaneous transluminal angioplasty of the renal artery. *Radiology* **153**, 77–84.

Thompson P.L., Mackay I.R., Robson G.S.M. & Wall A.J. (1971) Late radiation nephritis after gastric X-irradiation for peptic ulcer. *Quart. J. Med.* **40**, 145–55.

Upton, A.C. (1966) Pathologic effects of radiation. In: Schwartz E.E. (ed) *Biological Basis of Radiation Therapy.* J.B. Lippincott, Philadelphia, pp. 126–62.

VillaSanta U. (1972) Complications of radiotherapy for carcinoma of the uterine cervix. *Am. J. Obstet. Gynecol.* **114**, 717–26.

Von Hoff D.D., Rozencweig M. & Piccart M. (1982) The cardiotoxicity of anticancer agents. *Sem. Oncol.* **9**, 23–33.

Watson A.R., Rance C.P. & Bain J. (1985) Long term effects of cyclophosphamide on testicular function. *Br. J. Urol.* **291**, 1457–60.

Weiss H.D., Walker M.D. & Wiernik P.H. (1974) Neurotoxicity of commonly used antineoplastic agents (part 2). *N. Engl. J. Med.* **291**, 127–33.

Whitehead E., Shalet S.M., Morris Jones P.H., Beardwell C.G. & Deakin D.P. (1982) Gonadal function after combination chemotherapy for Hodgkin's disease in childhood. *Arch. Dis. Child.* **57**, 287–91.

Williams M.V. (1986) The cellular basis of renal injury by irradiation. *Br. J. Cancer.* **53** (Supplement VII), 257–64.

# *Index*